Essential Epidemiology

An Introduction for Students and Health Professionals

Third Edition

Penny Webb, MA (Cambridge), DPhil (Oxford), is a Principal Research Fellow and Group Leader at the QIMR Berghofer Medical Research Institute, Brisbane, and Honorary Professor in the School of Public Health, University of Queensland. She taught basic and intermediate epidemiology to public health students across Australia for 5 years and has worked as a visiting scientist at the International Agency for Research on Cancer, France, and Harvard University, USA. She has published more than 250 original research papers in the field of cancer epidemiology.

Chris Bain, MB BS (UQ), MPH, MSc (Harvard), formerly Reader in Epidemiology, University of Queensland, is currently a Visiting Scientist at the QIMR Berghofer Medical Research Institute and National Centre for Epidemiology and Population Health, Australian National University. He has taught epidemiology to public health and medical students for over 3 decades, and has co-authored a book on systematic reviews, as well as many research papers. He has had wide exposure to international epidemiological practice and teaching in the UK and US.

Andrew Page BA(Psych) Hons (Newcastle), PhD (Sydney) is Professor of Epidemiology in the School of Medicine at Western Sydney University, Australia. He has been teaching basic and intermediate epidemiology and population health courses to health sciences students for 10 years, and has published over 140 research articles and reports across a diverse range of population health topics. He has been a Research Associate at the University of Bristol and has also worked at the University of Queensland and University of Sydney in Australia.

Essential Epidemiology

An Introduction for Students and Health Professionals

Third Edition

Penny Webb
Principal Research Fellow,
QIMR Berghofer Medical Research Institute and
Honorary Professor,
University of Queensland, Brisbane, Australia.

Chris Bain
Visiting Scientist,
QIMR Berghofer Medical Research Institute,
Brisbane, Australia.

Andrew Page
Professor of Epidemiology,
School of Medicine,
Western Sydney University, Australia.

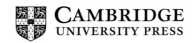

CAMBRIDGE
UNIVERSITY PRESS

University Printing House, Cambridge CB2 8BS, United Kingdom

Cambridge University Press is part of the University of Cambridge.

It furthers the University's mission by disseminating knowledge in the pursuit of education, learning, and research at the highest international levels of excellence.

www.cambridge.org
Information on this title: www.cambridge.org/9781107529151

First edition published in 2005
Second edition published 2011
Third edition 2017

Printed in Singapore by Markono Print Media Pte Ltd

A catalogue record for this publication is available from the British Library.

Library of Congress Cataloging-in-Publication Data
Names: Webb, Penny, 1963- , author. | Bain, Chris, 1947- , author. | Page, Andrew, 1974- , author.
Title: Essential epidemiology : an introduction for students and health professionals / Penny Webb, Chris Bain, Andrew Page.
Description: Third edition. | Cambridge ; New York : Cambridge University Press, 2017. | Includes bibliographical references and index.
Identifiers: LCCN 2016007893 | ISBN 9781107529151 (pbk. : alk. paper)
Subjects: | MESH: Epidemiologic Methods | Epidemiology
Classification: LCC RA651 | NLM WA 105 | DDC 614.4–dc23 LC record available at http://lccn.loc.gov/2016007893

ISBN 978-1-107-52915-1 Paperback

Additional resources for this publication at www.cambridge.org/9781107529151

Contents

Foreword

I am delighted to write the new foreword for the third edition of Essential Epidemiology.

This well known, highly respected and engaging book, aimed at the Masters level in Epidemiology, is a timely evolution from the earlier editions, bringing in new material and educational approaches (fully described in the authors' preface).

As someone who has been heavily involved in my own institution's under-graduate, masters, and doctoral level research and service training over many decades, and been external examiner for many other institutions, I see the value of this book to many international constituencies. The key audience will, of course, be those involved in Masters studies of Epidemiology, Public Health and related disciplines. However I would also recommend this book to those involved in undergraduate teaching of epidemiology, students and teachers, those in post-Master's training or practice, as well as those in the biomedical and social sciences who wish to understand and utilise the perspectives and principles of epidemiology.

The value of the book is that the authors have based it on many years of teaching students on the ground and the latest revision and refreshment ensures that it maintains relevance. Thus this book retains the major content of the earlier versions, with sound grounding in the core principles and practice of epidemiology, as well as incorporating new areas. It is vital that future epidemiological research is relevant to the challenges we face globally. The book continues to provide this wider perspective, as well as the more technical approaches that are used when merged with other fields such as genetics. This new edition also provides on-line further materials (including expanding on some trickier methodological topics) and full teaching materials (more on questions and answers, lecture slides), which allow students to engage in more active learning and teachers to draw on presentations which they can use and adapt.

As is clear I recommend this book strongly to those in relevant training and those involved in their education as an up to date, highly accessible and excellent resource.

Carol Brayne
Professor of Public Health Medicine
University of Cambridge

This book grew out of our collective experience of teaching introductory epidemiology both in the classroom and to distance students enrolled in public health and health studies programmes in the School of Public Health (formerly the Department of Social and Preventive Medicine and then School of Population Health), University of Queensland. It began life as a detailed set of course notes that we wrote because we could not find a single epidemiology text that covered all of the areas we felt were important in sufficient detail. As the notes were to be used primarily by distance students, we tried hard to make them accessible with lots of examples, minimal jargon and equations, and by engaging readers in 'doing' epidemiology along the way. Feedback from students and colleagues convinced us that the notes were both approachable and practical and the result is this text, which we offer as a practical introduction to epidemiology for those who need an understanding of health data they meet in their everyday working lives, as well as for those who wish to pursue a career in epidemiology.

The first revision of the text reflected evolution, not revolution. We listened to the feedback we received from instructors and students and tried to simplify and clarify some of the trickier bits of the original text while maintaining a very 'hands-on' approach. We added new material to reflect contemporary epidemiological practice in public health and re-ordered some of the existing elements to improve the flow and enhance the continuity between chapters. New and expanded topics included a look at how we measure the burden of disease, greater discussion of issues relevant to ethics and privacy, appendices covering life tables and calculation of confidence intervals for common epidemiological measures, and a glossary.

This, the third edition, reflects further evolution. With our new co-author Professor Andrew Page, and inspired by colleagues at a workshop on methods of teaching modern epidemiology convened by Professors Diana Safarti and John Lynch at the University of Otago, New Zealand in 2014, we have injected some more modern approaches to causal thinking, bias and confounding. These changes are most obvious in Chapter 4 (Study Design), which we have restructured to show more clearly how each design contrasts with the 'ideal' (counterfactual) experiment, Chapters 7 (Bias) and 8 (Confounding), and Chapter 10 (Causation). A series of constructive reviews from teachers using the book helped us to identify and correct some faults, convinced us to retain the infectious disease elements of the text but in a more focussed and practical form, and led us to add recommendations for 'further reading' for those who want deeper insights into some of the issues discussed. We have also refined the final chapter, which now builds on the experience of the earlier material to consider the role and value of epidemiology in translational research. Another major enhancement is the greatly expanded website, which provides the reader with access to additional examples and useful links, many of the references cited in the book (subject to copyright), additional questions with comprehensive worked answers and a 'Test Yourself' set of interactive multiple choice questions (and answers) for each of the main content chapters. For lecturers there are also more detailed sets of teaching slides for each chapter.

Our overall aims are, however, unchanged. Firstly, to give students a good understanding of the fundamental principles common to all areas of epidemiology, including the study of both infectious and chronic diseases as well as public health and clinical epidemiology, and to show the essential role of epidemiology in a broad range of health monitoring and research activities. Secondly, and perhaps more importantly, we have endeavoured to do this in a way that is both approachable and engaging, that minimises mathematical jargon and complex language without sacrificing accuracy, and that encourages study and stimulates epidemiological thought.

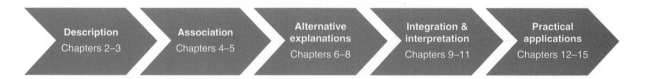

As previously, Chapter 1 is a general introduction that both answers the question 'what is epidemiology and what can it do?' and presents the main concepts that are the focus of the rest of the book. The next chapters are divided into five separate sections. The first covers the basic principles and underlying theory of epidemiology in a very 'hands-on' way. We start by looking at how we can measure disease and, new to this edition, the overall burden of disease in a population (Chapter 2), followed by a look at the role of descriptive epidemiology in describing health patterns (Chapter 3). We move on to look at the types of study that we use to identify potential causes of disease, including an expanded discussion of the potential of record linkage (Chapter 4) and how we quantify the associations between cause and outcome (Chapter 5). In the next section we look at the role of chance in epidemiology (Chapter 6), consider the thorny issues of error and bias (Chapter 7) and give a practical overview of the problem of confounding (Chapter 8). This leads to the third section, where we integrate this information in a practical look at how we read and interpret epidemiological reports (Chapter 9), think about assessing causation (Chapter 10), and finally synthesise a mass of information in to a single review to make practical judgements regarding the likelihood that a relation is causal (Chapter 11). In the final section we look at some specific applications of epidemiology, including its role in surveillance (Chapter 12), outbreak control (Chapter 13), prevention – including a discussion of how we can assess the impact of different preventive interventions on the health of a population (Chapter 14) and screening (Chapter 15). The greatly revised Chapter 16 then concludes by reviewing core concepts of the earlier material to address some of the challenges that face a modern epidemiologist who desires to improve health through 'translation' of research into practice.

Symbols

Throughout the book we have used **bold** typeface to indicate terms included in the glossary and the following symbols are used to define key elements within the text.

We strongly believe that the best way to learn anything is by actually doing it and so have included questions within the text for those who like to test their understanding as they go. Because we also know how frustrating it is to have to search for answers, we have provided these immediately following the questions for those in a hurry to proceed: The questions at the end of the chapters also have full worked answers at the end of the book.

We have used numerous real-life examples from all around the world to illustrate the key points and to provide additional insights in some areas. Extra examples that provide added interest and complement the main message in the text are given in boxes featuring this symbol.

Many books present clinical epidemiology as a separate discipline from public health epidemiology – a distinction that is strengthened by the fact that clinical epidemiologists have developed their own names for many standard epidemiological terms. In practice all epidemiology is based on the same underlying principles, so we have integrated the two approaches throughout the book but have also highlighted specific examples more relevant to the clinical situation. (Please note that this book does not offer a comprehensive coverage of clinical epidemiology; rather, we aim to show the similarity of the two areas where they overlap.)

We have deliberately tried to keep the main text free of unnecessary detail and equations, but have included some epidemiological 'extras'. This material is not essential to the continuity of the core text but provides some additional information for those who like to see where things have come from or want a more detailed perspective.

New to this third edition, we have identified areas where additional material is available online; www.cambridge.org/9781107529151. This material includes additional reading, links to the papers that we have cited and additional questions and answers.

Acknowledgements

If we were to name everyone who had contributed in some way to this book, the list would be endless. We would, however, like to acknowledge some of the great teachers (and their books) from whom we have learned most of what we know, and the books we have relied on heavily for our teaching. These include Brian MacMahon (*Epidemiology: Principles and Methods,* MacMahon and Pugh, 1970), Olli Miettinen, Charlie Hennekens (*Epidemiology in Medicine,* Hennekens and Buring, 1987), Ken Rothman (*Modern Epidemiology,* 1986), *Foundations of Epidemiology* (Lillienfeld and Lilienfeld, 1980), and *Epidemiology* (Gordis, 1996). We would also like to thank our colleagues and friends, especially the Fellows from the then School of Population Health, University of Queensland, and the staff and students from the then Cancer and Population Studies Group at the QIMR Berghofer Medical Research Institute, whose constructive feedback helped shape the first edition back in 1995.

Particular thanks go to our former colleague and co-author of the first edition, Sandi Pirozzo, who has since moved on to a rewarding new career post-epidemiology; we remain grateful for her prior contributions. Also to Adrian Sleigh (Australian National University) who wrote the original chapters on Outbreak Investigation and Surveillance and to Martyn Kirk (Australian National University) who extensively revised these chapters for this third edition. We are grateful to members of the former Burden of Disease group at the School of Public Health, University of Queensland, especially Theo Vos, Stephen Begg and Alan Lopez for their suggestions regarding our consideration of the 'Burden of Disease' for the second edition, and to Chalapati Rao (Australian National University) whose constructive feedback helped us to update Chapters 2 and 3 for this edition. The excellent critiques and suggestions we received from Michael O'Brien and Kate Van Dooren regarding the first edition helped improve the cohesion and internal 'sign-posting' of the book. We also thank Susan Jordan, Kate Van Dooren and Keren Papier, who helped pull everything together for the first, second and third editions, respectively. Finally, we would like to acknowledge the School of Public Health, University of Queensland, which provided the intellectual environment that led to us writing this book in the first place, the team from Otago University in New Zealand who provided very helpful feedback on the first edition, and the many users of the first two editions who provided the critical feedback that has directly led to this new and hopefully improved third edition.

Contributors

Martyn Kirk

Associate Professor, National Centre for Epidemiology and Population Health, Research School of Population Health, Australian National University, Canberra, Australia

Adrian Sleigh

Emeritus Professor, National Centre for Epidemiology and Population Health, Research School of Population Health, Australian National University, Canberra, Australia

Epidemiology is …

Box 1.1 Epidemiology is …

'The science of epidemics' (*Concise Oxford Dictionary*, 1964)

'The science of the occurrence of illness' (Miettinen, 1978)

'The study of the **distribution** and **determinants** of disease in humans' (MacMahon and Pugh, 1970)

'The study of the distribution and determinants of **health-related states or events** in specified populations, and the **application of this study to control of health problems**' (Porta, 2008)

'The study of the occurrence and distribution of health-related events, states and processes in specified populations, including the study of the determinants influencing such processes, and the application of this knowledge to control relevant health problems' (Porta, 2014)

So what is epidemiology anyway? As shown in Box 1.1, the *Concise Oxford Dictionary* (1964) defined it accurately, but not very helpfully, as 'the science of epidemics'. In 1970, MacMahon and Pugh came up with something a bit more concrete: 'the study of the *distribution* and *determinants* of disease'. Their definition succinctly identifies the two core strands of traditional epidemiology: *who* is developing disease (and *where* and *when*), and *why* are they developing it? The next definition, from the 2008 edition of the *Dictionary of Epidemiology* (Porta, 2008), takes things two steps further by broadening the scope to include health in general, not just disease, as well as highlighting the essential role of epidemiology in translating research findings into health policy and medical practice to control disease. The most recent definition (Porta, 2014) elaborates further still but, in doing so, loses some of the elegance of the earlier versions.

Epidemiology, therefore, is about measuring disease or other aspects of health, identifying the causes of ill-health and intervening to improve health; but what do we mean by 'health'? Back in 1948, the World Health Organization (WHO, 1948) defined it as '... a state of physical, mental and social well-being'. In practice, what we usually measure is physical health, and this focus is reflected in the content of most routine reports of health data and in many of the health measures that we will consider here. However, methods that attempt to capture the more elusive components of mental and social well-being are now emerging. Instead of simply measuring 'life expectancy', WHO introduced the concepts of 'health-adjusted life expectancy' (HALE) and subsequently 'disability-adjusted life years' (DALYs) to allow better international comparisons of the effectiveness of health systems. In doing so, they recognised that it is not longevity per se that we seek, but a long and healthy life. We will discuss these and other measures in more detail in Chapter 2.

Perhaps epidemiology's most fundamental role is to provide a logic and structure for the analysis of health problems both large and small or, as described by Wade Hampton Frost, epidemiology involves the 'orderly arrangement of [established facts] into chains of inference which extend more or less beyond the bounds of direct observation' (Frost, 1927). It emphasises the sound use of numbers – we have to count and we have to think. We have to think about what is worth counting and how best to count it, about what is practical and, importantly, about how well we (or others) finally measured whatever it was we set out to measure, and what it all means. Accurate measurement of health is clearly the cornerstone of the discipline, but we believe the special value of epidemiology flows from a way of thought that is open, alert to the potential for error, willing to consider alternative explanations and, finally, constructively critical and pragmatic.

We offer this book as an aid to such thought. It does not aim to turn you into a practising epidemiologist overnight, but will give clear directions if that is where you decide to go. Its primary goal is to help you interpret the mass of

Table 1.1 Numbers of people who became ill after eating various foods at a youth camp.

Food	People who ate the food		People who didn't eat the food	
	Total	Number ill	Total	Number ill
Friday dinner:				
Hot chicken	343	156	231	74
Peas	390	175	184	55
Potato fries	422	184	152	46
Saturday lunch:				
Cold chicken	202	155	372	75
Salad	385	171	189	59
Saturday dinner:				
Fruit salad	324	146	250	84

(Adapted from Hook *et al.*, 1996, with permission from John Wiley and Sons. © 1996 The Public Health Association of Australia Inc.)

epidemiological literature and the various types of health data that you may come across. We hope that you will see, by reading and by doing, that the fundamental concepts and tools of epidemiology are relatively simple, although the tasks of integrating, synthesising and interpreting health information are more challenging. But before we go any further, let us do some public health epidemiology.

A case of food poisoning

Epidemiology is a bit like detective work in that we try to find out why and how disease occurs. Our first example illustrates this. After an outbreak of food poisoning at a youth camp, the local public health unit was called in to identify the cause (Hook *et al.*, 1996). They first asked everyone at the camp what they had eaten prior to the outbreak and some results of this investigation are shown in Table 1.1.

Looking at the numbers in Table 1.1, it is difficult to see which of the foods might have been responsible for the outbreak. (Note that everyone is recorded as either having eaten or not eaten each food; and that most people will have eaten more than one of the foods.) More people became ill after eating potato fries than after eating cold chicken (184 versus 155) – but then more people ate the fries (422 versus 202). How then can we best compare the two foods? One simple way to do this is to calculate the *percentage* of people who became ill among those who ate (or did not eat) each type of food. For example, 156 out of 343 people who ate hot chicken became ill and

$$156 \div 343 = 0.45 = 45\%$$

So 45% of people who ate hot chicken became sick. This is known as the **attack rate** for hot chicken, i.e. 45% of hot chicken eaters were 'attacked' by food poisoning.

Calculate the attack rates for the other foods. Which food has the highest attack rate?

Although cold chicken has the highest attack rate (77%), not everyone who ate it (or, more precisely, who *reported* eating it) became ill and 20% or one in five people who did *not* eat cold chicken still became ill. This is to be expected; no matter what the cause of concern, it is rare that everyone who is exposed to it will show the effects (in this case, become ill). What can help here is to work out how much *more likely* people who ate a particular food were to become ill than those who did not eat it. For example, 45% of people who ate hot chicken became ill, compared with 32% of people who did not eat hot chicken. Hot-chicken eaters were therefore 1.4 times (45% ÷ 32% = 1.4) more likely to become ill than people who did not eat hot chicken. This measure gives us the risk of sickness in hot-chicken eaters *relative* to non-eaters, hence its name – **relative risk**.

Calculate the relative risk of developing food poisoning associated with each of the other food items. Which food is associated with the highest relative risk of sickness?

We can now conclude that the food item most likely to have been responsible for the outbreak was the cold chicken – people who ate this were almost four times as likely to become ill as those who did not. This is quite a strong relative risk; in comparison, eating any of the other foods was associated with no more than one and a half times the risk of disease. The relevant data, including the attack rates and relative risks, are summarised in Table 1.2, which is much more informative than the raw numbers of Table 1.1.

In identifying the cause of the outbreak you have just solved an epidemiological problem. The 'attack rates' and 'relative risks' that you used are simple to calculate and are two very useful epidemiological measures. We will discuss them further in Chapters 2 and 5 and they will appear throughout the book.

Subdisciplines of epidemiology

The outbreak investigation above is an example of what might be called *public health epidemiology*, or *infectious disease epidemiology*, with the first name reflecting the broad field of application and the second the nature of both the aetiological (causal) agent and the disease. It is quite common now to specify such subfields of epidemiology, which range on the one hand from *nutritional* through *social* to *environmental* and *eco-epidemiology*, and on the other from

Table 1.2 Numbers of people who became ill after eating various foods at a youth camp and attack rates and relative risks for each food.

Food	People who ate the food			People who didn't eat the food			Relative risk[a]
	Total	Number ill	Attack rate	Total	Number ill	Attack rate	
Friday dinner:							
Hot chicken	343	156	45%	231	74	32%	1.4
Peas	390	175	45%	184	55	30%	1.5
Potato fries	422	184	44%	152	46	30%	1.4
Saturday lunch:							
Cold chicken	202	155	77%	372	75	20%	3.8
Salad	385	171	44%	189	59	31%	1.4
Saturday dinner:							
Fruit salad	324	146	45%	250	84	34%	1.3

[a] Note, relative risks are calculated using the exact percentages and not the rounded values shown.
(Adapted from Hook *et al.*, 1996, with permission from John Wiley and Sons. © 1996 The Public Health Association of Australia Inc.)

cancer to *injury* or *perinatal epidemiology*: the former grouping being exposure-oriented and the latter focused on the particular disease or outcome. Nonetheless, the core methods and techniques of epidemiology remain common to all subdisciplines, so the contents of this book are relevant to all. Setting subspeciality boundaries largely reflects the explosion of knowledge in these areas, although some areas do present special challenges. For example, capturing a person's usual diet is remarkably challenging and the subsequent data analysis equally so; epidemiologists coming fresh to the field of nutritional epidemiology will need to develop experience and expertise in that specific area. You will meet examples from a wide cross-section of health research as you read on, and the common threads of logic, study design and interpretation will, we trust, become apparent.

It is of some interest to know a bit more about a few of the special epidemiologies. *Occupational epidemiology* has the longest history of all, with influential early observations of diseases linked to occupations such as mining appearing in the sixteenth century, and a systematic treatise on occupational diseases was published by Ramazzini back in 1700 (Rosen, 1958). Occupational health research in general, and epidemiology in particular, continue to contribute to enhancing workplace health today. Seminal contributions in the field include identification of the pulmonary (lung) hazards of asbestos for miners and construction workers (Selikoff *et al.*, 1965) and the work practices that led to an epidemic of a rare fatal cancer in workers in the polyvinyl chloride industry (Makk *et al.*, 1974). Company records of job tasks can provide measures of past exposure among employees, allowing researchers to look back in time and link, for example, past asbestos exposure to subsequent deaths in the workforce. (This type of study is a *historical cohort design* – see Chapter 4. It is only possible when there are good records of both exposure and outcome, usually death, and for this reason has proved particularly useful in occupational studies where such records often do exist.)

Far more modern are the subdisciplines of *molecular* and *clinical epidemiology*. The former aims to weld the population perspective of epidemiology with our rapidly increasing understanding of how variations in genes and their products affect the growth, form and function of cells and tissues. It thus has the potential to define genetic contributions to disease risk and can also provide biological markers of some exposures (e.g. changes to DNA following exposure to tobacco smoke). In contrast, clinical epidemiology differs from other branches of epidemiology in its focus on enhancing clinical decisions to benefit *individual patients*, rather than improving the health of *populations*. For this reason, clinical epidemiology is sometimes regarded as a separate discipline, a view encouraged by the fact that it has developed its own names for many standard epidemiological measures. The foundations are, however, identical to those of public health epidemiology and when appropriate we will discuss the two in parallel, highlighting any differences in language or approach along the way. There is also increasing interest in *lifecourse epidemiology*, which attempts to integrate events across the lifetime, often going right back to conception and sometimes to previous generations, to understand disease risk.

On epidemics

If we take the word 'epidemiology' itself, its origins from '*epidemic*' are clear. If we talk about an epidemic we immediately conjure up pictures of an acute outbreak of infectious disease but, both for practical and for etymological reasons, it seems reasonable to use the term to describe a notable excess of any disease over time. Many developed countries could, for example, be described as undergoing an epidemic of lung cancer over the last few decades (Figure 1.1). Notably the pattern of lung cancer over time differs for men and women; rates in men rose sharply between 1950 and 1980 but have been falling for some years now, while those in women rose later and started to fall more recently – a consequence of the fact that, as a group, women took up smoking more recently than men. To describe this excessive occurrence of disease (or death) as an 'epidemic' captures some of the urgency the numbers demand.

The derivation of the word 'epidemiology' itself is from the Greek *epi*, upon, *demos*, the people, and *logia*, study. Literally, therefore, it means the 'study

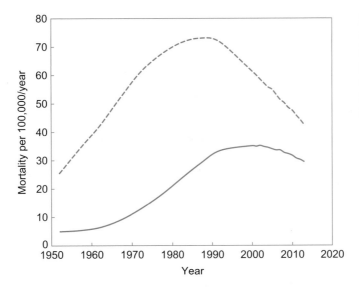

Figure 1.1 Time trends in lung cancer mortality rates in the USA (age-standardised to the 1970 US population) for white men (– –) and women (___). (*Drawn from*: CDC Wonder Database (CDC), accessed 26 February 2015.)

(of what is) upon the people'. Such study suggests a simple set of questions that have long lain at the heart of epidemiology.

- **What** disease/condition is present in excess?
- **Who** is ill?
- **Where** do they live?
- **When** did they become ill?
- **Why** did they become ill?

The first question reflects the need for a sound, common definition of a disease so that like is compared with like. Epidemiology is all about comparison – without some reference to what is usual, how can we identify excess? The next three questions form the mantra of descriptive epidemiology: '*person, place and time*'. As Figure 1.2 shows, an 'epidemic of premature mortality' occurred among young and middle-aged men in Russia in the mid-1990s and again in the early 2000s. This description captures the essence of the problem and prompts the next questions: what caused these epidemics? What changed in the circumstances of younger Russian men to reverse the pattern of falling mortality in the early 1980s and then cause it to almost double in less than 10 years? And why did this happen again in the late 1990s? Other data show that there were no such mortality changes in Western Europe, or among older Russian men or infants, or (to the same extent) in Russian women. This simple graph captures a public health disaster for Russia and prompts urgent causal speculation: *Why did this happen?* Solving and responding to this final question is critical for public health progress, but there is clearly no simple solution. In this case, a high proportion of the deaths were

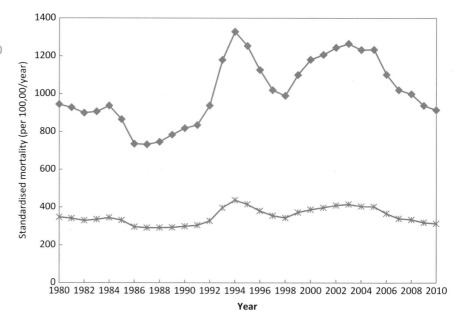

Figure 1.2 Changes in all cause mortality at ages 0–64 years in the Russian Federation from 1980 to 2010 (◆men, ✳women). (*Data from*: the European Health for All Database. WHO Regional Office for Europe, Copenhagen, Denmark, http://data.euro.who.int/hfadb/, accessed 27 February 2015.)

linked to excess consumption of alcohol during the 1990s: increases in mortality coincided with periods of economic and societal crisis, and rates fell when the economic situation improved (Zaridze *et al.*, 2009). The earlier decline during the 1980s coincided with an anti-alcohol campaign involving higher taxes and reduced production which led to sharp decreases in alcohol consumption in the short term, and lower rates of alcohol-related mortality and suicide (Pridemore and Spivak, 2003). This example highlights the importance of paying close attention to descriptive data that provide a 'community diagnosis' or take the public health 'pulse' of a nation. Much can be gleaned from apparently simple data to give a quite precise description of the overall health of a population or a more specific health event, as the following exercise shows.

An historical epidemic

Table 1.3 shows some data that relate to an actual human experience. It tells you how many people there were in various age, sex and socioeconomic groups and what percentage of these people died during the 'epidemic'. The challenge is to use these data to describe the event systematically in terms of **whom** this happened to (we have no data on place or time) and then to think about the sort of event that might have induced such a pattern.

Table 1.3 An historical event.

SES[a]	Adult males		Adult females		Children (both sexes)		Total population	
	Total	% Dead	Total	% Dead	Total	% Dead	Total	% Dead
High	175	67.4	144	2.8	6	–	325	37.5
Medium	168	91.7	93	14.0	24	–	285	58.6
Low	462	83.8	165	53.9	79	65.8	706	74.8
Other	885	78.3	23	13.0	0	–	908	76.7
Total	1690	80.0	425	25.6	109	47.7	2224	68.0

[a] SES, socioeconomic status.
(*Source*: www.anesi.com/titanic.htm, The *Titanic* casualty figures (and what they mean), accessed 29 April 2015.)

The following questions are designed to help you identify key features of the data.

1. What is distinctive about this isolated population with regard to:
   • the numbers of men and women (sex distribution),
   • the numbers of adults and children (age distribution), and
   • the numbers in each socioeconomic group (socioeconomic distribution)?
2. What strikes you about the percentage of people who died (the 'death rate')? Is this different for (a) adults and children, (b) men and women, (c) high and low socioeconomic status (SES) and (d) any particular combinations of the above?
3. How many times more likely were:
   • men to die than women, and
   • those of low SES to die than those of high SES?
4. To what historical event might these data refer?

Table 1.3 displays more complicated data than Table 1.2 because you had to consider the joint effects of three factors (sex, SES, and age) on mortality. The sequence of questions above underlines a general principle in describing such tables – i.e. to look at overall patterns first, then move on to more detail. We all see things in different ways, but until you develop your own style the approach shown in Box 1.2 may help you avoid getting lost in the array of possible relationships. You need first to grasp the size of the *whole group* under study and how many died; then check the overall patterns (the numbers and death rates[1]) across each 'exposure' separately (sex, SES, age).

---

[1] As you will see in Chapter 2, these are not technically 'rates' in the true sense of the word but it is convenient to call them rates as they are essentially identical in form to the attack rates in Table 1.2.

Box 1.2 An historical event

Things to note about the population include:

- the predominance of adult males (1690 ÷ 2224 = 76%), the much smaller proportion of adult females (19%), and the very few children;
- the substantial excess of persons of low SES (men and children in particular); and
- the total population (2224) is quite large – a village, small town, an army barracks . . . ?

Things to note about the 'death rates' include the following.

- The overall death rate is very high – more than two-thirds died.
- Overall, death rates increased with decreasing SES.
- The death rate in men (80.0%) was much higher than that in women (25.6%); the death rate in children was between these two.
- In men, the death rate was high in all socioeconomic classes, although those of high SES fared better than the rest; in women, the death rate was always lower than that for males of equivalent SES, but it increased strikingly from high to medium to low SES.
- The only children to die were of low SES.

Overall, the relative risk (RR) for men versus women is 80.0 ÷ 25.6 = 3.1
The RR for low versus high SES is 74.8 ÷ 37.5 = 2.0
The RR for women of low SES versus women of high SES is 53.9 ÷ 2.8 = 19.3
The RR for men of low SES versus women of high SES is 83.8 ÷ 2.8 = 29.9

A disaster has occurred, causing a high death rate that predominantly affected men (of all social classes) and, to a lesser extent, women and children of low social class. Overall there is a modest benefit of belonging to a higher social stratum, and among women this protection was exceptionally strong (a 19-fold higher risk of dying for low versus high SES).

Such substantial differences in risk reflect powerful preventive effects and in this instance it was a mix of social custom and the physical consequences of social stratification. The event was the sinking of the *Titanic*, where those of higher SES (the first-class passengers) were situated on the upper decks and were therefore closer to the lifeboats than those of medium and low SES (those travelling second and third class, respectively). The males gallantly helped the females and children into the lifeboats first. Those of 'other' SES were the crew.

For example, first look at the death rates for all adult males, ignoring their SES, or for all people of high SES, ignoring their age and sex. Only then consider the more complex joint effects such as the influence of SES on mortality among women.

In tackling this and the previous problem you have already done some serious epidemiology: you have *described* data, *interpreted* the patterns you observed and used *epidemiological measures* to help do this. We will build on this throughout the book, but first let's step back a little and see what other lessons we can learn from the past.

The beginnings[2]

The 'great man' approach has fallen out of favour in modern historical practice; however, linking historical events to people adds character so we will focus on some of the main players in this brief overview of the development of population health and epidemiology.

Good epidemiological practice and reasoning started long ago. Perhaps the first proto-epidemiologist (*proto* because he did not actually count anything) was Hippocrates of Cos (460–375 BC), who recognised that both environmental and behavioural factors could affect health (see Box 1.3).

The Dark Ages and Middle Ages (AD 500–1500) have little to say to us, other than in the development of causal reasoning, which we will set aside until later in the book (Chapter 10). The introduction of more quantitative methods into epidemiology and, in fact, into biology and medicine in general, has been attributed to John Graunt (1620–1674), a haberdasher and early Fellow of the Royal Society in London who published his *Natural and Political Observations Mentioned in a Following Index and Made Upon the Bills of Mortality* in 1662 (Graunt, 1662). He studied parish christening registers and the 'Bills of Mortality', and noted many features of birth and death data, including the higher numbers of both male births and deaths in comparison with females, the high rates of infant mortality and seasonal variations in mortality. He also provided a numerical account of the impact of the plague in London and made the first attempts to estimate the size of the population. In an attempt to define a 'law of mortality' he constructed the first life-table (Table 1.4). This summarised the health of a population in terms of the chance of an individual surviving to a particular age. Notice that at this time only three out of every hundred people reached the age of 66, and the majority of deaths occurred in early life. This technique was a forerunner of that used by life insurance companies for

---

[2] The material in this section is drawn from a mix of primary and secondary sources, with the latter including a number of texts, most helpful being those of Stolley and Lasky (1995) and Lilienfeld and Lilienfeld (1980).

Table 1.4 An historical example of a life-table.

Exact age (years)	Deaths	Survivors	Chance of living to that age (%)
0	–	100	
6	36	64	64
16	24	40	40
26	15	25	25
36	9	16	16
46	6	10	10
56	4	6	6
66	3	3	3
76	2	1	1
86	1	0	

(Adapted from Graunt, 1662.)

Box 1.3 On airs, waters and places

Whoever wishes to investigate medicine properly, should proceed thus: in the first place to consider the seasons of the year, and what effects each of them produces ... Then the winds, the hot and the cold, especially such as are common to all countries, and then such as are peculiar to each locality. We must also consider the qualities of the waters ... In the same manner, when one comes into a city to which he is a stranger, he ought to consider its situation, how it lies as to the winds and the rising of the sun; for its influence is not the same whether it lies to the north or the south, to the rising or to the setting sun. These things one ought to consider most attentively, and concerning the waters which the inhabitants use, whether they be marshy and soft, or hard, and running from elevated and rocky situations, and then if saltish and unfit for cooking; and the ground, whether it be naked and deficient in water, or wooded and well watered, and whether it lies in a hollow, confined situation, or is elevated and cold; and the mode in which the inhabitants live, and what are their pursuits, whether they are fond of drinking and eating to excess, and given to indolence, or are fond of exercise and labour ...

(Extracted from Hippocrates of Cos, 400 BC.)

calculating insurance premiums today, as well as a fundamental approach to measuring a population's health. As you will see, when we come back to consider life-tables in more detail in Chapter 2 (see also Appendix 5 for details of how to construct a life-table), things have improved considerably since

Graunt's time, with about 85 of every 100 men and 90 of every 100 women now making it to the age of 66 in developed countries.

During the nineteenth century, the collection and use of health statistics for what we now call 'descriptive epidemiology' continued to develop in England and also, briefly, in France. Of particular influence as a teacher was Pierre Charles-Alexandre Louis (1787–1872), who conducted some of the earliest epidemiological studies of treatment effectiveness when he demonstrated that bloodletting did not aid recovery from disease. Among his students was William Farr (1807–1883), physician, statistician and director of the Office of the Registrar General for England and Wales from 1837, its second year of operation. Farr studied levels of mortality in different occupations and institutions and in married and single persons, as well as other facets of the distribution of disease. He published these and other findings in the *Annual Reports of the Registrar General*, and the present UK system of vital statistics stems directly from his work.

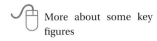 More about some key figures

John Snow (1813–1858), a physician and contemporary of Farr, was better known at the time for giving chloroform to Queen Victoria during childbirth, but is now remembered for his pioneering work in elucidating the mode of transmission of cholera (Snow, 1855). This remains a classic and exciting example of epidemiological detection and some of Snow's personal account of it is given below and again later in the chapter. His initial observations were based on a series of reports of individual cases of cholera and, in every instance, he was able to link the case to contact with another infected person (or their goods), thereby demonstrating that the disease could spread from person to person. He then surmised, contrary to popular belief at the time, that cholera could be transmitted through polluted water, a view that was strengthened by his observations linking a terrible outbreak of cholera around Broad Street, London, in 1854, to the local water pump (Box 1.4).

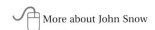 More about John Snow

Snow went to a lot of trouble to explain why some people developed cholera when they were believed *not* to have drunk the water from the Broad Street pump. He attributed these cases to the use of water from the pump in the local public houses, dining rooms and coffee shops. He was also able to explain why some groups of people did not develop cholera even though they lived in the affected area. If these low-risk groups (brewery workers, workhouse dwellers) had been users of the nearby Broad Street pump, Snow's hypothesis would have been in tatters. His findings among the 'exceptions' of both sorts thus bolster his arguments considerably: for the most part he found convincing explanations for why some people apparently at risk did not fall ill, and so too for the small group not living near the pump who did contract cholera. His openness to collecting all the facts, not just those that obviously supported his contention, is a salutary reminder of what constitutes good science – and that

Box 1.4 John Snow and the Broad Street pump (1854)

Within two hundred and fifty yards of the spot where Cambridge Street joins Broad Street, there were upwards of five hundred fatal attacks of cholera in ten days ... The mortality would undoubtedly have been much greater had it not been for the flight of the population ... so that in less than six days from the commencement of the outbreak, the most afflicted streets were deserted by more than three-quarters of their inhabitants.

There were a few cases of cholera in the neighbourhood of Broad Street, Golden Square, in the latter part of August; and the so-called outbreak, which commenced in the night between the 31st of August and the 1st of September, was, as in all similar instances, only a violent increase of the malady. As soon as I became acquainted with the situation and extent of this eruption of cholera, I suspected some contamination of the water of the much-frequented street-pump in Broad Street ... but on examining the water ... I found so little impurity in it of an organic nature, that I hesitated to come to a conclusion. Further inquiry, however, showed me that there was no other circumstance or agent common to the circumscribed locality in which this sudden increase of cholera occurred, and not extending beyond it, except the water of the above mentioned pump.

On proceeding to the spot, I found that nearly all the deaths had taken place within a short distance of the pump. There were only ten deaths in houses situated decidedly nearer to another street pump. In five of these cases the families of the deceased persons informed me that they always sent to the pump in Broad Street, as they preferred the water to that of the pump which was nearer. In three other cases, the deceased were children who went to school near the pump in Broad Street. Two of them were known to drink the water; and the parents of the third think it probable that it did so. The other two deaths, beyond the district which this pump supplies, represent only the amount of mortality from cholera that was occurring before the irruption took place ... [*Snow used a spot map to show the spread of cases in relation to this and other pumps.*] I had an interview with the Board of Guardians of St James's parish, on the evening of Thursday, 7th September, and represented the above circumstances to them. In consequence of what I said, the handle of the pump was removed on the following day.

Snow was also able to explain why some groups of people within the area did not develop cholera:

The Workhouse in Poland Street is more than three-fourths surrounded by houses in which deaths from cholera occurred, yet out of five

(*continued*)

Box 1.4 (*continued*)

hundred and thirty-five inmates, only five died of cholera, . . . The workhouse has a pump well on the premises, . . . and the inmates never sent to Broad Street for water. If the mortality in the workhouse had been equal to that in the streets immediately surrounding it on three sides, upwards of one hundred persons would have died. [*Note Snow's comparison of the 'observed' number of cases with the number 'expected'.*]

There is a Brewery in Broad Street, near to the pump, and on perceiving that no brewery men were registered as having died of cholera, I called on Mr Huggins, the proprietor. He informed me that there were above seventy workmen employed in the brewery, and that none of them had suffered from cholera . . . The men are allowed a certain quantity of malt liquor, and Mr Huggins believes they do not drink water at all . . .

The limited district in which this outbreak of cholera occurred, contains a great variety in the quality of the streets and houses; Poland Street and Great Pulteney Street consisting in a great measure of private houses occupied by one family, whilst Husband Street and Peter Street are occupied by the poor Irish. The remaining streets are intermediate in point of respectability. The mortality appears to have fallen pretty equally amongst all classes, in proportion to their number.

(Extracted from Snow, 1855.)

effective public health action requires realistic information about the problem at hand.

In addition to mapping the distribution of cases by place, Snow tabulated the numbers of cases and deaths over time. His time data are displayed graphically showing what is called an 'epidemic curve' in Figure 1.3.

When did the epidemic start? When did it end? What role did Snow's dramatic removal of the pump handle on 8 September play in interrupting its course?

The epidemic curve shows that the rise above the preceding baseline began on 30 August, with a dramatic increase over the next two days. And although the fall from the peak starts shortly thereafter, case numbers are still high for the next few days, not getting close to the preceding baseline until two weeks from the commencement. The epidemic had waned substantially before Snow's intervention on 8 September, probably largely due to the flight of much of the populace. However, because the graph shows the total *number* of cases occurring and does not take into account the size of the population, the *rate* of disease (the number of new cases occurring among the smaller number of people

Figure 1.3 The Broad Street cholera epidemic, 1854. (*Drawn from*: Snow, 1855.)

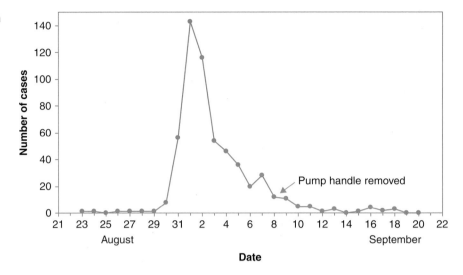

Pellagra, a disease that was common in poorer areas, is characterised by diarrhoea, dermatitis, dementia and ultimately death.

remaining in the area) could still have been fairly high. Snow's action may therefore truly have contributed to containment of the outbreak.

The second half of the nineteenth century saw the expansion of epidemiology in the direct service of public health in the UK, with a similar trend in the USA starting early the next century. Infectious diseases remained the core interest until the early 1900s, when Joseph Goldberger, a Hungarian physician working in the US Public Health Service, showed that pellagra was not infectious but of dietary origin and Wade Hampton Frost, another pioneer in the field, articulated the value of non-experimental epidemiology in discovering disease origins. Then in 1950, the publication of two case–control studies of lung cancer, by Richard Doll (epidemiologist) and Austin Bradford Hill (statistician) in the UK and Ernest Wynder (medical student) and Evart Graham (surgeon) in the USA, publicly marked the start of modern epidemiology.

Both papers (Doll and Hill, 1950; Wynder and Graham, 1950) showed that patients with lung cancer (*cases*) tended to smoke much more than people without lung cancer (*controls*). Doll and Hill then set out to confirm their findings using a different, prospective design (a *cohort study*, we will discuss the different types of study further in Chapter 4). They wrote to a large number of British doctors to find out how much they smoked and then 'followed' them (by mail and death records) over subsequent years to see what they died from. They again showed quite clearly that those who smoked cigarettes were much more likely to die of lung cancer than those who did not smoke, and the more they smoked the higher their risk (Figure 1.4). What is now known as the 'British Doctors Study' ran for more than 50 years (Doll *et al.*, 2004).

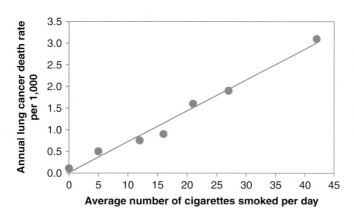

Figure 1.4 Age-standardised death rates from lung cancer in relation to the number of cigarettes smoked per day, British Doctors Study, 1951–1961. (*Reproduced from*: Doll and Hill, *British Medical Journal*, 1964;1:1399–1410, with permission from BMJ Publishing Group Ltd.)

Unfortunately, in spite of this and other clear evidence of the harmful effects of smoking, it was many years before attempts to discourage people from smoking were made, and it is only recently that tobacco companies have begun to admit that their products cause disease.

Twenty years after those key case–control studies came the publication of one of the first comprehensive epidemiology textbooks (MacMahon and Pugh, 1970). Widely influential at the time, it remains a benchmark for successors.

What does epidemiology offer?

You will have discerned parts of the answer to this question from what you have already read and done in reaching this point. Here we review the various elements more fully, and in doing so, effectively map the content of the rest of the book. This section outlines the broad purposes of epidemiology (which might be summarised as 'description', 'causal inference' and 'application') and the next aims to illustrate these through some concrete examples.

A large part of public health is about monitoring the health of a community, identifying health problems (who is becoming ill, where and when?), identifying what is causing the problems and then testing possible solutions to resolve or reduce the problem. Epidemiology is fundamental in providing the data needed to make public health judgements in each of these areas and the data come from studies of 'populations' (groups of people) of all sorts and sizes. Epidemiology largely deals with descriptions and comparisons of groups of people who may vary widely in their genetic make-up, behaviour and environments. The great challenge for epidemiologists is to deal with these multiple influences on health in a systematic and logical way in order to produce information of practical value to improve a community's health. How this challenge is met is what this book is all about.

Description of health status of populations

The observation and recording of health status makes it possible to identify sudden (and not-so-sudden) changes in the level of disease over time that might point to a need for action or further investigation. It also allows the setting of health targets, for example the *Millennium Development Goals* set by the United Nations (we will come back to discuss these in Chapter 2), and is essential to monitor progress towards these targets. Differences between groups of people in one area, between different geographical areas or at different time periods, can also give clues regarding the causes of disease (or health) in those groups. Such *descriptive statistics* are also important for health authorities and planners who need to know the nature and size of the health challenges faced by their communities.

Causation

In epidemiology and public health there is sometimes confusion over what is meant by **environmental factors**. We, and most others, use this term to include all non-genetic factors, including psychological, behavioural, social and cultural traits, as well as obvious environmental exposures such as air pollution.

Once a problem has been identified, we need to know what causes it, and probably the best-recognised use of epidemiology is in the search for the causes of disease. In some cases strong genetic factors have been identified, as for example with cystic fibrosis, a lung disease that occurs because of specific genetic defects. In other instances major environmental factors are crucial, such as asbestos in the development of lung mesothelioma (a rare form of lung cancer). In general, though, there is almost always some inter-action between genetic and environmental factors in the causation of disease. Epidemiological tools are central to the identification of modifiable factors that will allow preventive interventions.

Evaluation of interventions

Once we have identified a factor that causes disease, we then want to know whether we can reduce a population's exposure to this factor and so prevent the occurrence of disease – a 'primary' prevention programme (we will discuss prevention further in Chapter 14). As you will see in Chapter 4, epidemiology has a core role to play in this process and it is also key to the evaluation of different treatments for a particular disease (an aspect of both mainstream and clinical epidemiology) and assessments of the effectiveness of health services and policies.

Natural history and prognosis

Epidemiologists are also concerned with the course or *natural history* of a disease and the likely outcome or *prognosis*, both in individuals and in groups. Such knowledge has obvious value for discussing treatment options with individual patients, as well as for planning and evaluating interventions. Of particular interest is whether early disease is present for long before symptoms drive someone to seek medical attention. If it is and this 'subclinical' disease can be detected before the normal point of diagnosis and if, as a result, treatment is more effective, this opens the way for screening programmes that aim to improve treatment outcomes. (We will discuss screening further in Chapter 15.)

What do epidemiologists do?

How then are these objectives of epidemiological research attained? Let us look briefly at some more examples of what the practice of epidemiology can yield across some of its main dimensions.

Descriptive studies: person, place and time

By 'person'

In some countries there is concern over health differences between indigenous people and the rest of the population. Figure 1.5 shows Australian mortality data comparing Indigenous with non-Indigenous people. The bars show how many times higher mortality from circulatory, respiratory and infectious diseases and cancer is in Indigenous men and women in Australia compared to non-Indigenous Australians (the horizontal line at the level '1' indicates the point where mortality rates in Indigenous and non-Indigenous people would be equal).

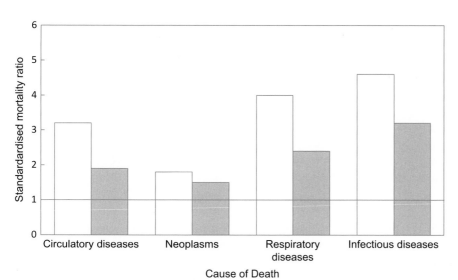

Figure 1.5 Age-standardised mortality ratios for selected diseases in the Indigenous compared to the non-Indigenous population in Australia, 2004–2008 (*drawn from*: AIHW, 2011). The bars indicate how much higher mortality was among Indigenous men (open bars) and women (solid bars) compared to non-Indigenous people.

How many times higher is mortality from circulatory diseases in Indigenous males than in non-Indigenous males?

What is the obvious striking fact about relative mortality in Indigenous people in general?

Mortality for circulatory diseases in Indigenous men is more than three times that in non-Indigenous men, while for women it is almost double that in non-Indigenous women. The data presented indicate a much worse health situation for Indigenous Australians than for the non-Indigenous population. (Note: these **standardised mortality ratios** are similar to the relative risk in the food poisoning example earlier. They show how many times more likely it was for an Indigenous Australian to die than a non-Indigenous Australian in 2004–2008. The process of standardisation also takes account of the fact that Indigenous Australians are, on average, younger than non-Indigenous people. We will discuss these measures further in Chapter 2.)

By 'place'

How 'healthy' is any given country in relation to the rest of the world – are things better or worse there compared with other countries? Figure 1.6 shows cardiovascular disease mortality rates in different countries. You can see that the UK, for example, is better off than Ireland, New Zealand, and particularly Finland and Hungary; but things could be better – as shown by the lower rates in the Netherlands, Portugal, France and Japan. What is it about the Japanese that makes them less likely to die of cardiovascular disease? If we can work this out then perhaps we could reduce cardiovascular mortality in the UK and elsewhere to the level seen in Japan (provided that the differences are not purely genetic). By studying patterns of disease and relating them to variations in risk factors for the disease we can come up with possible reasons why some people or places have higher rates of disease than others or why disease rates have changed over time.

By 'time'

What emerges if we look at the changing patterns of mortality in a country over time? The graph in Figure 1.7 shows mortality trends for selected conditions and groups over more than three decades (1979–2013) in the USA.

What are the most notable features of Figure 1.7?

The picture we see is mixed, some good news, some concerning. The most obvious health success story is the consistent downward trend in deaths from heart attacks, with about 100 fewer people in every 100,000 dying from them at the end of the period. A less dramatic decline is seen for motor vehicle

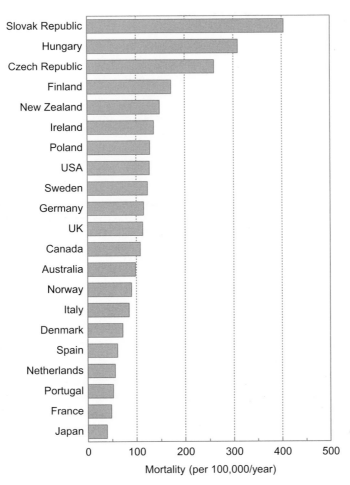

Figure 1.6 Ischaemic heart disease mortality for males and females in 2011, age standardised to the 2010 OECD population. (*Drawn from*: OECD, 2013.)

accidents. Deaths from AIDS rose until 1995 and have fallen since (an epidemic where perhaps the worst is past, at least for the USA). The same is true for lung cancer in men, although on this scale it is not striking. Most worrying was the steady rise in lung cancer deaths among women, although this has now levelled off.

However, these details don't give us the big picture. Some up, some down, some changing direction: what was happening to overall mortality in the USA during the period? Total mortality rates fell slightly from about 880 to 810 per 100,000 per year, but we would not be able to fit this information onto the same graph without losing almost all the details we noted above. We could, of course, draw a separate graph showing the total death rate, but we can do both by changing the scale of the vertical axis, as in Figure 1.8.

Figure 1.7 US mortality rates, 1979–2013, for heart attack (open diamonds), lung cancer in males (filled squares), lung cancer in females (filled triangles), motor vehicle accidents (open triangles), diabetes (filled circles) and AIDS (filled diamonds) (*drawn from*: CDC Wonder (CDC), accessed 27 February 2015).

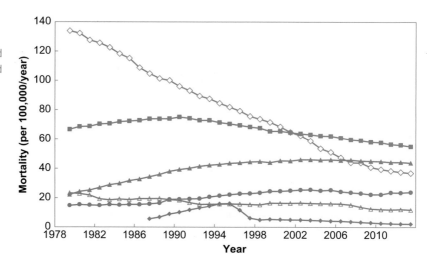

Figure 1.8 US mortality rates (log scale), 1979–2013 for all causes (open circles), heart attack (open diamonds), lung cancer in males (filled squares), lung cancer in females (filled triangles), motor vehicle accidents (open triangles), diabetes (filled circles), and AIDS (filled diamonds) (*drawn from*: CDC Wonder (CDC), accessed 27 February 2015).

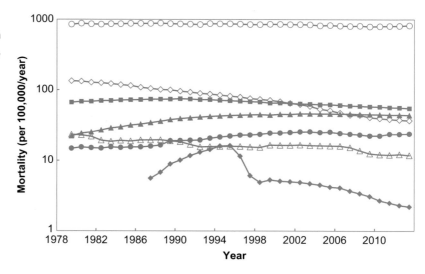

Instead of a linear scale (1, 2, 3, 4, . . .), we have now used a 'log' (logarithmic) scale (1, 10, 100, 1000, . . .) where the distance between 1 and 10 (a 10-fold difference) is the same as the distance between 10 and 100 (also a 10-fold difference), and so on. Now we can fit mortality rates as different as 2.2/100,000 (AIDS mortality in 2013) and 878/100,000 (all-cause mortality in 1980) on the same page. It also allows us to compare *relative* changes in mortality rates directly, with parallel slopes reflecting equal rates of change. The fall in heart attacks looks much less dramatic now: the drop is only about 2%–3% per year but, as Figure 1.7 showed, this led to a large absolute benefit,

Box 1.5 Smallpox

The elimination of smallpox had a major impact on the health of millions of people, especially in many of the poorest countries. Descriptive epidemiology played a major role by providing information about the distribution of cases (*jointly by person, place and time*) and levels of transmission, by mapping outbreaks and by evaluating control measures. In 1967, there were 10–15 million new cases and 2 million deaths from smallpox in 31 countries. By 1976, smallpox was being reported in only two countries and the last naturally occurring case was recorded in 1977. Elimination of this scourge was helped by simple but painstaking case-finding and counting (*'shoe-leather' epidemiology*) and by directing vaccination programmes to places and people still at risk.

The term ***shoe-leather epidemiology*** is sometimes used when the epidemiologist travels around to interview people (presumably wearing out their shoes in the process). It can be a critical aspect of public health epidemiology and could also be used to describe John Snow's work.

because the death rate was so high to start with. The rate of change for AIDS looks much steeper on a log scale because the percentage change is greater, but the absolute benefits are clearly much less. In public health we need to think on both relative and absolute scales: they tell us different things that are useful for different purposes. We will take this further in Chapter 5.

See Box 1.5 for a practical example of how simple descriptive epidemiology helped solve a major global health problem.

Analytic studies

Descriptive work like this may generate ideas about what is causing disease which can then be tested further in *analytic* studies, looking for associations between potential causal agents and diseases. This research is based on facts collected directly from groups of individuals, not large-scale population statistics. Are people with higher blood pressure more likely to develop coronary heart disease than those with normal blood pressure? Are people who smoke more likely to develop lung cancer than those who do not? Even more usefully, how *much* more likely is a smoker to develop lung cancer than a non-smoker? Does risk depend on the number of cigarettes smoked? That is, how *strong* is the effect of the exposure, and does it increase with higher levels of exposure? In the British Doctors Study mentioned earlier, Doll and Hill found that the risk of lung cancer increased steadily as people smoked more cigarettes (Figure 1.4). This adds weight to the idea that smoking cigarettes really does affect the chance that an individual will develop lung cancer. Box 1.6 describes another cohort study which has studied many exposures and diseases over the past three decades.

> ## Box 1.6 The Nurses' Health Study
>
> This cohort study of 120,000 US nurses was started in 1976 by Frank Speizer of the Channing Laboratory, Harvard Medical School. The study was initially funded for five years to study whether the oral contraceptive pill caused breast cancer, but the nurses are still being followed 40 years later. Hundreds of scientific papers have been published, covering scores of diseases and exposures and investigating their inter-relationships. The study has been particularly influential in the field of diet and disease (nutritional epidemiology), owing to diet questionnaires that the nurses have been completing since 1980. As with other long-term follow-ups of cohorts, such as the British Doctors Study of Doll and Hill, its success is jointly dependent on the enthusiasm and commitment of researchers and participants. For the latter this has extended to providing blood, toenail clippings (for measurement of trace metals) and samples of tapwater over the years. This human side to epidemiology does not feature much in textbooks, but is fundamental to successful fieldwork. (www.nurseshealthstudy.org)

Once we have found an association, the challenge is then to evaluate this in order to determine whether something really *causes* disease or is linked to it only secondarily. If we find that people with a peptic ulcer drink a lot of milk, does this mean that drinking milk causes ulcers, or simply that people with an ulcer drink milk to ease their pain? This latter situation is sometimes described as *reverse causality*. We will look more deeply at this challenge in Chapter 10.

Intervention studies

Finally, epidemiologists test new preventive measures, programmes or treatments to see if they actually do reduce ill health or promote good health. They also evaluate the effectiveness of these 'intervention' programmes after they have been implemented: do they deliver the benefits seen in the initial studies? Interventions can include different health-promotion strategies targeted at individuals or whole communities, or clinical trials of new drugs designed to prevent or cure disease. Does taking aspirin reduce your chance of having a heart attack? Which of several strategies is better at helping people give up smoking? Is one drug better than another for treating bronchitis?

A natural experiment

We will end this chapter with another example from John Snow's *On the Mode of Communication of Cholera* (1855) because, although this text is more than

150 years old, the methods he used and his combination of flair, skill, logic and dogged persistence remain the cornerstones of modern epidemiology. His work also exemplifies, in more detail than modern papers, the logical dissection of evidence about disease patterns to identify practical preventive strategies – which is still the key function of epidemiology – and it gives an excellent sense of the role and utility of epidemiology in practical public health.

In the early 1850s, London was cholera-free for a number of years and during that period one of the major water supply companies (the Lambeth Company) moved their waterworks out of London, thereby obtaining water free of the sewage of the city. During the next major cholera outbreak in 1853–1854, Snow was able to obtain information about the number of deaths occurring in the different subdistricts of London and he found that cholera mortality was lower in areas supplied by water from the Lambeth Company than in those supplied by the Southwark and Vauxhall water company which continued to take water from Battersea in the city. He did not stop there, but went on to conduct his 'Grand Experiment' (see Box 1.7).

Box 1.7 A grand experiment

Although the facts . . . afford very strong evidence of the powerful influence which the drinking water containing the sewage of a town exerts over the spread of cholera, when that disease is present, yet the question does not end here; for the intermixing of the water supply of the Southwark and Vauxhall Company with that of the Lambeth Company, over an extensive part of London, admitted of the subject being sifted in such a way as to yield the most incontrovertible proof on one side or the other . . . A few houses are supplied by one Company and a few by the other, according to the decision of the owner or occupier at that time when the Water Companies were in active competition . . . Each Company supplies both rich and poor, both large houses and small; there is no difference either in the condition or occupation of the persons receiving the water of the different Companies. Now it must be evident that, if the diminution of cholera, in the districts partly supplied with the improved water, depended on this supply, the houses receiving it would be the houses enjoying the whole benefit of the diminution of the malady, whilst the houses supplied with the water from Battersea Fields would suffer the same mortality as they would if the improved supply did not exist at all. As there is no difference whatever, either in the houses or the people receiving the supply of the two water Companies, or in any of the physical conditions

(*continued*)

Box 1.7 *(continued)*

with which they are surrounded, it is obvious that no experiment could have been devised which would more thoroughly test the effect of water supply on the progress of cholera than this which circumstances placed ready made before the observer.

The experiment, too, was on the grandest scale. No fewer than three hundred thousand people of both sexes, of every age and occupation, and of every rank and station, from gentlefolk down to the very poor, were divided into two groups without their choice, and, in most cases, without their knowledge; one group being supplied with water containing the sewage of London, and amongst it, whatever might have come from the cholera patients, the other group having water quite free from such impurity.

To turn this grand experiment to account, all that was required was to learn the supply of water to each individual house where a fatal attack of cholera might occur . . .

The Epidemic of 1854

When the cholera returned to London in July of the present year . . . I resolved to spare no exertion . . . to ascertain the exact effect of the water supply on the progress of the epidemic, in the places where all the circumstances were so happily adapted for the inquiry . . . I accordingly asked permission at the General Register Office to be supplied with the addresses of persons dying of cholera, in those districts where the supply of the two Companies is intermingled in the manner I have stated above . . . I commenced my inquiry about the middle of August with two sub-districts of Lambeth . . . There were forty-four deaths in these sub-districts down to 12th August, and I found that thirty-eight of the houses in which these deaths occurred were supplied with water by the Southwark and Vauxhall Company, four houses were supplied by the Lambeth Company, and two had pump-wells on the premises and no supply from either of the Companies.

As soon as I had ascertained these particulars, I communicated them to Dr Farr, who was much struck with the result, and at his suggestion the Registrars of all the south districts of London were requested to make a return of the water supply of the house in which the attack took place, in all cases of death from cholera. This order was to take place after the 26th of August, and I resolved to carry my inquiry down to that date, so that the facts might be ascertained for the whole course of the epidemic.

(continued)

Box 1.7 (*continued*)

The inquiry was necessarily attended with a good deal of trouble. There were very few instances in which I could at once get the information I required. Even when the water rates were paid by the residents, they can seldom remember the name of the Water Company till they have looked for the receipt. In the case of working people who pay weekly rents, the rates are invariably paid by the landlord or his agent, who often lives at a distance, and the residents know nothing about the matter. It would, indeed, have been almost impossible for me to complete the inquiry, if I had not found that I could distinguish the water of the two companies with perfect certainty by a chemical test. The test I employed was founded on the great difference in the quantity of chloride sodium [salt] contained in the two kinds of water, at the time I made the inquiry . . .

According to a return which was made to Parliament, the Southwark and Vauxhall Company supplied 40,046 houses from January 1st to December 31st, 1853, and the Lambeth Company supplied 26,107 houses during the same period; consequently, as 286 fatal attacks of cholera took place, in the first four weeks of the epidemic, in houses supplied by the former Company, and only 14 in houses supplied by the latter, the proportion of fatal attacks to each 10,000 houses was as follows. Southwark and Vauxhall 71, Lambeth 5. **The cholera was therefore fourteen times as fatal at this period amongst persons having the impure water of the Southwark and Vauxhall Company as amongst those having the purer water from Thames Ditton.**

(Excerpted from Snow, 1855.)

Conclusions

Again, we have a vivid picture of a master epidemiologist at work. Not satisfied that his hypothesis had been adequately tested, Snow identified the opportunity to conduct an even more rigorous test – his '*Grand Experiment*' – and in doing so he addressed the major epidemiological issues that still concern us today.

- He identified a situation in which people were unknowingly divided into two groups differing only in the source of their water, thereby creating what was effectively a **randomised trial** (we will look at the different types of epidemiological study in Chapter 4).
- In doing so, he realised the importance of ruling out other differences between the groups (e.g. sex, age, occupation, SES) that could explain any

mortality differences (a problem known as **confounding** that we will come back to in Chapter 8).

- He worked long and hard to acquire *accurate information* about both the water supply and the number of cholera deaths in each house – we will consider sources of data in Chapter 3 and will discuss the problem of error in Chapter 7.
- He *measured the **rates of** occurrence of cholera* in the two groups of houses served by the different water companies – we will look further at measures such as these in Chapter 2.
- He calculated *how many times more common* cholera deaths were in those houses receiving the contaminated water – we will come back to this measure (again a **relative risk**) in Chapter 5.
- He then integrated all of his information to reach the conclusion that cholera was indeed *caused* by contaminated water – Chapter 10.

He did not stop there, but went on to make a series of clear practical recommendations to prevent transmission of cholera in future – sensible measures including the need for cleanliness and sterilisation that are still practised today.

Snow's work therefore sets the scene for the chapters to come. Chapters 2–8 cover the basic principles and underlying theory of epidemiology in a very 'hands-on' way, leading to Chapters 9–11, which integrate this information in a practical look at how we read and interpret epidemiological reports, synthesise a mass of information in a single review and, finally, think about assessing causality. Chapters 12–15 then look at some specific applications of epidemiology and Chapter 16 concludes with a fresh look at epidemiology and how we can use it to help address the health concerns facing the world today.

But, before you move on, take a minute to stop and think. Imagine that someone asked you what epidemiology was and why it was useful. Could you now give them a satisfactory explanation in a few sentences?

REFERENCES

References

AIHW (Australian Institute of Health and Welfare). (2011). *The health and welfare of Australia's Aboriginal and Torres Strait Islander people, an overview 2011*. Cat. no. IHW 42. Canberra: AIHW.

CDC (Centers for Disease Control and Prevention), National Center for Health Statistics. Compressed Mortality File 1979–1998. CDC WONDER On-line Database, compiled from Compressed Mortality File CMF 1968–1988, Series 20, No. 2A, 2000 and CMF 1989–1998, Series 20, No. 2E, 2003. http://wonder.cdc.gov/cmf-icd9.html, accessed 8 Jan 2010 7:24:23 PM and Compressed Mortality File 1999–2006. CDC WONDER Online Database, released

October 2014. Data are from the Compressed Mortality File 1999–2013 Series 20 No. 2S, 2014, as compiled from data provided by the 57 vital statistics jurisdictions through the Vital Statistics Cooperative Program. http://wonder.cdc.gov/cmf-icd10.html, accessed 27 Feb 2015 12:40:22 AM.

Concise Oxford Dictionary, 5th edn. (1964). Oxford: Oxford University Press.

Doll, R. (1964). Mortality in relation to smoking: ten years' observations of British doctors. *British Medical Journal*, 1: 1399–1410, 1460–1467.

Doll, R. and Hill, A. B. (1950). Smoking and carcinoma of the lung. *British Medical Journal*, 2: 739–748.

Doll, R., Peto, R., Boreham, J. and Sutherland, I. (2004). Mortality in relation to smoking: 50 years' observations on male British doctors. *British Medical Journal*, 328: 1519–1528.

Frost, W. H. (1927). *Epidemiology. Nelson Loose-Leaf System, Public Health– Preventive Medicine*. Volume 2, Chapter 7. New York: Thomas Nelson & Sons. Re-printed in: Maxcy, K. F., ed. (1941). *Papers of Wade Hampton Frost, M.D. A contribution to epidemiological method*. New York: The Commonwealth Fund.

Graunt, J. (1662). *Natural and Political Observations Mentioned in a Following Index and Made Upon the Bills of Mortality*. London. www.neonatology.org/ pdf/graunt.pdf (accessed 29 April 2015).

Hippocrates of Cos. (400 BC). *On Airs, Waters, and Places*. Translated by Francis Adams. (http://classics.mit.edu).

Hook, D., Jalaludin, B. and Fitzsimmons, G. (1996). *Clostridium perfringens* food-borne outbreak: an epidemiological investigation. *Australian and New Zealand Journal of Public Health*, 20: 119–122.

Lilienfeld, A. M. and Lilienfeld, D. E. (1980). *Foundations of Epidemiology*, 2nd edn. New York: Oxford University Press.

MacMahon, B. and Pugh, T. F. (1970). *Epidemiology – Principles and Methods*. Boston: Little Brown.

Makk, L., Creech, J. L., Whelan, J. G. and Johnson, M. D. (1974). Liver damage and angiosarcoma in vinyl chloride workers – a systematic detection program. *Journal of the American Medical Association*, 230: 64–68.

Miettinen, O. S. (1978). *Course Notes – Principles of Epidemiologic Research*. Harvard School of Public Health.

OECD. (2013). *Health at a Glance 2013: OECD Indicators*, OECD Publishing. http://dx.doi.org/10.1787/health_glance-2013-en (accessed 29 April 2015).

Porta, M., ed. (2008). *A Dictionary of Epidemiology*, 5th edn. New York: Oxford University Press.

Porta, M., ed. (2014). *A Dictionary of Epidemiology*, 6th edn. New York: Oxford University Press.

Pridemore, W. A. and Spivak, A. L. (2003). Patterns of suicide mortality in Russia. *Suicide and Life-Threatening Behavior*, 33: 132–150.

Rosen, G. (1958). *A History of Public Health*. New York: MD Publications.

Selikoff, I. J., Churg, J. and Hammond, E. C. (1965). Relation between exposure to asbestos and mesothelioma. *New England Journal of Medicine*, 272: 560–565.

Snow, J. (1855). *On the Mode of Communication of Cholera*, 2nd edn. London: Churchill. www.ph.ucla.edu/epi/snow.html (accessed 29 April 2015).

Stolley, P. D. and Lasky, T. (1995). *Investigating Disease Patterns: the Science of Epidemiology*. New York: Scientific American Library.

WHO (World Health Organization). (1948). Text of the constitution of the World Health Organization. *Official Record World Health Organization* 2: 100.

Wynder, E. L. and Graham, E. A. (1950). Tobacco smoking as a possible etiologic factor in bronchiogenic carcinoma. A study of six hundred and eighty-four proved cases. *Journal of the American Medical Association*, 143: 329–336.

Zaridze, D., Maximovitch, D., Lazarev, A., *et al.* (2009). Alcohol poisoning is a main determinant of recent mortality trends in Russia: evidence from a detailed analysis of mortality statistics and autopsies. *International Journal of Epidemiology*, 38: 143–153.

RECOMMENDED FOR FURTHER READING

- Classic introductory epidemiology texts:
  MacMahon, B. and Pugh, T. F. (1970). *Epidemiology – Principles and Methods*. Boston: Little Brown.
  Lilienfeld, A. M. and Lilienfeld, D. E. (1980). *Foundations of Epidemiology*, 2nd edn. New York: Oxford University Press.
- For a very approachable introduction to the science of epidemiology:
  Stolley, P. D. and Lasky, T. (1995). *Investigating Disease Patterns: the Science of Epidemiology*. New York: Scientific American Library.

How long is a piece of string? Measuring disease frequency

Description	Association	Alternative explanations	Integration & interpretation	Practical applications
Chapter 2: Measuring health	Chapters 4–5	Chapters 6–8	Chapters 9–11	Chapters 12–15

Box 2.1 Who drinks the most beer?

According to the Brewers Association of Japan, the Chinese drink the most beer in the world (44,201 million litres in 2012, up from 28,640 in 2004) followed by the Americans (24,186 million litres). In contrast, the Czech Republic ranked a lowly 21st in terms of total consumption (1905 million litres) and Ireland didn't even make the top 25. This information may be useful for planning production, but do the Chinese and Americans really drink more beer than the rest of us? An alternative and possibly more informative way to look at these data is in terms of consumption *per capita*. When we do this, the USA falls to 14th position in the 'beer drinking league table' (77 litres per capita) and China falls way off the screen (a mere 33 litres per capita). The Czechs are now the champions (149 litres per capita), followed by Austria (108 litres) and Germany (106 litres) in 2nd and 3rd place and Ireland comes in 6th place (98 litres per capita). While Australia held the 4th spot in 2004 with an average of 110 litres per capita, by 2012 they had fallen to 11th on the table (83 litres).

(*Source*: www.kirinholdings.co.jp/english/news/2014/0108_01.html, accessed 2 May 2015.)

The goal of public health is to improve the overall health of a population by reducing the burden of disease and premature death. To do this we need to be able to quantify the levels of ill-health or disease in a population in order to monitor our progress towards eliminating existing problems and to identify the emergence of new problems. Many different measures are used by researchers and policy makers to describe the health of populations. You have already met some of these for example the attack rate, which was used to investigate the source of the food poisoning outbreak in the previous chapter. In this chapter we will introduce some more of the most commonly used measures so that you can use and interpret them correctly. We will first discuss the three fundamental measures that underlie both the attack rate and most of the other health statistics that you will come across in health-related reports, the **incidence rate**, **incidence proportion** (also called risk or **cumulative incidence**) and **prevalence**, and will then look at how they are calculated and used in practice. We will finish by considering some other more elaborate measures that attempt to get closer to describing the overall health of a population. As you will see, this is not always as straightforward as it might seem.

What are we measuring?

Before we can start to measure disease, we have to have a very clear idea of what it is that we are trying to determine. In general, the diagnosis of disease is based on a combination of *symptoms*, subjective indications of disease reported by the person themselves; *signs*, objective indications of disease apparent to the physician; and additional *tests*. Criteria for making a diagnosis can be very simple: the presence of antibodies against an infectious agent can indicate infection, and diagnosis of most cancers is fairly straight-forward on the basis of tissue histology (examination with a light microscope); but for some diseases, particularly mental health conditions such as depression, the diagnostic criteria are much more complex, involving combinations of signs and symptoms.

For health data to be meaningful, diagnostic criteria leading to a case definition have to be clear, unambiguous and easy to use under a wide range of circumstances. It is important to remember that different case definitions can lead to very different pictures. As shown in Figure 2.1, a study in the United Arab Emirates showed that the prevalence of gestational diabetes (diabetes during pregnancy) in a group of 3500 women was much higher using one set of criteria to diagnose diabetes (Carpenter's criteria, 30.4%) than another (O'Sullivan's criteria, 20.2%) (Agarwal and Punnose, 2002). Such differences obviously have major implications for health care planners. If you want to compare information from different reports the first thing to

From www.CartoonStock.com

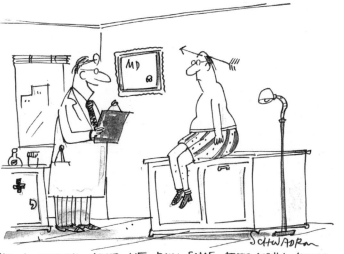

"DON'T WORRY. AFTER WE RUN SOME TESTS, WE'LL KNOW FOR SURE WHAT'S CAUSING YOUR HEADACHES."

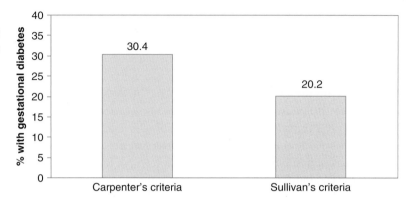

Figure 2.1 Percent of population with gestational diabetes according to two sets of diagnostic criteria. (*Drawn from*: Agarwal and Punnose, 2002.)

check is that you are comparing apples with apples – have they all measured the same thing using the same criteria? This can be a particular problem when trying to compare patterns of disease over time because changes in diagnostic criteria can lead to sudden increases or decreases in the number of cases recorded, and you will see a dramatic example of this in Chapter 3. It is also important to consider how good the measurements are, and we will look at this and the implications of poor measurement in more detail in Chapter 7. For the rest of this chapter, however, we will assume that we know what we want to measure and that we can measure it accurately.

The concepts: prevalence and incidence

Once we have defined what we mean by disease,[1] we can go on to measure how often it occurs.

In Table 2.1 we see the estimated number of people infected with HIV in the various regions of the world at the end of 2012, and the number of new cases of HIV infection that occurred during 2012. These data clearly show the huge burden borne by Sub-Saharan Africa, which has six times the number of cases of any other region, but what can they tell us about the relative importance of HIV in other regions? The East Asia and Western/Central Europe regions both had almost 900,000 people infected with HIV at the end of 2012. How can we describe and compare the burden of HIV in these populations more fully?

What percentage of people in Western and Central Europe were living with HIV at the end of 2012?

---

[1] Note that although much of our discussion will be in terms of measuring disease, the same principles apply to any dichotomous health outcome – that is, one that is either present or absent.

Table 2.1 Estimates of the number of people living with HIV and the number of new HIV infections around the world in 2012.

Region	Population (×1000)	People living with HIV (end of 2012)	New HIV infections (2012)
Sub-Saharan Africa	867,000	25,000,000	1,600,000
East Asia	1,554,400	880,000	81,000
Oceania	34,200	51,000	2100
South and Southeast Asia	2,286,000	3,900,000	270,000
Eastern Europe & Central Asia	278,900	1,300,000	130,000
Western and Central Europe	608,200	860,000	29,000
North Africa & Middle East	319,500	260,000	32,000
North America	348,800	1,300,000	48,000
Caribbean	36,300	250,000	12,000
Latin America	557,000	1,500,000	86,000
TOTAL	**6,890,300**	**35,301,000**	**2,290,100**

(Data source: UNAIDS, 2013 and Population Reference Bureau, 2012.)

What percentage of people in Western and Central Europe became HIV-positive during 2012?

At the end of 2012, 860,000 of the 608,200,000 people in Western and Central Europe or 0.14% of the population were living with HIV. During 2012, another 29,000 people or 0.0048% of the population became infected with HIV. Now 0.0048% is a very small number. It simply tells us that there were 0.0048 new HIV infections for every 100 people during 2012, so an alternative way to present the same information would be to multiply the numbers by 1000 and say that there were 4.8 new infections in every 100,000 people ($4.8/100,000$ or $4.8/10^5$).[2]

What you calculated above were, first, the **prevalence** of *existing* HIV infections in Western and Central Europe at the end of 2012 and, second, the **incidence** of *new* HIV infections in the same region during 2012. These measures give us two different ways of quantifying the amount of disease in a population. Table 2.2 shows the same information for each of the regions. These data confirm the high levels of HIV infection in Sub-Saharan Africa and show us that, despite the relatively low number of new cases in the Caribbean, the small population there means that the incidence is also high. The data

---

[2] If you are not familiar with this nomenclature, the superscript number is simply a shorthand way to say how many zeros the number has. So, 10^2 would be 100, 10^5 is 100,000 and 10^6 is one million (1,000,000).

Table 2.2 The prevalence and incidence of HIV infection around the world in 2012.

Region	Population (×1000)	People living with HIV (end of 2012)	Prevalence (%)	New HIV infections (2012)	Incidence (per 100,000/year)
Sub-Saharan Africa	867,000	25,000,000	2.88	1,600,000	184.5
East Asia	1,554,400	880,000	0.06	81,000	5.2
Oceania	34,200	51,000	0.15	2,100	6.1
South and Southeast Asia	2,286,000	3,900,000	0.17	270,000	11.8
Eastern Europe & Central Asia	278,900	1,300,000	0.47	130,000	46.6
Western and Central Europe	608,200	860,000	0.14	29,000	4.8
North Africa & Middle East	319,500	260,000	0.08	32,000	10.0
North America	348,800	1,300,000	0.37	48,000	13.8
Caribbean	36,300	250,000	0.69	12,000	33.0
Latin America	557,000	1,500,000	0.27	86,000	15.4
TOTAL	**6,890,300**	**35,301,000**	**0.51**	**2,290,100**	**33.2**

(Data source: UNAIDS, 2013 and Population Reference Bureau, 2012.)

also show us that although the actual *numbers* of cases in East Asia and Western/Central Europe are similar, the *prevalence* per 100 people (%) is much lower in East Asia (0.06%) than in Western and Central Europe (0.14%). Like the beer example in Box 2.1, these data emphasise the need to take the size of a population into account when comparing it with others.

We will now look at these measures in more detail.

Prevalence

The prevalence of a disease tells us what proportion of a population actually has the disease at a specific point in time: an estimated 0.14% or 140 of every 100,000 people in Western and Central Europe were living with HIV at the end of 2012. This is a snapshot of the situation at a single point in time and, for this reason, it is sometimes called the 'point' prevalence. Note that you may also see references to 'period prevalence' which measures the proportion of the population that had the disease *at any time during a specified period*. This is a complex measure that combines the prevalence (everybody who had the disease at the start of the period) and incidence (all of the new cases of disease during the period).

> **Percentages** can be confusing because there is often more than one way in which they can be calculated and this can lead to problems with interpretation – see Box 2.2 for some additional guidance.

> *Prevalence* measures the amount of a disease in a population at a given point in time:
>
> $$\text{Prevalence} = \frac{\text{Number of people with disease at a given point in time}}{\text{Total number of people in the population at that time}} \quad (2.1)$$

Box 2.2 A note about percentages

Imagine a study that gave the following results:

	Asthma	No asthma	Total
Non-smokers	40	360	400
Smokers	30	170	200
Total	70	530	600

There are two ways that we can look at these data. One way would be to calculate the percentages of (a) non-smokers and (b) smokers who have asthma – these are row percentages because we use the total of each row, the number of non-smokers or smokers, as the denominator (note: the *denominator* is the bottom half of a fraction and the *numerator* the top half):

	Asthma	No asthma	Total
Non-smokers	40 ÷ 400 = 10%	360 ÷ 400 = 90%	400 = 100%
Smokers	30 ÷ 200 = 15%	170 ÷ 200 = 85%	200 = 100%

This tells us that 10% of non-smokers and 15% of smokers have asthma.

Alternatively, we could use the same data to calculate the percentages of people with and without asthma who smoke – these are column percentages because now we use the total of each column, the number of people with or without asthma, as the denominator:

	Asthma	No asthma
Non-smokers	40÷70 = 57%	360 ÷ 530 = 68%
Smokers	30÷70 = 43%	170 ÷ 530 = 32%
Total	70 = 100%	530 = 100%

This tells us that 43% of people with asthma and only 32% of people without asthma are smokers.

It is very important to decide first which percentages are most relevant for a particular situation and then to calculate and interpret the percentages correctly. Saying that 43% of people with asthma are smokers (correct) is not the same as saying that 43% of smokers have asthma (incorrect; 15% of smokers have asthma).

Prevalence measures are just one number (the number of people with disease) divided by another number (the total number of people in the population). They have no units, and are mostly reported simply as a proportion or a percentage (2.9% of Sub-Saharan Africans were living with HIV at the end of 2012), but may also be shown as cases/population, for example 370/100,000

Rounding: If the first number that is cut off is between 0 and 4 you round *down* and if it is between 5 and 9 you round *up*. Here we rounded 2.8835 *up* to 2.9, but if it had been 2.8435 we would have rounded down to 2.8. In practice it is rarely necessary to show results to more than two or three 'significant' figures (e.g. 2900, 2.9, 0.0029 are all rounded to 2 significant figures), unless we are confident the additional numbers are both accurate and important.

North Americans were living with HIV at the end of 2012. Note that a more precise answer for the proportion of Sub-Saharan Africans with HIV is 0.02883506... or 2.883506% but, for simplicity, we have *rounded* this to one decimal place giving 2.9%. Although you will often see the term 'prevalence rate', this is not a true rate because a rate should include units of time. An example of a true rate is the use of distance travelled *per hour*, i.e. kph or mph, to measure the speed of a car. The time point at which people are counted should, however, always be reported when giving an estimate of prevalence. This is often a fixed point in calendar time, such as 31 December 2015, but it can also be a fixed point in life, for instance, birth or retirement. For example, if 1000 babies were born alive in one hospital in a given year and, of these, five babies were born with congenital abnormalities, we would say that the prevalence of congenital abnormality *at birth* was 5/1000 live births in that year. Prevalence can be expressed per 100 people (per cent, %) or per 1000 (10^3), 10,000 (10^4) or 100,000 (10^5). It doesn't matter as long as it is clear which is being used.

In practice, it would be rare to identify all prevalent cases of disease at one precise point in time; e.g. a blood pressure survey may take weeks or months to conduct, given limited numbers of researchers, amounts of equipment and availability of those being measured. The exact size of the population may also not be known on a given day and this might well be based on an estimate or projection from the most recent census data.

Incidence

The **incidence** of disease measures how quickly people are developing the disease and it differs from prevalence because it considers only *new* infections, sometimes called *incident cases*, that occurred in a specific time period. During 2012, 1.6 million people in Sub-Saharan Africa or 0.18% of the population were newly diagnosed as HIV-positive. Another way of saying this is that the incidence of HIV infection was 184.5/100,000 per year (Table 2.2). You will find that people use the term 'incidence' on its own to mean slightly different things – some use it for the *number* of new cases (i.e. 1.6 million), some for the *proportion* of people who are newly infected (i.e. 0.0018 or 0.18%) and some for the *rate* at which new infection has occurred (i.e. 184.5 new cases per 100,000 people *per year*). To avoid confusion we will describe the latter measure as the **incidence rate** which, unlike measures of prevalence, is a true rate because it includes a measure of time.

$$\text{Incidence rate} = \frac{\text{Number of people who develop disease } \textit{in one year}}{\text{Average number of people in the population } \textit{in the same year}}$$

$$(2.2)$$

We will look further at how to calculate these measures later, but first let us consider the concept of the 'population at risk' and the relationship between prevalence and the incidence rate.

Population at risk

In the example above it is probably not unreasonable to assume that everyone in the population might be at risk of contracting HIV, although, obviously, some groups will be more 'at risk' than others; but what if the disease of interest were something like cervical cancer? To use the whole population to calculate rates of cancer of the cervix (the neck of the uterus) would be inappropriate, because a man could never develop the disease. We would calculate a *sex-specific* rate by dividing the number of cases by the number of *women* in the population. However, many women will have had a hysterectomy (removal of the uterus). They are then no longer at risk of developing cervical cancer and so, strictly speaking, should not be included in the population at risk. In practice, published rates of both cervical and endometrial cancer (cancer of the lining of the uterus) rarely allow for this so it is difficult to compare the rates of these cancers between countries that have very different hysterectomy rates. We discussed above the importance of making sure that different reports used the same definition of disease (i.e. they counted the same thing in the numerator); it is also crucial to ensure that the denominators represent equivalent populations (e.g. they are similar in age, sex distribution, etc.).

The relationship between incidence and prevalence

If two diseases have the same incidence, but one lasts three times longer than the other, then, at any point in time, you are much more likely to find people suffering from the more long-lasting disease. Very crudely (and assuming that people do not move into or out of the area), the relationship between prevalence (P) and the incidence rate (IR) depends on how long the disease persists before cure or death (average duration of disease, D):

$$P \approx IR \times D \tag{2.3}$$

where $\approx$ means approximately equal to. (Box 2.3 shows a more accurate version of this formula.)

For example, in the USA in 2009, the incidence of hepatitis A was relatively high with an estimated 21,000 new infections (CDC Division of Viral Hepatitis, 2009) and almost one-third of the population may have been infected at some time. However, because it is an acute infection and people recover fairly quickly, the prevalence of hepatitis A infection at any one point in time would be quite low. In contrast, hepatitis C infection is less common (approximately 16,000 new infections in 2009) but most of those infected develop a chronic infection and are infected for life. This means that the prevalence of hepatitis C is much higher with between 2.7 and 3.9 million Americans estimated to be living with chronic infection.

Hepatitis A infection rates have been falling in the USA since the introduction of infant and child vaccination, while reported cases of **hepatitis C** have increased.

> ## Box 2.3 More about the relationship among prevalence, incidence and duration
>
> The relationship $P \approx IR \times D$ is approximately true in what is called a *stationary* population where the number of people entering the population (immigration and birth) balances the number of people leaving (emigration and death). A second requirement is that the prevalence of disease must be low (less than about 10%). This is the case for many diseases, but a more general formula that does not require the disease to be rare is
>
> $$\frac{P}{1 - P} \approx IR \times D \tag{2.4}$$
>
> where P is the prevalence of disease expressed as a proportion and $1 - P$ is the proportion of *non-diseased* people; e.g. if the prevalence (P) is 2% or 0.02 then $1 - P$ is 0.98.

If a new treatment were developed for a disease, what effect would this have on the prevalence and incidence of the disease?

If the new treatment meant that people were cured more quickly and so were ill for less time, then the prevalence would fall. However, if the disease had previously been fatal and the new treatment meant that people lived longer with the disease, then the prevalence would increase. In general, a new treatment will not affect the incidence of a disease. The only exception to this rule might be for an infectious disease: if people were ill and thus infectious for less time, they might pass the infection to fewer people and so the incidence would fall.

As you can see, the prevalence of a disease reflects a balance of several factors. If the incidence of a disease increases then the prevalence will also increase; if the duration of sickness changes then the prevalence will change. This means that the prevalence of a disease is generally not the best way to measure the underlying forces driving the occurrence of the disease – we must use the incidence rate for this. Nonetheless, prevalence is useful for measuring diseases that have a gradual onset and long duration such as type-2 diabetes and osteoarthritis, and also for capturing the frequency of congenital malformations at birth. Both prevalence and incidence are of direct value for describing the overall disease burden of a population and, together with simple counts of the numbers of cases of disease, are fundamentally important for assessing health care needs and planning health services.

Measuring disease occurrence in practice: epidemiological studies

As we discussed above, the occurrence of disease can be quantified by looking at the **prevalence** or the **incidence rate**. We will now consider these further, together with an alternative way of measuring incidence known as the **incidence proportion** (or risk or **cumulative incidence**). These three fundamental measures form the basis of *descriptive epidemiology*, which seeks to answer the first four of the five core questions that you met in Chapter 1: What (diseases are occurring)? Who (is getting them)? Where? and When? The measures can all be calculated from routinely collected data (as in the HIV example above) or from studies conducted specifically to measure the incidence or prevalence of disease, and they are widely used in health reports around the world. We will come back to the use of routine data below and for now will concentrate on how we measure the occurrence of disease in an epidemiological study.

To measure the *prevalence* of disease we need to conduct a *survey*, or what is often called a **cross-sectional study**, in which a random sample (or cross-section) of the population is questioned or assessed to ascertain whether they have a particular condition at a given point in time. To measure the *incidence* of disease we need to start with a group (or *cohort*) of people who are free of the disease of interest but who are 'at risk' of developing it. We then follow them over time to see who actually develops the disease (a **cohort study**; e.g. the British Doctors Study mentioned in Chapter 1).

When we conduct a research study we can specify exactly who is in the study and can usually collect individual data for all (or most) of those people. We can therefore identify who is 'at risk' and calculate quite accurate measures of disease incidence (or prevalence). We can also relate the occurrence of disease to its potential causes to answer the final question, Why?, and we will consider this aspect further in Chapter 5.

Consider, for example, a study conducted in a hypothetical primary school with 100 pupils. Imagine that, on the first day of the new term, nine children had a cold. Over the next week another seven children developed a cold.

What percentage of children had a cold on the first day of term?

What percentage of the children who didn't have a cold on the first day of term developed one during the next week?

The first measure that you calculated is the **prevalence** of the common cold in this group of children: 9 out of 100 children or 9% had a cold on the first day of term. The second measure is known as the **incidence proportion** or risk of colds: out of 91 children 'at risk' of developing a cold (i.e. they did not have one already), 7 or 7.7% developed one during the first week of term. The denominator (population at risk) is 91 in this case because 9 of the 100 children already had a cold and were not therefore 'at risk' of catching another at the same time. As its name suggests, the incidence proportion measures the proportion, or percentage, of people (children in this case) who were at risk of developing a cold and who did so during the period of the study (one week). Note that it is always important to specify the time period – a risk[3] of 5% in 1 year would be very different from a risk of 5% in 20 years. The incidence proportion is sometimes known as the **attack rate**, especially when it refers to a short time period as, for example, in the context of an outbreak of infectious diseases like the food poisoning example in Chapter 1.

This example was simple because the common cold is just that, very common, and we were only interested in the children for one week. Imagine that we were trying to measure the incidence of a much rarer disease such as cancer. We would obviously need a much larger group of people and we would need to follow them for much longer to see who developed the cancer. In this situation it is very difficult to keep track of people and we would inevitably lose some from the study group and not know what happened to them. Another problem is that people will die from other 'competing' causes and so they will no longer be at risk of developing the cancer. In this situation, calculations of the incidence proportion may be inaccurate (or will become so over time) because we will not know exactly who has developed the disease. In practice, we can calculate this measure only when we have a clearly defined group of people who are all (or almost all) followed for the specified follow-up period.

When this is not the situation we use a different method to calculate an **incidence rate**. Instead of simply counting the actual *number* of people at risk of disease, we count up the *length of time* they were at risk of disease. Imagine that we followed a group of 1000 men for 5 years and that during this time 15 of them had a non-fatal heart attack. This gives us an incidence proportion or risk of 1.5% for the 5-year period. During this period the men have lived a total of $1000 \times 5 = 5000$ years of life or **person-years**. We could have obtained the same number of person-years by following a group of 5000 men for 1 year each, or a group of 500 men for 10 years each. Alternatively, we could have followed some men for one year, some for two years, some for three years, etc., to arrive at the same total of 5000. We are no longer so focussed on the actual number of people who were at risk of the disease, but rather on the total person-time[4] (number of person-years) they were at risk. This not only gives us a much more accurate measure of how quickly disease is occurring among those at risk, but it also gives us much greater flexibility. Assuming that we still

---

[3] Because the term 'incidence proportion' can be unwieldy, we will also use 'risk' to describe this measure.

[4] Person-time can be measured in person-years as in this example or any other measure of time, e.g., person-months, person-days, depending on the time scale of the study.

saw 15 heart attacks during our 5000 person-years (py), we could calculate the **incidence rate** as 15 per 5000 *person-years* or, more usually, 3 per 1000 or 300/100,000 person-years.

> The **incidence rate** is also sometimes called the incidence density.

The **_incidence proportion_ (IP)** (also known as cumulative incidence or risk) measures the *proportion of people* who develop disease *during a specified period*:

$$IP = \frac{\text{Number of people who develop disease in a specified period}}{\text{Number of } people \text{ at risk of getting the disease}} \quad (2.5)$$
$$\text{at the start of the period}$$

The **_incidence rate_ (IR)** measures *how quickly* people are developing a disease:

$$IR = \frac{\text{Number of people who develop disease in a specified period}}{\text{Total } person\text{-}time \text{ when people were at}} \quad (2.6)$$
$$\text{risk of getting the disease}$$

Note that, although Equation (2.6) looks slightly different from Equation (2.2), they are measuring the same thing – if you are unsure about this, see Box 2.4 for an explanation of why this is true. We will also come back to this under 'Crude incidence and mortality rates' on page 49.

Box 2.4 Calculating incidence rates

As you saw above, the 'person-time' method for calculating an incidence rate (Equation (2.6)) is particularly useful in research studies when different people have been followed for different lengths of time. However, at the population level we may be dealing with millions of people and it is clearly not feasible to calculate the person-time that each is at risk. Instead we usually calculate the incidence rate for a single year and work on the assumption that everyone in the population is at risk for the whole of that year (Equation (2.2)). The fundamental concept is, however, the same – if there are 500,000 people in the population and we assume they are all at risk for one year that is the same as 500,000 person-years. The only distinction is that the 'routine rates' calculated using Equation (2.2) are based on population averages, whereas the 'epidemiological rates' calculated using Equation (2.6) are based on adding together carefully measured units of individual person-time to give a precise denominator. The resulting incidence rates are also presented slightly differently: routine incidence rates are usually described per 100,000 *people per year*, whereas

(continued)

Box 2.4 (*continued*)

in epidemiological studies using individual data they are usually shown per 100,000 *person-years*. You will find that some people differentiate the rates calculated based on person-time by describing them as **incidence density**; however, we, as most others, will refer to both as incidence rates because they are effectively measuring the same thing.

In practice, it will usually only be possible to calculate the incidence rate one way. If data are available for individual people who have been followed for different lengths of time then we use Equation (2.6). If we only have summary data for a population then we use Equation (2.2).

Incidence rates versus incidence proportion

The distinction between an *incidence proportion* or risk and an *incidence rate* can be confusing. An analogy that we have found helpful is to think of these measures in terms of driving a car.

- The *incidence rate* is equivalent to the average *speed* of a car at a particular point in time, e.g. 60 km/hour.
- The *incidence proportion* is analogous to the *distance* travelled by a car during a specified interval of time, e.g. 60 km in one hour.

The *distance* a car travels depends both on its average *speed* and on the length of time it travels for. If a car travels at an average speed of 60 km/hour then it will cover 30 km in 30 minutes, 60 km in one hour, and so on. When we consider a time interval of one hour, the total distance travelled (60 km in one hour) looks very similar to the average speed because this is expressed per hour (60 km/hr). Distance and speed are, however, fundamentally different.

In the same way, the incidence rate describes the 'speed' at which new cases of disease are occurring, and therefore reflects what is sometimes called the underlying *force of morbidity*. As its name suggests, the incidence proportion measures the proportion of a group who develop the disease over a particular time and is thus a function both of the underlying incidence rate and of the length of follow-up. If the incidence rate is 10 per 100,000/year then the incidence proportion will be 10 cases in 100,000 (= 0.0001 or 0.01%) in one year, 20 cases in 100,000 (= 0.0002 or 0.02%) in two years, and so on. As with the car example, when we consider a time interval of one year, an incidence proportion expressed as 10 per 100,000 people *in one year* looks much like an incidence rate (10 per 100,000 *per year* or *person-years*) because we usually

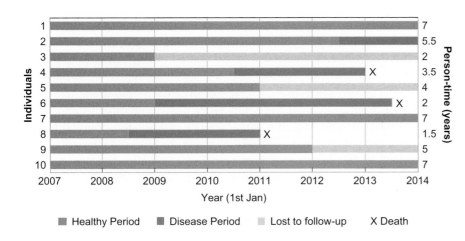

Figure 2.2 A hypothetical follow-up study.

show incidence rates per year. It is important to recognise that, as with distance and speed, the measures are different. A good way to help avoid confusion is to ensure that the incidence proportion is expressed as a proportion (e.g. 0.0001) or percentage rather than 'per 100,000'.

Example

Imagine that we identified a group of 10 healthy people on 1 January 2007 and that we decided to follow these people for seven years to see who developed a particular disease. Figure 2.2 shows the hypothetical experience of these people: four developed the disease of interest and three of them died, and another three were 'lost to follow-up' (e.g. they moved away or died of some other disease). Let us now look at how we would calculate the different measures of disease occurrence in this group.

Prevalence

Remember that prevalence tells us the proportion of the population who were sick at a particular point in time (Equation (2.1)). For example, on 1 January 2010, two people were sick out of the nine people left in our group on that date (one was lost to follow-up), so

Prevalence = 2 ÷ 9 = 22%

What was the prevalence of the disease on 30 June 2011?

On 30 June 2011 two people were sick but there were only seven people left in the group on that date (one had died and two had been lost to follow-up), so

Prevalence = 2 ÷ 7 = 29%

Incidence proportion (cumulative incidence)

This tells us the proportion of a population 'at risk' of developing a disease who actually became ill during a specified time interval (Equation (2.5)). It is also the probability or average *risk* that an individual will develop the disease during the period: if 30% of people in a population develop a disease then each individual has a 30% chance of developing it themselves. It is important to note that this is the average risk for the population, the risk for any individual is either zero (they won't develop the disease) or one (they will).[5] With the exception of some rare genetic diseases such as Huntington's disease where all those who carry the aberrant gene will eventually develop the disease, this individual risk is usually unknown or unknowable, making accurate predictions for individuals in the clinical setting almost impossible.

In the example, 4 of the 10 people who were at risk at the start of the study developed the disease, but three were lost to follow-up and we do not know whether they developed the disease. This means that we cannot accurately calculate the incidence proportion or risk at seven years, but a *minimum estimate* would be

IP = 4 ÷ 10 = 40% in seven years

This is assuming that none of those lost to follow-up developed the disease. If any of them had developed the disease then the true risk would have been higher than 40%. The *maximum estimate* of the incidence proportion would assume that all three of the missing people developed the disease:

IP = 7 ÷ 10 = 70% in seven years

Note that we could calculate an accurate incidence proportion at two years – because we do have complete follow-up to that point:

IP = 1 ÷ 10 = 10% in two years

One type of study in which the study group is clearly defined and loss to follow-up is usually minimal is a **clinical trial** (see Chapter 4) and this means that the incidence proportion is an appropriate and common measure of outcome in this type of study. However, the field of clinical epidemiology has developed its own terminology for what we call the incidence proportion (see Box 2.5).

Incidence rate

Although we do not know what happened to three people in the group, we do know that they had not developed the disease before they were lost to follow up. We can use this information to help us calculate the incidence rate or what

---

[5] Note that risk can be measured on a scale from 0 to 1, or from 0 to 100%; a risk of 30% is therefore equal to a risk of 0.3.

Box 2.5 The incidence proportion in clinical trials

You will find that in clinical trials what we have called the incidence proportion or risk may be called the **experimental event rate (EER)** when it describes the risk in the intervention or treatment group, and the **control event rate (CER)** in the control or placebo group.

For example, a group in the USA investigated whether four weeks of aspirin treatment would reduce the risk of blood clots in patients being treated with antibiotics for infective endocarditis (an infection of the lining of the heart that usually affects the heart valves). In total 115 patients were enrolled in the study and assigned at random to receive aspirin ($n = 60$) or placebo ($n = 55$). During the study, 17 patients in the aspirin group (EER or $IP_{Intervention} = 17 \div 60 = 28.3\%$) and 11 in the placebo group (CER or $IP_{Control} = 11 \div 55 = 20.0\%$) experienced blood clots (Table 2.3). The authors concluded that aspirin treatment did not reduce the risk of clots (Chan et al., 2003).

Table 2.3 Results of an RCT evaluating aspirin use for infective endocarditis.

	Total patients	Number with blood clots	Event rate (incidence proportion of blood clots)
Aspirin	60	17	28.3%
Placebo	55	11	20.0%

(From Chan et al., 2003.)

is sometimes called the incidence density (Equation (2.6)). This is the number of new cases of disease (four) divided by the total amount of *person-time* at risk of developing the disease. An individual is at risk of developing the disease until the actual moment when they do develop it (in practice, when they are diagnosed) or until they are lost to follow-up.[6] In this example, individual number one would contribute seven years of person-time; individual number two would contribute five and a half years; individual number three would contribute two years, and so on.

---

[6] For this example we assumed that those lost to follow-up were no different from those who remained in the study. In practice this may not be true, e.g., people who are sicker may be more likely to drop out, and in this situation the rate we calculate may be biased. We will come back to discuss this problem in Chapter 7.

What is the total amount of person-time at risk?

What is the incidence rate for this disease per 100 person-years?

The total amount of person time is

$7 + 5.5 + 2 + 3.5 + 4 + 2 + 7 + 1.5 + 5 + 7 = 44.5$ person-years

So the incidence rate is

4 cases ÷ 44.5 person-years = 0.09 cases/person-year or 9 cases/100 person-years

Measuring disease occurrence in practice: using routine data

In practice, much of our information about the occurrence of disease comes from routine statistics, collected at a regional, national, or international level (we will discuss some of the sources of these data in Chapter 3), and in this format they comprise the core of many published reports. The data are not based on specific information about *individuals*, but relate the number of cases of disease (or deaths) in a *population* to the size of that population (often an estimate from a census). This can lead to problems when we try to relate the occurrence of disease to potential causes. For example, if a region has a very high level of unemployment and also has a high incidence of suicide, it might be tempting to jump to the conclusion that being unemployed drives people to commit suicide. However, we have no way of knowing from routine statistics whether it is the same people who are unemployed who are committing suicide. (This dilemma where we try to extrapolate from an association seen at the population-level to draw conclusions about the relation in individuals is often called the **ecological fallacy** (or **cross-level bias**) and we will discuss it again in Chapter 3.)

A second drawback of routine data relates to the fact that in public health we often want to measure the *incidence* of disease – how quickly are people becoming ill? Unfortunately, it is often difficult to obtain reliable information about incidence because few illnesses are captured reliably in routine statistics. Some diseases, such as HIV infection and cancer, are 'notifiable' in many countries and, therefore, all cases *should* be reported to a central body; however, these examples are the exceptions rather than the rule, and such data are not available for most diseases. Furthermore, even where reporting is mandated it does not always occur in practice. When HIV first came to world attention, and again during the 2003 SARS (severe acute respiratory syndrome) outbreak, some countries suppressed the real numbers of cases for both political and economic reasons. We will take up some of these issues in more detail when we discuss surveillance in Chapter 12.

As a result, many common measures that you will come across will be measures of mortality because death and cause of death are regularly and reliably recorded in many, but certainly not all, countries. Incidence and mortality rates have exactly the same form, but for incidence we count new cases of a disease whereas for mortality we count deaths. Mortality data are obviously uninformative for many diseases that are not usually fatal – things like osteoarthritis, non-melanoma skin cancers, psoriasis and rubella (German measles), to name but a few. However, even for diseases that can be fatal, mortality figures might not mirror the underlying incidence of disease, for example if a more effective treatment is introduced. Mortality data can also lag well behind changes in incidence, delaying identification of changes over time that may be important for planning or for providing clues as to the causes of the disease.

Crude incidence and mortality rates

As you saw above, when we conduct an epidemiological study we calculate the incidence rate as the number of cases of disease divided by the total *person-time* at risk of disease (where this is summed over all of the individuals in the study). This method is particularly useful when different people have been followed for different lengths of time, but at the population level we may be dealing with millions of people and it is clearly not feasible to calculate the person-time that each is at risk. Instead we usually work on the assumption that everyone is at risk for the whole of the year that we are interested in.

When we are working with routine data, therefore, we calculate the incidence rate by dividing the total number of new cases of a specific disease (or the number of deaths) in a specified period, usually one year, by the average number of people in the population during the same period (Equation (2.2)). This is then usually multiplied by 100,000 (10^5) and presented as a rate per 10^5 people per year. The size of the population will, inevitably, change over a period of a year, so ideally we would use the number of people in the population in the middle of the year or the average of the size of the population at the start and at the end of the period of interest. Incidence rates may be calculated for a broad disease group (e.g. cancer) or a more specific disease (e.g. breast cancer). Similarly, mortality rates may include deaths from all causes (sometimes called *all-cause* mortality) or only those from a specific cause. These basic rates are called **crude rates** because they describe the overall incidence or death rate in a population without taking any other features of the population into account (in contrast to **standardised rates** – see below).

Table 2.4 Crude mortality rates (per 100,000 per year) for ischaemic heart disease (IHD) in males from selected countries, 1995–1998.

Country	Crude IHD mortality rate (per 10^5/year)
Germany	211
Australia	168
Canada	160
Singapore	118
Spain	116
Japan	50
Brazil	47

(Data source: Global Cardiovascular Infobase, www.cvdinfobase.ca, accessed 23 September 2003.)

Describe the data shown in Table 2.4.

Comment on the order of the countries – is this helpful to understanding what is going on? How else might the data have been ordered?

Table 2.4 shows crude mortality rates for ischaemic heart disease (IHD) in men in seven countries in 1995–1998. We see that Germany, Australia and Canada had high mortality rates, with intermediate rates in Singapore and Spain and low rates in Japan and Brazil. The countries are ordered from the highest rate to the lowest, making it easier to compare the rates between them. If, for example, they had been ordered alphabetically or by geographic region, this would have made the comparison of rates harder. A good table should be structured to convey the most important messages as simply as possible.

Can we conclude from these data that men were three to four times as likely to die from IHD in Western countries such as Germany, Australia and Canada than in countries like Japan and Brazil?

If not, why not?

Age-specific incidence and mortality rates

Table 2.4 describes the total burdens that the different health systems have to cope with, but a major disadvantage of crude rates is that they are just that – crude. Most importantly, they do not take into account the fact that different populations have different age structures and the risk of becoming ill or dying varies with age. Many diseases are more common among older people

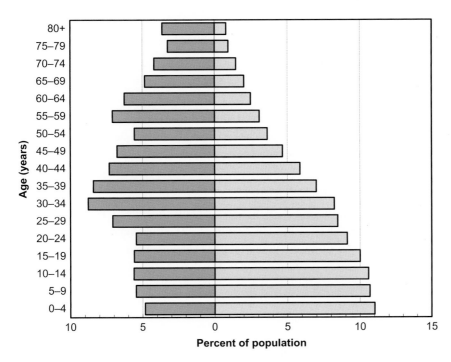

Figure 2.3 Age distribution of the population in Germany (1998, dark bars) and Brazil (1995, light bars). (*Drawn from*: Global Cardiovascular Infobase, www.cvdinfobase.ca, accessed 23 September 2003.)

and the older a person is, the greater their risk of dying. Developed countries like Germany have a high proportion of older people, whereas less-developed countries like Brazil have a much greater proportion of young people, at a relatively lower risk of dying. Their contrasting population structures are shown in Figure 2.3. In the example above it turns out that we are trying to compare countries with very different age structures, so a crude comparison of IHD mortality has limited meaning if we are trying to assess the comparative 'cardiovascular health' of these countries (see also Box 2.6).

One obvious way to avoid this problem is to calculate separate rates for different age groups (*age-specific rates*). The rate in a particular age group can then be compared between countries. This process can be extended to calculate separate rates for other groups, for instance men and women (*sex-specific rates*), and for different racial or socioeconomic groups. Table 2.5 extends Table 2.4 to show selected age-specific mortality rates for the seven countries.

What do the age-specific rates shown in Table 2.5 tell us about the relative cardiovascular health in these countries?

If we compare the age-specific rates, we can see that in each country the rate is much higher in the older age group. We can also see that, while the crude rates for Singapore and Spain are similar, the age-specific rates are

> ## Box 2.6 Cardiovascular diseases simplified
>
> You will find that, when we use examples relating to cardiovascular diseases, the conditions often have different names and abbreviations. Cardiovascular diseases are grouped and described in many different ways, emphasising the need to be sure that you know what the numbers you are looking at represent. The following is a simplified summary of some commonly used terms:
>
> Myocardial infarction (MI): heart attack
> Ischaemic heart disease (IHD): heart attack (MI) or angina
> Coronary heart disease (CHD): essentially identical to IHD
> Cardiovascular disease (CVD): includes CHD, stroke, and other cardiac and vascular diseases (note that CVD can also be used as an abbreviation for cerebrovascular disease, i.e. stroke and transient ischaemic attack, but we will not use it in this way)

about twice as high in Singapore, which actually has the highest rates of all the countries in both age groups. Brazil has also moved up in the IHD rankings, although it is still doing better than Germany and Australia, while Japanese men have notably low rates at all ages.

Standardised incidence and mortality rates

If age-specific rates are presented for a large number of different age groups, as well as for both sexes, we end up with a lot of numbers to compare and interpret (we only showed two age groups in Table 2.5 for simplicity). An alternative is to summarise or combine these age-specific rates using a process called standardisation. **Direct standardisation** involves calculating the overall incidence or mortality rate that you would have expected to find in a 'standard' population if it had the same age-specific rates as your study population. (The details of how to do this are shown in Appendix 1.) The same methods can also be used to standardise for other factors that differ between populations that you want to compare, for example sex or race, because disease rates often differ markedly between men and women and those from different ethnic backgrounds.

The **age-standardised rates** can then be compared across the populations (assuming that the disease is defined in the same way in each) because the problem of different age patterns has been removed (Table 2.6). You will notice that, in countries with an older population, the standardised rate is

Table 2.5 Crude and age-specific mortality rates (per 100,000 per year) for IHD in males from selected countries, 1995–1998.

Country	Crude rate (per 10^5/year)	Age-specific rates (per 10^5/year)	
		45–54 years	55–64 years
Germany	211	76	245
Australia	168	68	222
Canada	160	73	239
Singapore	118	100	346
Spain	116	59	156
Japan	50	20	60
Brazil	47	64	183

(Data source: Global Cardiovascular Infobase, www.cvdinfobase.ca, accessed 23 September 2003.)

Table 2.6 Crude and age-standardised mortality rates (per 100,000 per year) for IHD in males from selected countries, 1995–1998.

Country	Crude IHD mortality rate (per 10^5/year)	Age-standardised rate (per 10^5/year)
Germany	211	121
Australia	168	111
Canada	160	108
Singapore	118	121
Spain	116	65
Japan	50	29
Brazil	47	60

(Data source: Global Cardiovascular Infobase, www.cvdinfobase.ca, accessed 23 September 2003.)

much lower than the crude rate, but in Brazil this pattern is reversed, and the standardised rate is higher than the crude rate because Brazil has a much younger population than the standard population used for this comparison. The age-standardised rates give a more accurate picture of the relative levels of cardiovascular health in the seven countries than the crude rates did because they take into account the larger numbers of older people in the more developed countries. It is important to stress, however, that for any individual population the actual rates (crude or age-specific) are of much greater utility for health planning.

A note about standard populations

It is important to add a word of caution at this stage. There are many different 'standard' populations and, in practice, you can age-standardise to *any* population. You will often come across rates that have been standardised to the 'world' population which reflects the average age structure of the whole world. Other common standard populations reflect the typical age structure of either 'developed' or 'developing' countries. If the aim is to compare rates in different groups within the same country then it is common practice to use the overall age structure of that country as the standard population. To some extent the choice is arbitrary, but it is important to note that if you standardise to two very different populations you will get very different standardised rates, and the relationships between different populations may change. For this reason, it is always important to note what standard population has been used.

For example, when we standardised IHD mortality in Germany to the world standard population the age-standardised rate was $121/10^5$ per year. If we had standardised to the younger 'African' standard population, it would have been only $60/10^5$ per year, whereas if we had standardised to the older 'European' standard population it would have been $198/10^5$ per year. In this example we were comparing populations around the world, so it was appropriate to use the world standard population. If all the countries had been in Europe or Africa then the European or African standard populations might have been more appropriate.

In 2001, the World Health Organization (WHO) proposed a new world standard population to reflect the general ageing of populations around the world. (This and examples of other common standard populations are provided in Appendix 2.) However, what seems like a logical updating of information has major ramifications for anyone looking at time trends in the occurrence of disease because rates cannot usefully be compared if they have been standardised to different populations (see Box 2.7).

Measuring risk using routine statistics

Routine statistics may also be used to estimate the incidence proportion and, in this situation, it is usually described as a risk. It gives the probability or risk that someone will develop disease (or die) within a given time period, and this time period can be anything from a few days to a lifetime (a lifetime is commonly taken as ages 0 to 74 years). For example, men in Australia have a lifetime risk of lung cancer of 3.8% or, in other words, 3.8% of Australian men will develop lung cancer before their 75th birthday (AIHW, 2015). An alternative way to look at the same information is to say that the average *lifetime risk* of lung cancer in Australian men is '1 in 26' or, in other words, 1 in every 26 Australian men will develop lung cancer before their 75th birthday. Note that these measures assume that someone remains 'at risk' of lung cancer until their 75th birthday

> As people are living longer, some now calculate **lifetime risk** to age 85. An Australian male has a 7.9% risk or 1 in 13 chance of developing lung cancer before his 85th birthday.

and they also do not take into account any other factors, such as smoking. Clearly, the lifetime risk will be much higher for a smoker than for a non-smoker and for personalising risk, for example in the doctor's surgery, smoking-specific risks would be much more informative, but special research studies with individual exposures are needed to provide such data. (The methods for calculating risk and lifetime risk for routine data are shown in Appendix 3.)

Other measures commonly used in public health

We will now consider some other measures that are used commonly in public health to assess different aspects of disease burden. Many of these descriptive measures are fundamental to health planning and service provision. They are expressed in a variety of ways – some are ratios, some percentages, i.e. per 100 population, while others are shown as rates per 1000, 10,000 or 100,000

Box 2.8 Rates, ratios and proportions

A **ratio** is simply one number divided by another number. For example, the number of beers drunk in one year divided by the number of people in the population (beers per capita) or the number of cases observed divided by the number of cases expected.

A **proportion** is a special type of ratio in which everything or everyone in the numerator is also counted in the denominator. For example, the number of people who develop disease divided by the total number of people in the population (those with and without disease). A proportion can never be less than 0 (if no-one is affected) or greater than 1 (if everyone is affected). It can also be expressed as a percentage between 0 and 100%. All proportions are ratios – not all ratios are proportions.

A **rate** should contain some measure of time, for example 60 km *per hour*, 17/100,000 *per year*. Unlike a proportion, it has no upper limit.

population (see Box 2.8 for clarification of the differences between rates, ratios and proportions). In some cases different people will use the same term to describe a slightly different measure. The definitions that we give are as in *A Dictionary of Epidemiology* (Porta, 2014) and are probably those most commonly used. Whenever you come across these rates it is advisable to check exactly what the numbers being compared are, and what the size of the reference population is – whether the rate refers to 100, 1000 or 100,000 events or people.

Standardised incidence and mortality ratios

Figure 1.5 in Chapter 1 showed standardised mortality ratios (SMRs) for Indigenous compared to non-Indigenous Australians. These come from an alternative way of standardising rates called **indirect standardisation** (see Appendix 4). In this example the standardisation is for age, but the same process is commonly used to adjust for sex, and/or to compare data from different time periods. The actual number of deaths 'observed' in a population (e.g. deaths from cancer in Indigenous men) is compared with the number of deaths that would have been 'expected' if the death rates in the Indigenous population had been the same as those for the non-Indigenous population. The SMR is calculated by dividing the observed number of deaths (O) by the expected number (E). This measure tells us how much more common death from cancer is in Indigenous people than in the non-Indigenous population (about 1.6 times in this case). We can do exactly the same thing with disease

Box 2.9 Direct vs. indirect standardisation

It can be hard to get your head around the difference between direct and indirect standardisation. When we standardise for age using **direct standardisation** we calculate the overall *rate* that we would see in a 'standard' population if it had the same age-specific rates of disease as our study population. We can then compare rates that have been directly age-standardised to the same standard population because any age differences between the original populations have been removed.

In contrast, when we use **indirect standardisation** we calculate the *number of cases* we would have expected to see in our study population if it had the same age-specific rates of disease as a standard population (often the general population). We then compare this expected number of cases to the number of cases that actually occurred in the study population (the 'observed' number) and calculate a standardised incidence (or mortality) ratio by dividing the observed number of cases by the expected number.

Table 2.7 summarises the differences between the two methods; although these are presented in terms of age-standardisation, the same issues apply if we are standardising for sex, race or any other factors.

incidence to calculate a standardised incidence ratio (SIR). SIRs are also commonly reported by cancer registries, which are among the few sources of reliable incidence data at the population level.

The SMR and SIR are similar to the relative risk that you met in Chapter 1. Remember also that Snow used observed and expected numbers of deaths to show that cholera mortality in the workhouse near the Broad Street pump was unexpectedly low (Box 1.4). Strictly speaking, they are *measures of association* because they compare disease incidence or mortality in one population with that in a reference population and, as such, would fit more logically into Chapter 5. We have included them here because of the parallels between the processes of direct and indirect standardisation (see Box 2.9).

> **SMR and SIR:** while we (and others) use the term standardised incidence ratio or SIR, some people call this a standardised *morbidity* ratio and thus use SMR to describe both standardised mortality and morbidity ratios.

The proportional (or proportionate) mortality ratio (PMR)

This is a measure of the relative importance of a particular cause of death in a given population. A PMR looks like an SMR, but is used when there is insufficient information to calculate an SMR (usually because information is available only about those who have died, so it is not possible to calculate mortality rates). It is calculated by dividing the *proportion* of deaths due to a specific cause in a group of interest by the *proportion* of deaths due to the same cause in a comparison group. A PMR is commonly multiplied by 100, so a PMR of

Table 2.7 Direct versus indirect standardisation for age.

	Direct Standardisation	Indirect Standardisation
Information required	Age-specific rates in *study* population Age distribution of *standard* population	Age-specific rates in *standard* population Age distribution of *study* population Total number of cases (deaths) in *study* population
Measure calculated	Age-standardised incidence (mortality) rate	Standardised incidence (mortality) ratio, SIR (SMR)
Advantages and disadvantages	Good for comparing large populations where the age-specific rates are reliable; *less good for small populations because the age-specific rates may be unstable* Allows comparisons between the standardised rates for different populations	Can be used when the age-specific rates in the study population are unknown or unreliable, for example when the population is small *Two SIRs and SMRs cannot be directly compared because they are both calculated relative to a separate third population*
Uses	Commonly used to compare rates across different countries or between large subgroups within a country, for example men versus women	Often used to compare incidence or mortality in smaller subgroups of a population, for example veterans from a particular armed conflict, to the general population. *Although direct standardisation could be used in this situation, if the subgroup is relatively small, the age-specific rates may not be very reliable and indirect standardisation is preferred*

100 means that the proportions of deaths due to a specific cause are the same in the study and comparison groups, and a PMR of 200 indicates that twice as many of the deaths in the study group are due to the specific cause. Proportional mortality ratios are most commonly used in occupational studies. For example, a study of deaths among electrical workers on construction sites in the USA found that 127 of the total of 31,068 deaths (0.4%) were due to electrocution. This value was almost 12 times as high (PMR = 1180) as the proportion of such deaths that would be expected in the general US population (Robinson *et al.*, 1999). Proportional mortality ratios have fairly limited utility because they cannot easily be compared across different populations. They are usually calculated only when no population data are readily available and precise mortality rates cannot be calculated.

The case–fatality ratio (CFR)

The CFR (often called the case–fatality *rate*, although, strictly speaking, it is an incidence proportion and not a rate because it does not contain a measure of time, see Box 2.8 above) is the proportion of people with a given disease or condition who die from it in a given period. It is a common measure of the short-term severity of an acute disease and allows a direct assessment of the effectiveness of an intervention. For example, the CFR for myocardial infarction (heart attack) is usually measured over a period of 28 days. When deaths occur over a longer time period then it is more appropriate to consider the survival rate (see below). The CFR is usually expressed per 100 cases, i.e. as a percentage. As an example, the overall CFR in the 2003 SARS epidemic was estimated to be 14%–15%, i.e. approximately one in every seven people who contracted SARS died. However, this average ratio hides the fact that, while patients under the age of 25 were unlikely to die (CFR = 1%), approximately half of patients over the age of 65 died (CFR = 50%). (Note that the mortality from SARS occurred so quickly that the particular time period the CFR refers to is generally not specified.)

Survival rate and relative survival rate

As we discussed above, the CFR is an appropriate measure for short-term mortality (a month or so) but is less useful for conditions in which death may occur further down the track. For conditions such as cancer, mortality is often expressed in terms of the proportion of patients who are still alive a specified number of years after diagnosis – the **survival rate**. This proportion is often adjusted to allow for the fact that, depending on the age group being considered, some people would have been expected to die anyway from causes other than their cancer and this is known as the **relative survival rate**. A relative survival rate of 100% thus indicates that mortality does not differ from that experienced by the general population. In developed countries, five-year relative survival rates are often used to compare and report outcomes for patients with different types of cancer and to show changes over time. As an example, five-year relative survival rates for breast cancer are about 75%–80%, compared with only about 15% for lung cancer.

Global health indicators

In Table 2.6 we saw that age-standardised rates of heart disease were higher in Germany and Singapore than in Spain and Brazil which, in turn, had higher rates than Japan, but this is only one disease; how does the overall health of these populations compare? The measures that we have looked at so far have focussed on either morbidity (incidence) or mortality and many are only really useful for describing a single disease or group of diseases at a time. They can tell us how rates of cancer or mortality from heart disease vary between countries or over time, but they are less useful if we want to look at the overall

> ## Box 2.10 Millennium Development Goals
>
> In 2000, the heads of state from 149 countries participating in the United Nations Millennium Summit adopted the Millennium Declaration which set out to achieve what are now known as the Millennium Development Goals by 2015. The eight goals encompass 18 targets and 48 indicators:
>
> 1. Eradicate extreme poverty and hunger
> 2. Achieve universal primary education
> 3. Promote gender equality and empower women
> 4. Reduce child mortality
> 5. Improve maternal health
> 6. Combat HIV/AIDS, malaria and other diseases
> 7. Ensure environmental sustainability
> 8. Develop a global partnership for development
>
> www.un.org/millenniumgoals/

health of a population at a particular point in time and see how it compares with other time periods and/or populations. In this section we will look at some of the measures that are commonly used by bodies such as WHO to monitor different aspects of health, and particularly those that have been used to track progress towards the *Millennium Development Goals* (MDG, see Box 2.10). Some are simple mortality measures similar to those you have already met, but they obviously tell us nothing about the many states of ill-health short of death. To assess these we need measures that can account for the severity of disease and when it occurs in life. A number of measures have been developed to help solve this problem as organisations such as WHO attempt to measure not only disease occurrence, but also its consequences such as pain, disability and loss of income. These measures bring us closer to measuring the overall 'health' of a population according to the WHO definition and are being used increasingly by national and regional health departments for planning and resource allocation.

Mortality indicators

Cause-specific mortality rates like those you met earlier are used to monitor progress towards MDG-6 which seeks to reduce the impact of HIV and AIDS, malaria and other diseases – between 2000 and 2012, malaria mortality rates fell by 42% (United Nations, 2014). Other critical indicators of the general health of a community include measures of mortality relating to early life, and

Table 2.8 Mortality indicators.

Measure	Deaths (numerator)	Population at risk (denominator)	Notes
Maternal mortality ratio	Deaths among women from causes related to childbirth in 1 year (WHO defines this as deaths up to 42 days after birth, but sometimes deaths up to 1 year are included)	Number of live births in the same year	Strictly speaking the denominator should be *all* pregnant women, but this information is not recorded directly
Stillbirth or fetal death rate	Number of stillbirths in 1 year where a still birth is usually a fetal death after 28 weeks gestation although other time points may also be used (e.g. 20 weeks)	Live births + fetal deaths in the same year	Sometimes calculated as the ratio of the number of fetal deaths to the number of live births (excluding fetal deaths). This is often called the *fetal death ratio*
Neonatal mortality rate	Deaths in children aged less than 28 days	Number of live births in the same year	Only live births are included in the denominator because only babies born alive are at risk of dying before the age of 28 days
Infant mortality rate	Deaths in children up to 1 year of age	Number of live births in the same year	Probably the most widely used single indicator of the overall health of a community
	WHO defines and calculates this as the probability of dying between birth and age 1, per 1000 live births		
Child or under-five mortality rate	Deaths in children up to 5 years of age	Ideally the number of children under 5 in the population; often the number of live births in the same year	An alternative to the child death rate, the latter version is preferable in countries where it is hard to enumerate the population of young children
	WHO defines and calculates this as the probability of dying by age 5, per 1000 live births		
Adult mortality rate	*WHO defines and calculates this as the probability of dying between ages 15 and 60, per 1000 population*		

Table 2.8 shows a number of these which are integral to monitoring progress towards MDG-4 and MDG-5. By 2012–2013, major improvements had been seen in both areas, with infant and maternal mortality rates having fallen by almost 50% and 45%, respectively, since 1990 (United Nations, 2014).

The underlying concept of each rate is the same – it is the ratio of the actual number of deaths that occur in one year to the total population 'at risk of death'

Technically, these **mortality rates** are *proportions* or *ratios* rather than true *rates* because they do not have units of time – see Box 2.8; they are, however, commonly described as rates and we will also use this terminology.

in the same year. Because it is not always possible to obtain an accurate figure for the number of people at risk, an approximation is sometimes used. For example, any woman who is pregnant is at risk of maternal death, but the number of women who are pregnant in a given year is not routinely recorded, so in practice this is estimated by taking the number of live births in one year. It is also worth noting that the *infant mortality rate* is the number of infant deaths (age 0–1 year) relative to the number of live births in the same year. This means that the children in the numerator (deaths) are not the same as those in the denominator (births) because many of those who die will have been born in the previous year. This is not a problem if the birth rate is fairly stable.

For each indicator we have given the most standard definition(s) but, as you will see, there are some variations. For example, the *stillbirth* (or *fetal death*) *rate* should be calculated as the ratio of stillbirths to the number of live births *plus* the number of stillbirths. This is because all of these children (live plus stillbirths) were at risk of being stillborn although not all of them were. This measure is, however, sometimes presented as a *stillbirth* or *fetal death ratio* where only live births are counted in the denominator. WHO in particular tends to use this variant (WHO, 2014a). Because the number of live births will be less than the number of live births plus stillbirths, the fetal death or stillbirth ratio will always be slightly larger than the stillbirth rate. WHO also calculates infant and under-five mortality rates slightly differently, defining them as the *probability of dying* before the age of one or five, respectively (WHO, 2014b). This reinforces how important it is to check exactly what the numbers refer to in order to make sure that you are always comparing like with like.

Describe the data shown in Figure 2.4 and comment on the scale used for the graph.

Figure 2.4 shows the enormous variation in infant mortality rates around the world, reflecting the great disadvantages under which many countries still labour. It also shows the very strong inverse correlation between GDP (gross domestic product) and infant mortality – the more wealthy a country, the lower the infant mortality rate. In a poor country like Sierra Leone the rate is more than 70 per 1000 live births or, in other words, 7% of babies die before their first birthday. This compares with less than 3 per 1000 in Japan and Singapore. The use of log scales for the axes (a log–log plot), where each increment represents a 10-fold increase in GDP or infant mortality, allows us to show the 35-fold difference in mortality rates and the 100-fold range in GDP on a single graph. (A study like this that compares different populations is called an **ecological study**, we will discuss these in more detail in Chapter 3.)

It is, however, important to remember that all of these measures just give an average picture for the whole population. Low average rates can often hide much higher rates in some subgroups of the population. This is particularly

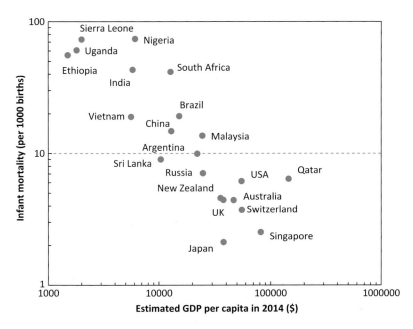

Figure 2.4 Infant mortality rates in relation to GDP in 20 countries around the world. (*Drawn from*: The World Factbook 2013–14. Washington, DC. Central Intelligence Agency, 2013. https://www.cia.gov/library/publications/the-world-factbook/index.html, accessed 23 May 2015.)

true in countries that include more than one ethnic group. For example, as you saw in Chapter 1, in Australia the Indigenous population has mortality rates that are several times higher than those of Australians as a whole, and in the USA in 2010 infant mortality was considerably higher among births to non-Hispanic black women (11.5 per 1000 live births) than for non-Hispanic White or Asian and Pacific Islander mothers (5.2 and 4.3 per 1000, respectively) (Mathews and MacDorman, 2013).

Life expectancy

Another mortality-based measure that accounts for the *timing* of death is **life expectancy**, the average number of years that an individual of a given age is expected to live *if current mortality rates continue*. For example, a boy born in the Russian Federation in 2012 has a life expectancy of 63 years, compared with 80 years for a boy born in Japan (WHO, 2014a). Because they cannot take account of future changes in incidence and/or treatment of diseases, estimates of life expectancy are largely hypothetical. Mortality rates have been falling over time and, until recently, the expectation has been that this trend would continue into the future. Life expectancy figures therefore almost certainly underestimate the actual number of years someone could expect to live. However, the HIV epidemic and other national phenomena, such as that seen for Russian men in Figure 1.2, have already reversed this situation in some countries; and this could become more generally true with the increasing 'obesity epidemic' in many westernised countries predicted to lead to higher mortality rates and thus lower life expectancy in future (Olshansky *et al.*, 2005).

Life expectancy can be presented for any age, but is used most commonly to describe life expectancy at birth or at age 60 as an indicator of adult health. It is calculated using a 'life-table' similar in principle to that shown in Table 1.4. The starting point is a hypothetical group of newborns (usually 100,000) and age-specific mortality rates are then used to estimate the number that would be expected to die at each year of life. The total number of years of life expected for the entire cohort can then be added up and the life expectancy at birth is this total divided by 100,000. Life expectancy at other ages is estimated by adding up the number of years of life after the age of interest and dividing by the number of people in the cohort who had reached that age (see Appendix 5 for the detailed calculations). If we draw a graph of the number or proportion of people expected to survive to each age we get what is called a survival curve. Figure 2.5 shows the survival curves for Australian men and women in 2011–2013, illustrating the survival advantage that women still have over men.

Disability-free life expectancy

There is little point in working to extend life expectancy if the additional years of life are lived in very poor health. This concept is illustrated by the survival curves shown in Figure 2.6. As in Figure 2.5, the top line shows the proportion of people surviving at each age, but now the lower line shows the smaller proportion of people who are still in full health at each age. The combined areas A and B represent total life expectancy, but only a proportion of that life, the area A, is lived in full health, while area B indicates life lived with some

Figure 2.5 Survivorship curve for Australian males and females in 2011–2013. (*Drawn from*: Australian Bureau of Statistics, 2014.)

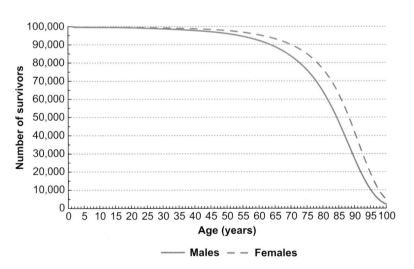

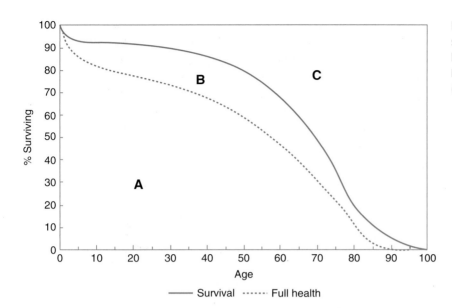

Figure 2.6 Survivorship curves showing years of life lived in full health (A), years lived in less than full health (B), and years of life lost (C). (*Adapted from*: Murray *et al.*, 2000.)

degree of disability. Area C represents the potential years of life lost and the combined areas C and B represent the total health gap – the loss both of years of life and years of health. So how can we measure this?

One solution is to refine the calculations of total life expectancy to calculate **disability-free life expectancy**, which takes into account not only age-specific mortality rates but also the prevalence of disability at that age. This measure effectively adjusts the number of years of life expected for an individual at a given age by the probability that those years will be lived with some degree of disability. One advantage of this measure is that it is relatively simple to calculate and, as a result, it is quite widely used. However, its disadvantages are that, first, an arbitrary decision has to be made as to what level of disability will lead to someone being classified as disabled and, second, years of life lived with disability are not counted at all and thus are effectively considered as bad as being dead.

Years of life lost (YLL)

Life expectancy measures what is being achieved and is sometimes described as a measure of **health expectancy**. An alternative approach is to measure what is being lost and this type of indicator is sometimes described as a **health gap** (Lopez *et al.*, 2006, p. 47). One such measure, the **years of life lost** (YLL), also referred to as expected years of life lost (EYLL), looks not at the number of years someone can expect to live, but instead at the numbers of years of potential life they have lost if they die before a certain age. This age is frequently taken to be the life expectancy of the population or, if many populations are to be compared, an average global value, but YLL can also be calculated in relation to a predefined age, often taken as 65 or 70 years, in which case it is known as the **potential years of life lost** (PYLL). The YLL for a population is calculated by counting the total number of deaths from a specific cause in each age group and then multiplying this by the average number of years of life lost as a result of each of these deaths. For example, if life expectancy were 80 years, a death from coronary heart disease at age 60 would contribute 20 years of life lost compared with 30 years for a death at age 50. Thus, although there are fewer deaths among younger people, each contributes a greater number of YLL than the deaths in the elderly.

One advantage this measure has over life expectancy is that it is possible to count the YLL due to specific causes of death such as cancer or heart disease and thus to target those conditions with the highest YLL. In addition, the years of life lost due to each cause of death can be summed to give the total years of life lost. It is, however, important to be aware that, unlike life expectancy measures, the YLL depend on the size of the population. Assuming two populations have similar life expectancy and mortality rates, the YLL for the larger population will always be greater than that for the smaller population, although it is possible to get around this by calculating average YLL to facilitate comparisons between populations.

Quality-adjusted life years (QALYs)

The problem of how best to integrate measures of morbidity and mortality also arises in clinical trials. Before introducing a new treatment, it is important to know that it will either increase life expectancy, improve quality of life, or both. A treatment that improves both survival and quality of life is clearly worth having, but how can we compare two drugs if one increases survival but at the expense of worse quality of life? This challenge led to the development of the concept of a **quality-adjusted life year** (QALY). Quality-adjusted life years weight each year of life by the perceived quality of that life from a value of one for perfect health down to zero for death. One QALY would thus represent a year of life in perfect health while 0.5 QALY could represent 6 months lived in perfect health or 12 months with 50% disability (or ill-health). The QALYs gained from a new radical treatment that increases life expectancy by 10 years but is associated with major side effects might thus be lower than those from a less-effective drug that increases life expectancy by only 8 years but does not have any major side effects. It is, however, important to note that *these measures are entirely dependent on the* *magnitude of the weights assigned to different health conditions* and this process is necessarily highly subjective.

Health-adjusted life expectancy (HALE)

By combining QALYs with measures of life expectancy we can calculate **health-adjusted** or **healthy life expectancy** (HALE), which represents the equivalent number of years an individual can expect to live *in full health*. A health-adjusted life expectancy of 60 years might therefore represent an expectation of 50 years life in full health plus an additional 20 years at 50% or 30 years at 33% of full health.

Table 2.9 shows data on life expectancy and healthy life expectancy for a number of different countries. Notice that healthy life expectancy is consistently 5–12 years less than life expectancy. This difference is a function both of the expected number of years of life at less than full health and of the extent of disability. Because life expectancy at birth is partly dependent on mortality in the first year of life, it is inevitably much lower in lower-income countries, which tend to have much higher neonatal and infant mortality rates than do high-income countries. Once an individual has survived the first few years of life in a low-income country, however, their chances of living to old age are then much greater and the difference between high- and low-income countries becomes less marked. As an example, see the apparent paradox in Nigeria. Healthy life expectancy at birth for a man in 2012 was only 53 years; but, if a man makes it to 60, he can then expect about another 15 years of

Table 2.9 Life expectancy at birth and age 60 (years), healthy life expectancy at birth (years), and adult mortality rates in 2012 (from WHO, 2014a).

	Life expectancy at birth		Life expectancy at age 60		Healthy life expectancy at birth	Adult mortality rate (per 1000)	
	Males	Females	Males	Females		Males	Females
Australia	81	85	24	27	73	75	44
India	64	68	16	18	57	242	160
Japan	80	87	23	29	75	82	43
Nigeria	53	55	15	16	46	371	346
Russian Federation	63	75	14	20	61	339	127
Switzerland	81	85	24	27	73	67	40
United Kingdom	79	83	22	25	71	90	56
Unites States of America	76	81	21	24	70	130	77

healthy life. Notice also that, while in most countries women can expect to live about 2–5 years longer than men, the high mortality rates among young Russian men (Figure 1.2) mean that the difference in the Russian Federation is 12 years.

Disability-adjusted life years (DALYs)

The concept of a **disability-adjusted life year** or DALY was developed to facilitate attempts to quantify the global burden of disease (World Bank, 1993; Murray *et al.*, 2012). Like YLL, DALYs estimate loss of life, but they have the major advantage that they count not only years of life lost completely due to premature death but also years of health lost through disability. As for QALYs, the extent of disability is weighted from zero to one, although the weights go in the opposite direction – from zero for a year spent in perfect health to one for a year lost to death. These weights were defined by an international panel of health experts based on data from population surveys. One DALY can be thought of as one lost year of healthy life. Thus, if a person lives with a moderate disability for 10 years, this might equate to the loss of

Table 2.10 The 10 leading causes of mortality and DALYs in the world, 2012.

Mortality	Deaths (millions)	% of total deaths	Burden of disease	DALYs (millions)	% of total DALYs
Ischaemic heart disease	7.4	13.2	Ischaemic heart disease	165.7	6.0
Stroke	6.7	11.9	Lower respiratory infections	146.9	5.4
Chronic obstructive pulmonary disease	3.1	5.6	Stroke	141.3	5.2
Lower respiratory infections	3.1	5.5	Preterm birth conditions	107.2	3.9
Trachea, bronchus and lung cancers	1.6	2.9	Diarrhoeal diseases	99.7	3.6
HIV/AIDS	1.5	2.8	Chronic obstructive pulmonary disease	92.4	3.4
Diarrhoeal diseases	1.5	2.7	HIV/AIDS	91.9	3.6
Diabetes	1.5	2.7	Road injury	78.7	2.9
Road injury	1.3	2.3	Unipolar depressive disorders	76.5	2.8
Hypertensive heart disease	1.1	2.0	Birth asphyxia/trauma	74.6	2.7

Data source: WHO Global Health Estimates 2014 Summary Tables www.who.int/healthinfo/global_burden_disease/en/, accessed 24 May 2015.

Table 2.11 The top 10 causes of DALYs in the world, by income level, 2010.

Risk factor	Developing countries DALYs (millions)	% of all DALYs	Developed countries DALYs (millions)	% of all DALYs
Dietary risks	165.6	7.9	64.5	16.8
High blood pressure	124.3	5.9	49.3	12.8
Smoking	112.0	5.3	44.9	11.7
Household air pollution from solid fuels	105.7	5.0	2.4	0.6
Alcohol use	62.5	3.0	34.7	9.0
High body mass index	55.2	2.6	38.4	10.0
High fasting plasma glucose	68.6	3.3	20.4	5.3
Childhood underweight	77.3	3.7	<0.1	0.01
Ambient particulate matter pollution	65.6	3.1	10.6	2.7
Physical inactivity and low physical activity	46.9	2.2	22.4	5.8

(Data source: IHME, 2013, accessed 7 May 2015.)

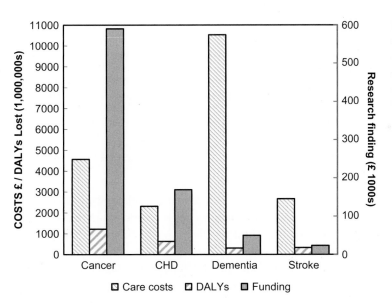

Figure 2.7 Health and social care costs and disability-adjusted life-years (DALYs) for cancer, coronary heart disease (CHD), dementia and stroke in relation to research funding in the UK in 2007–2008. (*Drawn from*: Luengo-Fernandez *et al.*, 2012.)

5 years of healthy life or five DALYs. Like the measures of potential years of life lost, DALYs are a health gap indicator and have the useful property that they can be calculated separately for different diseases (see Table 2.10) or for different causes of disease (Table 2.11). Measurements of DALYs are

More about the GBD project

increasingly used to estimate the burden of various diseases or exposures in different countries, as for example in the Global Burden of Disease (GBD) project (Murray *et al.*, 2012) and the World Health Reports produced by WHO (WHO, 2014a), and to identify priorities for health intervention. Like QALYs, they are highly dependent on the magnitude of the weights assigned to different health conditions.

The use of measures like DALYs highlights the enormous burden of ill-health due to some common but non-fatal conditions such as unipolar depressive disorders that do not feature at all on lists derived from mortality-based indicators. It also highlights the enormous burden of ill-health attributable to some entirely preventable risk factors such as smoking and alcohol use. DALYs can also give a very different sense of priorities for disease control from conventional rates (see Figure 2.7 and Box 2.11). Dementia, for example, puts an enormous burden on the health system, yet far greater financial resources tend to be given to research into high-profile conditions such as cancer.

Box 2.11 Suicide rates: are we winning or losing?

Suicide is a major cause of premature mortality in many countries, but is the situation becoming better or worse? Data from the UK show that:

- between 1981 and 1998, suicide rates in men and women aged 15 and over *fell by 18%*; and
- between 1981 and 1998, the years of potential life lost due to suicide *increased by 5%*.

How do we interpret these apparently conflicting data? The answer is that the major drop in suicide rates has occurred among the older age groups (45 years and over) and suicide rates in younger men have actually increased over the same time period. Suicide in a younger person leads to greater loss of potential life, so although the overall suicide rates are falling, this average effect hides an increasing loss of life among young men.

These data underline how different measures of health capture different things and can give very different pictures of the health of a population. A politician hoping to demonstrate improvements in mental health could legitimately claim that suicide rates were falling, while an advocate for more funding for mental health could equally legitimately cite the increase in years of life lost.

(Gunnell and Middleton, 2003.)

Table 2.12 A summary of measures of disease occurrence.

Measure	Definition	Formula	Units
Prevalence (P)	The *proportion* of the population with disease at a specific point in time	$$\frac{No.\ people\ with\ disease\ at\ a\ given\ point\ in\ time}{Total\ number\ of\ people\ in\ the\ population\ at\ that\ time}$$	% or proportion (e.g. 0.01) (or per 1000, 10,000, 100,000, etc.)
Incidence Proportion (IP) or Risk	The *proportion* of people who develop disease during a specified period. Synonyms: *Cumulative Incidence, Attack Rate, Experimental and Control Event Rate* (in the treated and control groups in a clinical trial)	$$\frac{No.\ who\ develop\ disease\ in\ a\ specified\ period}{No.\ at\ risk\ of\ the\ disease\ at\ the\ start\ of\ the\ period}$$	% or proportion (or per 1000, 10,000, 100,000, etc.)
Incidence Rate (IR)	The *rate* at which disease is occurring, measured from individual data in a study. Synonym: *Incidence density*	$$\frac{No.\ who\ develop\ disease\ in\ a\ specified\ period}{No.\ person\text{-}years\ at\ risk\ of\ getting\ the\ disease}$$	per 100,000/person-years (or per 1000, 10,000 person-years, etc.)
	The *rate* at which disease is occurring, measured from population data, may be *crude, specific* (e.g. age-specific) or *standardised* (direct standardisation)	$$\frac{No.\ people\ who\ develop\ disease\ in\ one\ year}{Average\ no.\ in\ the\ population\ in\ the\ same\ year}$$	per 100,000/year (or per 1000, 10,000/year, etc.)
Standardised Incidence or Mortality Ratio (SIR/SMR)	Compares incidence or mortality to a standard population using *indirect* standardisation	$$\frac{Observed\ number\ of\ cases\ (deaths)}{No.\ expected\ for\ a\ standard\ population}$$	A ratio, sometimes a percentage
Proportional Mortality Ratio (PMR)	Compares the *proportion* of deaths to a standard population (can be used when information is only available for deaths)	$$\frac{Proportion\ of\ deaths\ from\ a\ specific\ cause}{Proportion\ expected\ for\ a\ standard\ population}$$	A ratio, sometimes a percentage
Case Fatality Ratio (CFR)	The proportion of people who die from a disease in a specified (usually short) time period (actually an *incidence proportion*)	$$\frac{No.\ who\ die\ from\ disease\ in\ a\ specified\ period}{Total\ no.\ with\ disease}$$	A percentage (or per 1000, 10,000, 100,000, etc.)

Summary

As you have seen, a plethora of measures are used to try to quantify the health of a population and each has their advantages and limitations. Some measure only limited aspects of health but are commonly used because they are easy to calculate, whereas other more complex measures come closer to capturing our ideal notion of 'health' but are much harder to calculate and thus not so easily applied in practice. All measures have their uses and selection of the most appropriate measure for any given situation will depend almost entirely on the question being asked. You should now be able to interpret most measures of disease and health that you come across (the key features of the main incidence and mortality measures are summarised in Table 2.12). It is still important to be very careful when comparing measures of disease across different groups of people because many other factors can complicate the comparisons. We will discuss some of these issues in the following chapters.

Questions

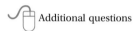 Additional questions

1. For each of the following scenarios, calculate a measure of the incidence of disease and identify what type of measure it is:
   (a) One thousand healthy women were followed for 8 years and 15 developed high blood pressure.
   (b) A large group of elderly men was followed for a total of 5000 person-years and 75 of the men had a stroke during the duration of the study.
   (c) In a community with a population of 50,000 people, 27 developed diabetes during a 1-year period.
2. Two thousand women aged 55 years were given a health check and 100 were found to have high blood pressure. Ten years later, all 2000 women attended a second check and another 300 women had developed high blood pressure.
   (a) What was the prevalence of high blood pressure in the women (i) at age 55, and (ii) at age 65?
   (b) How many women were 'at risk' of developing high blood pressure at the start of the 10-year period?
   (c) What was the incidence of high blood pressure in these women? Is this an incidence proportion or an incidence rate?
   Assume that, on average, each of the 300 women who developed high blood pressure did so half-way through the 10 year follow-up period.
   (d) Calculate the total number of person-years at risk (of developing high blood pressure) during the 10 years.
   (e) What was the incidence rate of high blood pressure in these women?

3. Community A and community B both have crude mortality rates for ischaemic heart disease of 4 per 1000 population per year. The age-adjusted mortality rate for ischaemic heart disease in community A is 5 per 1000 population and the age-adjusted rate for ischaemic heart disease in community B is 3 per 1000 population. Which of the following is correct?
   (a) community A has a younger population than community B
   (b) community A has an older population than community B
   (c) diagnosis is more accurate in community A
   (d) diagnosis is more accurate in community B
4. Look back to Table 2.10. What does this tell us about the relative import-ance of chronic obstructive pulmonary disease and lower respiratory infections as causes of mortality and ill health and explain the patterns you see.

REFERENCES

 References

Agarwal, M. M. and Punnose, J. (2002). Gestational diabetes: implications of variation in diagnostic criteria. *International Journal of Gynecology and Obstetrics*, 78: 45–46.

Anderson, R. and Rosenberg, H. (1998). Age standardization of death rates: implementation of the Year 2000 standard. *National Vital Statistics Reports*, vol. 47, no. 3. Hyattsville, MD: National Center for Health Statistics.

Australian Bureau of Statistics. (2014). Life Tables, States, Territories and Aus-tralia, 2011–2013. ABS Publication 3302.0.55.001. http://www.abs.gov.au, accessed 23 May 2015.

AIHW (Australian Institute of Health and Welfare). (2015). *Australian Cancer Incidence and Mortality (ACIM) books: Lung cancer*. Canberra: AIHW. Accessed via www.aihw.gov.au/acim-books, accessed 30 May 2015.

CDC (Centers for Disease Control). Division of Viral Hepatitis. *Viral Hepatitis Surveillance United States, 2009*. www.cdc.gov/hepatitis/statistics/, accessed 22 May 2015.

Chan, K.-L., Dumesnil, J. G., Cujec, B., *et al.* for the Investigators of the Multi-center Aspirin Study in Infective Endocarditis. (2003). A randomized trial of aspirin on the risk of embolic events in patients with infective endocarditis. *Journal of the American College of Cardiologists*, 42: 775–780.

Gunnell, D. and Middleton, N. (2003). National suicide rates as an indicator of the effect of suicide on premature mortality. *Lancet*, 362: 961–962.

IHME (Institute for Health Metrics and Evaluation). (2013). *GBD Compare*. Seattle, WA: IHME, University of Washington. vizhub.healthdata.org/gbd-compare, accessed 7 May 2015.

Lopez, A. D., Mathers, C. D., Ezzati, M., *et al.* (eds). (2006). *Global Burden of Disease and Risk Factors*. World Bank and Oxford University Press.

Luengo-Fernandez, R., Leal, J. and Gray, A. M. (2012). UK research expenditure on dementia, heart disease, stroke and cancer: are levels of spending related to disease burden? *European Journal of Neurology*, 19: 149–154.

Mathews, T. J. and MacDorman, M. F. (2013). Infant mortality statistics from the 2010 period linked birth/infant death data set. *National Vital Statistics Reports*, vol. 62, no. 8. Hyattsville, MD: National Center for Health Statistics.

Murray, C. J. L., Salomon, J. A. and Mathers, C. (2000) A critical examination of summary measures of population health. *Bulletin of the World Health Organization*, 78: 981–994.

Murray, C. J. L., Vos, T., Lozano, R., *et al.* (2012). Disability-adjusted life years (DALYs) for 291 diseases and injuries in 21 regions, 1990–2010: a systematic analysis for the Global Burden of Disease Study 2010. *The Lancet*, 380: 2197–2223.

Olshansky, S. J., Passaro, D. J., Hershow, R. C., *et al.* (2005). A potential decline in life expectancy in the United States in the 21st Century. *New England Journal of Medicine*, 352: 1138–1145.

Population Reference Bureau. (2012). *2012 World Population Data Sheet*. PRB. http://www.prb.org/pdf12/2012-population-data-sheet_eng.pdf, accessed 13 March 2015.

Porta, M. (ed.) (2014). *A Dictionary of Epidemiology*, 6th edn. New York, NY: Oxford University Press.

Robinson, C. F., Petersen, M. and Palu, S. (1999). Mortality patterns among electrical workers employed in the U.S. construction industry, 1982–1987. *American Journal of Industrial Medicine*, 36: 630–637.

United Nations. (2014). *The Millenium Development Goals Report*. New York, NY: United Nations.

UNAIDS. (2013). *Report on the Global AIDS Epidemic 2013*. Geneva: UNAIDS. http://www.unaids.org/en/resources/campaigns/globalreport2013/global report, accessed 13 March 2015.

World Bank (1993). *Investing in Health: World Development Report 1993*. New York, NY: Oxford University Press.

WHO (World Health Organization). (2014a). *World Health Statistics 2014*. Geneva: World Health Organization. http://www.who.int/gho/publications/world_health_statistics/2014/en/, accessed 2 May 2015.

WHO (World Health Organization). (2014b). *World Health Statistics 2014. Indicator Compendium*. Geneva: World Health Organization. http://www.who.int/gho/publications/world_health_statistics/2014/en/, accessed 2 May 2015.

Who, what, where and when?
Descriptive epidemiology

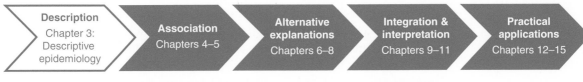

Description	Association	Alternative explanations	Integration & interpretation	Practical applications
Chapter 3: Descriptive epidemiology	Chapters 4–5	Chapters 6–8	Chapters 9–11	Chapters 12–15

The rates and measures that we explored in Chapter 2 provide a variety of ways to describe the health of a population and thus also enable us to compare patterns of health and disease between populations and over time. This allows us to answer the core questions relating to disease burden that are the essential first step in setting health planning and service priorities. As we discussed in Chapter 1, this *descriptive epidemiology*, concerned as it is with 'person, place and time', attempts to answer the questions 'Who?', 'What?', 'Where?' and 'When?'. This can include anything from a description of disease in a single person (a case report) or a special survey conducted to measure the prevalence of a particular health issue in a specific population, to reports from national surveys and data collection systems showing how rates of disease or other health-related factors vary in different geographical areas or over time (time trends).

Although descriptive data may be collected specifically to answer a defined question, they often come from governments, health care providers and statistical agencies that routinely collect vast amounts of information. Summary data – often the various forms of rate which you met in Chapter 2 – can be accessed from published reports and, increasingly, from online databanks. In some cases it is also possible to obtain information from which the rates are calculated at the individual level. These descriptive data are essential to identify health problems and for health planning and, although they cannot usually answer the question 'Why?', they may provide the first ideas about causality and thus generate hypotheses that can then be tested in more formal 'analytic' studies that we will discuss in Chapter 4. As you will come to see in later chapters, descriptive studies also play a critical and often under-appreciated role in monitoring the effects of large-scale interventions.

In this chapter we will look in more detail at some of the most common types of descriptive data and where they come from. However, before embarking on a data hunt, we first need to decide exactly what it is we want to know, and this can pose a challenge; to make good use of the most relevant descriptive data, *it is critical to formulate our question as precisely as possible.* If we want to know about youth suicide, are we interested in the suicide rate, the number of hospitalisations for attempted suicide, or the proportion of teenagers who have considered suicide? Mortality data are probably readily available from a number of sources, but the accuracy of the underlying certification of this cause of death may be problematic. Hospital admission data may also be accessible, but might not capture suicide attempts that are dealt with in the emergency room and not admitted. Furthermore, separating individuals from events can be tricky – are a lot of youths making a single suicide attempt each, or are there a smaller number who have made multiple attempts? The resulting policy implications are quite different. In contrast, to find out what proportion of youths have suicidal thoughts we would probably need to conduct a special survey, as this information is unlikely to be captured in routine statistics.

Case reports and case series

The identification of a new or recurring health problem often begins with a *case report* or *case series*. These are detailed descriptions, usually by a doctor or group of doctors, of one or more cases of a disease that are unusual for some reason. This might be because the disease has not been seen before or the cases may have occurred either in individuals who would not normally be expected to develop that disease, or in an area where the disease had not previously been reported or was thought to have been controlled. The cases might also be reported in conjunction with a previous exposure to something that, it is speculated, may have caused the disease.

The selective nature of these reports and the limited amount of information they contain mean that they provide little evidence of causality and cannot say much about patterns of disease occurrence. However, they can help identify potential health problems such as the outbreaks of Ebola, severe acute respiratory syndrome (SARS), bird flu and swine flu that the world experienced during the last decade (we will discuss these further in Chapter 13). They may also stimulate interest in an area, leading to more detailed studies, and in this regard some have been seminal in advancing knowledge (Box 3.1). However, if we want to know how big the problem is or even if the occurrence is really anything out of the ordinary, we need more comprehensive information about the frequency of occurrence of the event of interest in the population.

Vital statistics and mortality data

As you saw in Chapter 2, most of the measures we use in descriptive epidemiology relate the number of events of interest that occurred to the number of people in the population – for example, the number of new cases of HIV per 100,000 people in a given country in a given year. In this section we will look at some of the sources of routine data that provide information about the size of a population and key vital statistics such as birth and death rates before we move on to consider other more specialised sources of data that provide information about other health events. We will note some of their advantages and disadvantages, give examples of the uses to which they can be put, and provide links to some of the most useful sources. Table 3.1 summarises some of the more common mortality and morbidity data collection and reporting systems.

> Events such as births, marriages and deaths are collectively known as **vital statistics**, from the Latin *vita* meaning life.

Census data

A census is a regular procedure for systematically counting and collecting information about everyone in a given population. It is this emphasis on 'everyone' that differentiates it from a survey which would normally only collect data for a sample of people. Early records of national censuses include

Box 3.1 Case reports and case series that were instrumental in the early identification of health problems

- The classic description of a series of infants born with congenital cataracts, some with additional cardiac abnormalities, in Australia in 1941. This led a Sydney doctor to postulate a causal link between a severe epidemic of rubella (German measles) that had occurred six to nine months before the children were born and the subsequent abnormalities (Gregg, 1941). It is now well known that if a woman develops rubella during pregnancy it may affect her unborn baby.

- A case report published in the UK in 1961 described the development of a pulmonary embolism in a 40-year-old pre-menopausal woman, five weeks after she had started using an oral contraceptive (OC) to treat endometriosis (Jordan and Anand, 1961). Because pulmonary embolism is rare in women of that age, the authors suggested that it might have been caused by the OC, particularly as it was a novel exposure at that time. A report of one case could not provide conclusive evidence that it was the OC rather than some other characteristic of the patient that led to the embolism – but it did pave the way for more detailed studies. These have consistently shown that there is an association between the use of OCs and the risk of this condition.

- A report of a series of five cases of *Pneumocystis carinii* pneumonia that occurred in young, previously healthy, homosexual men in three Los Angeles hospitals in a six-month period during 1980–81 (CDC, 1981). Until then, this disease had been seen almost exclusively in the elderly, the severely malnourished and those on anti-cancer chemotherapy whose immune systems were suppressed. This cluster of cases in young men suggested that the men were suffering from a previously unknown disease, possibly related to sexual behaviour. We now know this as AIDS.

the biblical account of the census conducted in Israel around the time of Jesus' birth and the Domesday Book compiled by William the Conqueror in England in 1086. In both cases the goal of the census was to facilitate the collection of taxes. Sweden was the first European country to establish a regular population census in 1749. Census data provide information about the number of people in the population and their age and sex as well as information about where people have come from, where they live, family structure, education and

Table 3.1 Some common health data collections and reporting systems.

Data collection or reporting system	Source of raw data	Summary data published	Individual-level data sometimes available[a]
Census	Census forms (self-reported); completion required by law	Population estimates, overall and in subgroups	–
Civil registration or vital statistics systems (national)	Birth, marriage and death certificates; often required by law	Fertility and mortality rates	Date and cause of death (through a National Death Index or Register)
Health and demographic surveillance systems (regional)	Regular surveys *of the same population*	Vital statistics and a variety of other data	–
Disease registries (e.g. cancer registries, injury registers)	Pathology reports, testing laboratories, hospital and medical records; sometimes required by law	Incidence, mortality and survival rates, prevalence	Diagnosis, date, disease characteristics and demographics;[b] mortality data may also be available
Notifiable disease systems (e.g. AIDS, SARS, TB, other infectious diseases)	Laboratories, medical practitioners and hospitals	Numbers of cases, incidence rates	Diagnosis, date, disease characteristics and demographics
Hospital administrative systems	Hospital discharge sheets and databases, medical records	–	Diagnosis, date, medications prescribed, investigations and procedures performed, costs and demographics
Other administrative health systems, e.g. prescribing and insurance databases	Prescriptions, investigations and medical procedures performed	Health service use and costs	Date, medications prescribed, investigations and procedures performed, costs
Demographic and Health Surveys (morbidity, risk factors, needs, service use, etc.)	Special surveys, sometimes national, often repeated at regular intervals *with a different sample of the population each time*	Special reports	De-identified grouped data sometimes available
Special surveillance systems[c]	e.g. 'sentinel' primary care practices or disease registers (UK GP data base), MONICA (international CHD)	Varied	Varied

[a] With appropriate consent/approvals.
[b] Basic demographic information such as age, sex, and last known address.
[c] See Chapter 12 for a more detailed discussion of surveillance systems.

Demography, the study of the characteristics of human populations such as population size, growth and distribution and vital statistics such as births and deaths, has many parallels to descriptive epidemiology.

employment. The United Nations recommends that countries conduct a census at least every 10 years and provides guidelines regarding the information that should be collected in a census in order to standardise practice (United Nations, 2008). Census data usually provide the best estimates of the number of people in the population, both overall and by key characteristics such as age, country of birth, area of residence and level of education, and they are usually readily available in summary form through the relevant national statistics office.

Civil registration systems

While censuses provide valuable snapshots of a population at isolated points in time, they inevitably miss events that occur between census years. *Civil registration* refers to the ongoing compulsory recording of the occurrence and characteristics of events such as births, marriages and deaths within a population. In most countries, the registration of these events is a legal requirement and the resulting birth, marriage and death certificates are legal documents. So, for example, when someone dies, a medical practitioner must complete a medical certificate that usually includes basic demographic information about the individual, including name, date of birth, ethnicity and gender, as well as the date and cause(s) of death. This goes to the Registrar who registers the death and issues a legal death certificate. Information about the cause of death is coded according to the WHO International Classification of Diseases or ICD (World Health Organization, 2015) and used to compile national mortality statistics. Again, Sweden was one of the first countries to establish a nationwide population register and, as a result, Statistics Sweden has national statistics spanning a period of more than 250 years (e.g. see Figure 3.1). Elsewhere, the General Register Office of England and Wales has records of births, marriages and deaths dating back to 1837 with data from Australia, New Zealand, the USA and Canada available from the late nineteenth century. These data form the basis of many of the mortality-based measures that you met in Chapter 2 and historical information is often made available to individuals for genealogy research. Access to more recent records is tightly controlled but sometimes possible for approved medical research (e.g. see National Death Registers, below). Complete coverage, accuracy and timeliness are critical for quality vital statistics and good population statistics are essential to measure and track health indicators such as the Millennium Development Goals that you met in Chapter 2.

Describe the changes in life expectancy by age and sex over time shown in Figure 3.1 and comment on the patterns.

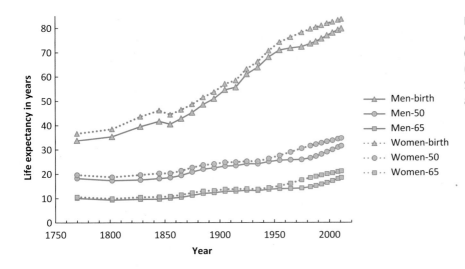

Life expectancy at birth increased by about 45 years compared to increases of only 10–15 years for life expectancy at ages 50 and 65. Why is this?

In the late eighteenth century, average life expectancy in Sweden was only about 35 years for men and women, although then, as now, women could expect to live slightly longer than men. This young average age was a consequence of the very high mortality rates in babies and children at the time and improvements in this area led to much of the large gains in average life expectancy, particularly between 1850 and 1950. However, even in 1800, if an individual survived their childhood years and made it to their 65th birthday they could then expect to live to about 75. Now, most deaths in a country like Sweden occur over the age of 65; thus, someone who reaches that age can still only expect to live until about 85, a much more modest improvement.

National death registers

Recognising the enormous value of the information, particularly the mortality data, collected by their registries of births, marriages and deaths, many countries with a comprehensive civil registration system now also operate a national death register or index to facilitate health research. These electronic registers hold information about the name, date of birth and sex of every individual who has died since the register began, as well as their date, place and cause of death and they allow *bona fide* researchers conducting scientifically and ethically approved studies to obtain death information for individuals in their studies. In some countries it is also possible to get approval to 'link' these data to other health data sets; we will discuss this further in Chapter 4.

Verbal autopsy

In many lower-income countries the vital registration systems are less well-developed than in high-income countries and, although the fact of death is registered, information about cause of death may not be available. In these areas an alternative method used to capture information about causes of death, particularly among children, is the **verbal autopsy**. These 'autopsies' are conducted by a structured interview with the family members about the circumstances of their relative's death. This information can then be used to classify the cause of death according to defined rules and criteria. For example, until recently up to 40% of the 400,000 deaths each year in Thailand were classified to poorly defined conditions, and there were concerns regarding the accuracy when specific causes were assigned. To obtain more reliable information about the patterns of mortality in Thailand, researchers conducted almost 10,000 verbal autopsies and compared the results to those obtained from the vital registration system. This showed that for some conditions mortality rates were at least double those estimated from vital registration data, while life expectancy was approximately two years lower (Porapakkham *et al.*, 2010). An even larger project, the Million Death Study (MDS, Centre for Global Health Research, 2015) is ongoing in India where, despite the introduction of laws mandating birth and death registration in 1969, some states still have low rates of death registration. The MDS, which is monitoring almost 14 million people in 2.4 million nationally representative households from 1998 to 2014, uses verbal autopsies to assign a probable cause to any deaths that occur. The resulting data help identify areas with excess mortality so that action can be taken to reduce preventable deaths. While initially used primarily in the research setting, there is now a push to incorporate verbal autopsies into the routine death registration process in countries with less-developed vital registration systems, and WHO and other groups are working to develop a standard instrument for verbal autopsy.

Health and demographic surveillance systems

In many sub-Saharan African countries and some countries in Asia, the civil registration and vital statistics systems are incomplete or non-existent. In the absence of a comprehensive national system, Health and Demographic Surveillance Systems (HDSS) have been established to monitor vital events within a defined region. Some of these systems have been in existence for several decades, for example the Niakhar HDSS which was first established in a rural area of Senegal in 1962 and now includes 30 villages with a combined population of approximately 43,000 (Delaunay *et al.*, 2013). As well as collecting standard vital statistics, the HDSS often collect additional information about locally relevant health issues, such as the vaccination status of children and cases of vaccine-preventable diseases or other diseases such as malaria. Unlike the Demographic and Health Surveys that we will discuss below, the key feature of a HDSS is that it follows the *same group of people over time*.[1]

In 1998, the International Network for the Demographic Evaluation of Populations and their Health (INDEPTH; www.indepth-network.org[2]) was established to bring together the existing HDSS sites and encourage new sites to join (Sankoh and Byass, 2012). In 2014 there were 49 member centres from 22 countries including 36 from 15 countries in sub-Saharan Africa. Use of the verbal autopsy is common in the HDSS regions and the INDEPTH Network has been closely involved with WHO in developing standardised forms for this.

Challenges in using mortality Data

As we noted above, death registration is a legal requirement in most countries. The registration of a death therefore establishes the *fact* that someone has died with virtual certainty. Unfortunately, the information is less reliable when the *cause* of death is of interest, rather than the simple fact that a death has occurred. This can be a consequence either of misdiagnosis (e.g. if a doctor does not know a person's full medical history) or of mis-specification on the form. The sample certificate shown in Figure 3.2 shows the challenge of getting the sequence and content right. Look at the instructions on completing the 'cause of death' section: it will often not be easy, and those dying at older ages tend to have a number of coexisting diseases. How should the practitioner sequence the diagnoses of an overweight woman who has had diabetes for 20 years and high blood pressure for 10 years and who dies of pneumonia 1 year after suffering a stroke? Such a scenario is not uncommon, so we can be left with considerable uncertainty about the actual cause of death even on inspection of the original form. Indeed, in research studies where people are followed up for mortality, considerable extra effort often needs to be made in collecting clinical and pathology records in order to ensure accuracy in assigning cause of death. This can never be the case for routine vital statistics collections (it is far too expensive), so reports of mortality rates based on death certificates need to be used circumspectly. Generally only a single cause is extracted from the death certificate for each person who has died, that which is thought to be *underlying* any subsequent conditions. Multiple cause of death coding has recently been introduced in some countries but, while this

---

[1] This characteristic means the HDSS have many parallels with the cohort studies that we will discuss in Chapter 4.

[2] The web addresses given throughout this chapter and elsewhere in the book are current as of mid-2016 but, although most have been stable for some time, web addresses can change.

Medical Certificate of the Cause of Death

To the Registrar-General

I hereby certify that

(name in full)

aged   years, date of birth   __/__/__   who usually resided at

Postcode   was attended and last

seen by me on   __/__/__   (or by* Dr.   on   __/__/__

*if not attended by certifying medical practitioner within 3 months prior to death, insert name of medical practitioner who last attended deceasedand date)

and I am informed that he/she died on   __/__/__   at

(town, place etc of death)

Cause of Death (print clearly and do not abbreviate)

Duration of last illness

Disease or condition directly leading to death
(This means the disease, injury or complication which caused death – NOT ONLY, for example, the mode of dying such as "heart failure", "asphyxia", etc)

1a

due to, or as a consequence of

1b

due to, or as a consequence of

Antecedent causes - *morbid conditions, if any giving rise to the above cause, stating the underlying condition last*

1c

due to, or as a consequence of

1d

Other significant conditions
Contributing to the death, but not related to the diseases or condition causing it

2

Date and type of operation in the last 4 weeks   __/__/__

Was a Coroner consulted before issuing this certificate?

No, death not subject to the provisions of the Coroners Act

Yes, issue of this certificate agreed to by   , Coroner

Signature of Medical Practitioner   Date   __/__/__

Initials and Surname (BLOCK Letters)

Professional Qualifications

Figure 3.2 A typical form completed to record a death.

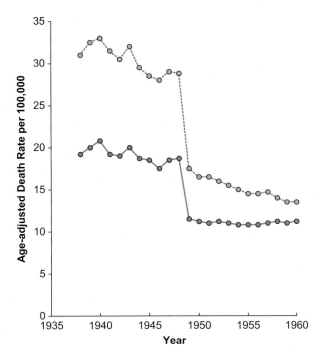

Figure 3.3 Age-adjusted mortality rates for diabetes by gender (females, open circles; males filled circles) in the USA, 1938–1960, Whites only. (From *Methods in Observational Epidemiology*, 2nd edition, by Kelsey, Thompson and Evans (1996), Figure 3.2, p. 51. By permission of Oxford University Press, USA.)

may alleviate the problem of coding multiple conditions, it introduces another – the question of how to report and use this extra information.

Figure 3.3 shows diabetes mortality rates over time in the USA. What explanations can you think of for the sudden change that occurred between 1948 and 1949? Which do you think is most likely?

We saw in Chapter 1 (Figures 1.7 and 1.8) that US death rates for a number of causes have been declining over time, but none as dramatically as seen here in Figure 3.3, where the mortality rate for diabetes appeared to halve between 1948 and 1949 before plateauing at the new level.[3] This *could* be due to a spectacular new treatment (but insulin is still the mainstay, as it was in the 1940s), or to fewer cases of diabetes occurring (but no good means of preventing diabetes had been identified). So we are forced to consider artefacts in the data as a possible explanation. Here the dramatic shift in diabetes mortality was due to a coding change in the International Classification of Diseases (ICD), such that, when diabetes and coronary heart disease occurred together, diabetes was no longer listed as the underlying cause.

---

[3] During this period most deaths would have been from type 1 or insulin-dependent diabetes that is usually diagnosed at younger ages. Unlike type 2 diabetes, which is associated with overweight and obesity and is increasing in incidence, type 1 diabetes is not related to obesity.

Cause of death coding is particularly challenging for suicide as it may be hard to differentiate between intentional self-harm and accident. While the reported number of suicides has fallen in Australia since 1997, the numbers of deaths coded as accidents involving asphyxia or firearms, methods suggestive of suicide, increased. Overall, the authors suggested suicide cases were undercounted by between 11% and 16% (De Leo *et al.*, 2010).

Not surprisingly, some diseases are recorded more accurately on death certificates than others. One that is rapidly fatal is likely to be clear-cut, whereas with a long-term disease there is more chance of another illness occurring and being recorded on the death certificate instead. For example, many people like the woman described above would not have diabetes recorded anywhere on their death certificates. Similarly, diseases that are easily diagnosed tend to be more accurately recorded than those that require more complex diagnostic procedures; in the absence of an autopsy (and they are now uncommon), death from a motor vehicle accident would clearly be easier to recognise than one from pancreatic cancer. In an Australian study it was found that the overall accuracy of death certificates was only 77% compared with autopsy records, although cancers were accurately reported in 90% of cases (Maclaine *et al.*, 1992). A similarly high concordance for cancers was found in a UK study linking death certificates and hospital records, but chronic diseases such as diabetes and hypertension were correctly listed as an underlying cause only about half of the time (Goldacre, 1993). More recent studies have continued to report considerable levels of discrepancy between the cause of death listed on a death certificate and that assigned based on an independent review of the medical records (Rampatige *et al.*, 2014).

Certain diseases may also be under-reported because of a reluctance to record the information. This might be either because of the potential stigma attached to the patient, as in the case of a death from suicide or AIDS, or because of the possibility that blame might be attached to the physician. The UK research found that conditions generally regarded as 'avoidable' causes of death were frequently omitted from the death certificate; for example, fractured neck of femur (broken hip) in the elderly was recorded in only one-quarter of cases.

Morbidity data

Although mortality data can provide valuable information about the health of a population, they are clearly more useful for conditions associated with a high death rate and provide little or no information about the many conditions that are not normally fatal. Unfortunately, it is much harder to find reliable morbidity data. The scope of information is enormous and little is captured in a systematic way. As a result, it is rarely simple to obtain complete information at a local level, and the problems escalate dramatically when trying to make comparisons between regions or countries. Having said that, attempts are made to record some aspects of morbidity in a routine way and these sources can provide valuable information (see Table 3.1).

Disease registries

Cancer is the only disease group for which good morbidity data are widely and routinely available. Some countries, most notably in Scandinavia, have cancer registries that cover the whole country and have been operating for many decades. In others, such 'population-based' registries are newer and less well-established or, as in the USA, cover only part of the population. However, coverage is generally increasing, and a wealth of data on incidence, mortality and survival is available at regional, national and international levels. In some jurisdictions cancer is a legally notifiable disease, whereas in others (e.g. the UK) comprehensive identification of cases has come about gradually due to a combination of enthusiastic local registries and increasing awareness of the value of good morbidity data for planning and evaluating services. Cancer is an ideal candidate for such monitoring due to its relatively clear-cut diagnosis, usually based on a single simple record (a pathology report of histology). Rapid advances in technology now allow much of this information to be transferred electronically from the pathologist to the registry. An added benefit is that cancer registries around the world collaborate through the International Association of Cancer Registries and the International Agency for Research on Cancer (IARC) to compile detailed information about cancer incidence and mortality at a global level. These data are made widely available through the 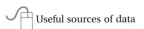 Useful sources of data publications 'Cancer Incidence in Five Continents' and the 'GLOBOCAN' project, both accessible through the IARC website (see Box 3.4).

Many health authorities also keep registers of notifiable infectious diseases, although their prime purpose is for real-time surveillance to allow rapid response to emerging epidemics. (We will come back to discuss *surveillance* in more detail in Chapter 12.) Data for these registers usually come from medical practitioners and pathology laboratories, often under legal compunction. Despite this, and in contrast to cancers, most such diseases are poorly reported. Exceptions are those conditions which are perceived to be more severe, presenting either an acute challenge to a health system (SARS, AIDS) or a long-standing threat, such as tuberculosis. WHO publishes summary statistics for a number of infectious diseases including cholera, meningococcal meningitis and the conditions covered by the Millennium Development Goals including HIV and AIDS, malaria and tuberculosis through their Global Health Observatory. Although other disease registries exist (or have existed) to meet local health or research needs, they cover only a small minority of conditions. For example, when it was noted that mortality from coronary heart disease (CHD) had started to fall in some countries in the late 1960s, it was not obvious what was driving this. Cardiologists of course claimed that better treatment in the newly introduced coronary care units meant that fewer patients were dying (lower case fatality). It was also possible that the number of new cases (incidence) was falling due to changes in smoking and dietary patterns, but no directly relevant data were available to clarify the public health debate. WHO responded in the early 1980s by encouraging the establishment of a series of registers around the world to capture international trends in CHD incidence (the MONICA programme). These provided a wealth of data on CHD incidence, risk factors and mortality (Tunstall-Pedoe *et al.*, 1999), leading to the conclusion that both falling incidence and better clinical outcomes had contributed to the drop in death rates. However, now that their job is finished, most of the MONICA sites have stopped active monitoring. Other conditions that are sometimes covered by registries include injury (e.g. the Australian Spinal Cord Injury Register) while Australia, Sweden and Norway amongst others operate a Diabetes Register that covers all or part of the population.

Health records

> In the UK, NHS Digital provides information on a wide range of health indicators (www.digital.nhs.uk).

Governments, health care providers and health insurers have to maintain good records for administrative and financial reasons and these also generate essential information about service provision and health care quality and delivery. Hospital records can provide useful information on conditions that require hospitalisation. Although detailed patient records may only exist in paper format, making it necessary to go through individual files by hand to collect the required information, many countries now require hospitals to keep electronic records of all patients seen, the conditions they were diagnosed with, and any treatment provided. These data should be fairly reliable, although varying degrees of misdiagnosis, mis-recording and mis-coding are inevitable. A further limitation occurs where there is no unique patient identifier because aggregate admissions will be greater than the number of people admitted to hospital (because some will go to hospital more than once). Choosing the right numerator for a morbidity rate can thus be a challenge. There may also be local idiosyncrasies that affect the utility of the data. For example, in Australia, funding for public hospitals is provided at a state level so each state maintains an 'Admitted Patients Database' with detailed information about inpatients treated in public hospitals in the state. In contrast, reimbursement for procedures performed in private hospitals is the responsibility of the national government and information about these is held in a separate national database (the Medical Benefits Scheme, MBS). It is therefore important to consider whether data obtained will be representative of the general population or whether any conclusions will be restricted to the specific individuals from whom the data were obtained, for example those treated in a private hospital in the case of the Australian MBS data.

It is also important to remember that hospital databases can only provide information about those admitted to hospital. For conditions such as heart attacks that almost always require hospitalisation, they may provide good information on the levels of disease in the community. For conditions commonly treated outside hospital or that do not require an overnight stay, however, the hospital-based population will not be typical: rather, it will be biased towards those with more severe disease, or towards those groups of society more likely to be hospitalised. Information about the potentially greater burden of conditions treated by family practitioners or in the home is harder to obtain, although some of this information is now becoming more accessible. As an example, the Clinical Practice Research Datalink in the UK (www.cprd.com) contains over 13 million patient records from 650 primary care practices.

A wide range of other health data may also be available, for example in some countries it is possible to access electronic data regarding medications prescribed at a regional and/or national level. These may only be available in the form of summary statistics but, with appropriate scientific and ethical approvals, it is sometimes possible to access individual-level information for research. We will discuss the use of these and other health databases for data linkage further in Chapter 4.

Prevalence surveys

If we want to measure the prevalence of a disease that is not captured by other routine statistics, or another aspect of health – for example, conditions such as obesity, health-related behaviours (e.g. smoking, sun-exposure, diet) or use of health services – it may be necessary to conduct a special survey. This might vary in size and complexity from a simple face-to-face survey of people attending a specific location or event, for example shoppers at a mall, to a national mail- or telephone-based survey of several thousand people carefully selected to represent the whole population. Whatever the purpose, it is important to remember that the information collected will only be directly relevant to the people who were surveyed. If the goal is to apply this information to a wider population, such as everyone living in the local community, it is essential to ensure that the sample of people who were actually questioned (the *study population*) is as representative of the community (the *target population*) as possible. The best way to ensure this is to select them at random from the population such that everyone has an equal chance of being selected. However, this is not as easy to do in practice as it might seem (see Box 3.2).

Many countries now conduct regular demographic and health surveys to collect information at a national level. A major advantage of these government-led surveys is that legislation may exist to compel people to take part, thereby greatly reducing the potential for bias. These spot checks on the overall health of a community are crucial to expanding our understanding of health burdens, needs and services beyond the hospital sector. They can also be used to monitor changes in the heath of a nation or region over time. In recent decades

> A group of people recruited from e.g. a shopping mall is often called a **convenience sample** because the people are chosen for practical reasons (it is easy to stop them to ask a few questions). While the information they give may tell us about people who shop at that mall on that day and at that time, it may not be relevant to the rest of the population.

Box 3.2 Sampling

In practice it is rarely, if ever, possible to survey everyone in the population that we are interested in and the people who actually end up completing the survey may only be a very small minority (see Figure 3.4). If, for example, we define the **target population** as the population living in Australia, then we would like to have a list of everyone who lives in Australia to select people from – the **sampling frame**. One option is the national electoral roll (enrolment to vote is required by law in Australia), but this roll only includes Australian citizens (so misses those who are permanent residents but have not taken Australian citizenship), and it does not include anyone under the age of 18. Also, because the list is usually only updated prior to a general election, the information it holds may be inaccurate if people have died, moved house or changed their name. Then, even if we select a random sample of people from the electoral roll (although not straightforward, it is still possible to get access to lists of names and addresses from the Australian electoral roll for approved health research), not all of these people will agree to take part in our survey (in practice, only 10%–20% of those approached via the elect-oral roll now agree to take part in a research study). The types of people who agree to take part in surveys are often very different from those who do not want to take part, so the final **study population** may, therefore, differ quite markedly from the Australian population as a whole. This means that the information we get from them may not accurately reflect the true prevalence in the whole population. We will discuss this issue of *selection bias* in more detail in Chapter 7.

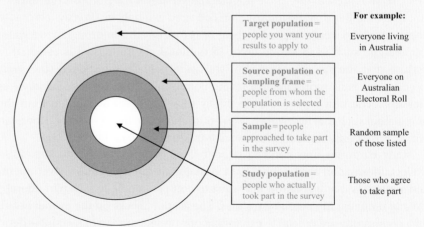

Figure 3.4 Sampling.

Box 3.3 The US National Health and Nutrition Examination Surveys (NHANES)

NHANES is probably the largest and longest-running national source of objectively measured health and nutrition data. It was born out of the National Health Survey Act of 1956, which provided for the establishment of a continuing National Health Survey to obtain information about the health status of individuals residing in the USA, and responsibility for this was given to the National Center for Health Statistics (NCHS). It was originally known as the National Health Examination Survey (NHES) and the first wave was conducted in 1959–62 (see Table 3.2). Subsequent waves focussed on children and then adolescents before the NHES was combined with the National Nutrition Surveillance System, which had been established in 1969, to create the current series of NHANES in 1971, and this is still running in 2016. The NHANES populations are carefully selected to reflect the multifaceted US population, and they have given rich descriptions of many prevalent conditions.

(Data source: http://www.cdc.gov/nchs/nhanes.htm, accessed 31 August 2014.)

Table 3.2 The US National Health and Nutrition Examination Surveys.

Survey	Years	Population	Size (approximate)
NHES I	1959–1962	Age 18–79	7,800
NHES II	1963–1965	Age 6-11	7,400
NHES III	1966–1970	Age 12–17	7,500
NHANES I	1971–1975	Age 1–74	32,000
NHANES II	1976–1980	Age <1–74	28,000
Hispanic (H) HANES	1982–1984	Age <1–74	16,000
NHANES III	1988–1994	Age > 2 months	34,000
NHANES Continuous	Annual from 1999, data released in 2-year cycles from 1999–2000	All ages	5,000 p.a.

they have become a feature of broad-based 'community diagnosis' and health planning, using a wide range of sampling and data-capture designs including telephone and face-to-face interviews, and sometimes very detailed physical examinations. One of the longest running examples is the National Health and Nutrition Examination Surveys (NHANES) conducted in the USA since 1956 (see Box 3.3); and since 1991, 5000–15,000 adults have been interviewed every

Figure 3.5 Estimated prevalence of diabetes (light bars) and prediabetes (dark bars) among Chinese adults in 2010, by age group. (*Drawn from*: Xu *et al.*, 2013.)

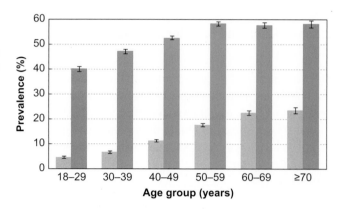

year for the Health Survey for England (HSE) (Mindell *et al.*, 2012). These undertakings are very expensive, so in both cases the investigators have increased the value of the baseline information by asking participants to consent to follow-up to identify risk factors for subsequent morbidity (requiring further personal contact or through linkage to cancer registration data) and mortality (by linking to centrally held death records). Similar surveys are now conducted in many other countries.

Figure 3.5 shows some contemporary data that will be important for future health care planning.

How is the prevalence of diabetes related to age?

What additional data are needed for a comprehensive planning response?

We see that, in 2010, the prevalence of diabetes in China rose markedly with age, affecting almost one quarter of the population over the age of 70 years.[4] This is a very heavy clinical load to manage: diabetes is a metabolic disease with many consequences, including heart and kidney damage, and adequate numbers of doctors, nutritionists and podiatrists must be provided and their care integrated. For a better view of the future health care burden (and the potential for prevention) we need to know time trends both in diabetes and for its risk factors. The very high prevalence of prediabetes, even among the young, foreshadows a major challenge as it suggests the prevalence of diabetes may increase markedly in the future (Xu *et al.*, 2013).

To a large extent, studies such as these are purely descriptive and their aim is primarily to survey a sample of the population in order to determine the prevalence of the factors of interest in the community, often to aid health

[4] In this study the diagnosis of diabetes was based on the ADA criteria using results from clinical tests, but a limitation of many prevalence surveys is their reliance on self-reporting by participants.

planning. Sometimes, however, the breadth of information collected allows much more in-depth analysis of the relationships between health behaviours and conditions. For example, the Australian National Health Survey collects a vast array of information from participants about their health behaviours such as alcohol consumption, smoking and physical activity and about health conditions including diabetes, injury and mental health problems. This allows us to look at the relation between behaviour and health. For example in 2004–05, people who reported high levels of psychological distress were more likely to be physically inactive than those with low levels of distress, or, in other words, the prevalence of inactivity was much higher in those with distress (48%) than those without distress (31%) (ABS, 2006). A study like this that looks at the relation between two aspects of health in a 'cross-section' of the population is often described as a **cross-sectional study** and we will discuss these further in Chapter 4.

> Good **prevalence data** are also essential to estimate the proportion of disease attributable to different risk factors; we will come back to this in Chapters 5 and 14.

Demographic and health surveys

Since 1984, the United States Agency for International Development has collaborated with agencies in low- and middle-income countries to conduct nationally representative surveys through the Demographic and Health Survey (DHS) program (www.dhsprogram.com). Unlike the HDSS described above, the key characteristic of these surveys is that they collect information from a different sample of the population at each time point and the content of the surveys often changes from year to year. As at late 2014, more than 300 surveys had been conducted in more than 90 countries. These surveys have a focus on measures of fertility, maternal and child health, nutrition and health behaviours as well as mortality, and they provide an additional resource for monitoring vital statistics as well as a range of population health indicators (Corsi *et al.*, 2012). The data have also been combined with information from UNICEF (the United Nations Children's Fund) for the *Countdown to 2015: Maternal, Newborn and Child Survival* project, which was established in 2005 to stimulate and monitor progress towards the Millennium Development Goals, particularly Goals 4 and 5 which focus on child and maternal health (Requejo *et al.*, 2014). This project now provides profiles for each of the 75 countries that together account for more than 95% of all maternal and child deaths.

Creative use of existing data

The many sources of data on mortality, morbidity and other factors relevant to health are, inevitably, of varying reliability, quality and completeness. This is true not only across different countries (note that our emphasis here is on the better-developed data systems), but also within any country, because all public data sets will have some problems, and some of them will have many.

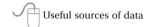
Useful sources of data

> ## Box 3.4 Good sites for accessing and visualising international health data
>
> - WHO Global Health Observatory (www.who.int/gho/en/) provides access to data, graphs, and maps showing a wide range of health-related information from the World Health Organization.
> - IHME (the Institute for Health Metrics and Evaluation) (www.healthdata.org/gbd) has a series of visualisation tools that allow you to interact with and view data from the Global Burden of Diseases (GBD) project.
> - The Global Cancer Observatory (gco.iarc.fr) provides access to graphs, charts and maps via GLOBOCAN and the Cancer Incidence in Five Continents database from the International Agency for Research on Cancer.
> - Gapminder World (www.gapminder.org) uses moving graphs to show how a wide range of socioeconomic and health indicators have changed over time in different countries.

Any comparisons should be made only with a good understanding of the accuracy and completeness of the raw data underlying the summary rates. Another thing to remember is that the data will almost certainly have been collected for a reason other than your question of interest and therefore might not be in the ideal form for your purpose. For example, the definition of who is a 'case' might not fit your criteria exactly; the data could have been collected for age groups that do not correspond to those you want to know about, and so on. It is always important to balance these disadvantages against the major advantage of using existing data – someone else has already done the hard work to collect it. New ways of accessing and displaying this information are continually appearing and Box 3.4 shows some current examples.

Although, as we said at the start of the chapter, descriptive epidemiology is mainly concerned with 'who, what, where and when' we can also use simple descriptive information to start to link exposures and health outcomes to try to determine 'why' disease occurs. For example, Figure 3.6 shows trends in lung cancer mortality over time in Hungary, the UK and the USA.

What does this graph tell us about lung cancer? Why might rates have risen in Hungary between 1980 and 1995 but fallen in the UK and USA? Do we need any other information before we can draw any conclusions from this information?

Figure 3.6 suggests that lung cancer mortality rates in the UK have fallen dramatically since the early 1970s, whereas in the USA they are gradually falling after having peaked in the 1980s. In contrast, the rates in Hungary rose markedly in the 1980s and only started to fall in the late 1990s. However,

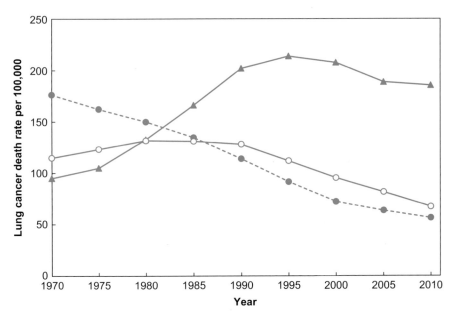

Figure 3.6 Age-standardised death rates from lung cancer among men aged 40–69 years in Hungary (triangles), the USA (open circles) and the UK (filled circles). (Data source: WHO Cancer Mortality Database (WHO, 2014; United Nations, 2012), http://www-dep.iarc.fr/WHOdb/WHOdb.htm, accessed 24 May 2015.)

before we accept that these are real differences, we must consider whether there might be an alternative explanation for the observed patterns. Is lung cancer diagnosed in the same way in each country? Have either the method of diagnosis or the criteria for diagnosis changed over time and have they changed differently in the three countries? Does lung cancer mortality mirror the incidence of lung cancer (i.e. is lung cancer really more common in Hungary?), or are the mortality rates higher in Hungary simply because treatment is less effective and the case–fatality ratio higher? Are lung cancer mortality rates in the UK and USA falling because the incidence is falling or because treatment has improved? If this is a real effect, does the fall in rates in the western countries reflect the reduction in cigarette smoking?

Data of this type leave us with many questions but few definitive answers. However, if we can relate them to changes in other factors that might influence mortality they can add support to a hypothesis. For example, by plotting a graph of per-capita cigarette consumption over time and comparing this with lung cancer mortality rates (Figure 3.7), we find that the rise in lung cancer mortality in the USA parallels increasing cigarette sales, but it occurred 20–30 years later. This represents the two to three decades that it takes smoking to cause lung cancer and kill someone. The fact that lung cancer rates started to fall again 20–30 years after the decline in smoking adds further weight to the hypothesis that smoking causes lung cancer: if this fall had not occurred then the hypothesis would have failed a critical test – removal of the cause should reduce the incidence of disease. So, although these data do not prove that smoking causes lung cancer, they add weight to the belief that it could. If we found that an

Figure 3.7 Cigarette sales and lung cancer mortality rates in males, age-standardised to the world population (cigarette consumption data from www.infoplease.com, lung cancer mortality rates from WHO Mortality Database, http://www-dep.iarc.fr/WHOdb/WHOdb.htm, accessed 16 January 2010).

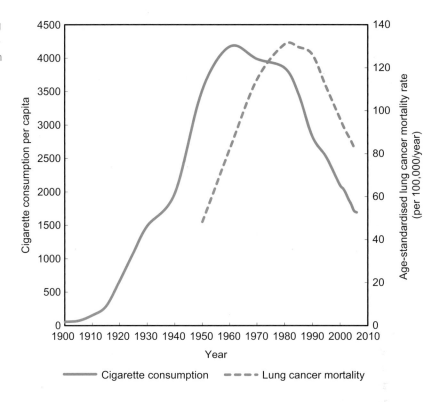

Figure 3.7 Cigarette sales and lung cancer mortality rates in males, age-standardised to the world population (cigarette consumption data from www.infoplease.com, lung cancer mortality rates from WHO Mortality Database, http://www-dep.iarc.fr/WHOdb/WHOdb.htm, accessed 16 January 2010).

increase in cigarette consumption in Hungary occurred much later than the increases seen in the UK and USA, this would strengthen the belief even further.

Migrant studies

Another creative use of descriptive data comes from what are often called *migrant studies*. One of the challenges we face when we try to interpret differences in disease rates between countries is separating the effects of nature and nurture. Do Japanese women have very low rates of breast cancer compared with White American women because they are Japanese (i.e. because of a different genetic predisposition) or because they live differently (i.e. have different environmental exposures, such as diet)? For some populations we are fortunate to have what could be called 'natural experiments' when large numbers of people have migrated from a country with a low risk of a particular disease to a high-risk country, or vice versa, which can help to answer these questions. For example, large numbers of Japanese have migrated to Hawaii and California, and Table 3.3 shows SMRs comparing mortality rates in these migrants, their offspring and the US white population to the Japanese population in Japan.

Remember from Chapter 2 that a **Standardised Mortality Ratio** (SMR) of 100 indicates no difference; an SMR of 120 suggests mortality is 20% higher than in Japan, etc.

Table 3.3 SMRs for selected cancer sites and cardiovascular diseases among Japanese migrants to the USA (1959–62), their offspring (1959–62), and US Whites (1959–61) compared to Japan (1960–61) (data from Haenszel and Kurihara, 1968).

	Standardised Mortality Ratios (SMR)			
Cause of death	Japanese in Japan	Japanese migrants to USA	Offspring of migrants in USA	White US population
All cancer	100	128	78	104
Stomach cancer	100	72	38	17
Colon cancer	100	135	129	140
Breast cancer	100	166	136	591
Degenerative heart disease	100	266	165	481
Stroke	100	32	24	37

Describe the data shown in Table 3.3. Do you think the differences between breast cancer rates in Japan and the USA are due more to genetics or lifestyle?

Table 3.3 shows that the mortality rates of colon cancer, breast cancer and heart disease among the migrants have moved away from the low levels in Japan towards the higher levels of the USA; the converse is seen for stomach cancer and stroke mortality rates, which are both lower in the USA than in Japan. For colon cancer and stroke these changes happened very quickly, with the migrants themselves assuming rates similar to the white US population; for stomach cancer the decline happened over the first generations after migration; while for breast cancer and heart disease, the changes have been less marked. If these diseases were largely genetic in origin then the rates could not have changed so quickly when the migrants moved to the USA. This strongly implicates the importance of the environment in increasing or decreasing the migrants' risk of disease, and has led to enthusiasm for the idea that diet plays an important causal role in these diseases. However, the only specific causal hypothesis that is directly tested by such data is that large-scale international variation in these diseases is not primarily genetic in origin.[5]

Ecological or correlation studies

Figure 3.8 shows the relation or correlation between the prevalence of infection with *Helicobacter pylori* (a bacterium that infects the stomach) and stomach

---

[5] Note that a minority of women do develop breast cancer because they have a mutation in a gene known to influence breast cancer risk; the most important of these are known as *BRCA1* and *BRCA2*.

Figure 3.8 An ecological study comparing the prevalence of serum antibodies to *H. pylori* (a gastric infection) and gastric cancer mortality rates in 46 rural Chinese counties. (*From*: Forman *et al.*, 1990, reprinted by permission of John Wiley & Sons, Inc. © 1990 Wiley-Liss, Inc.)

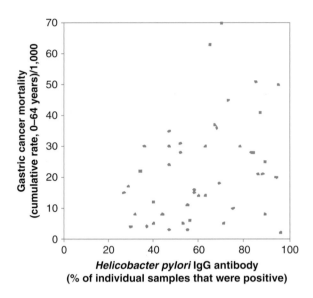

cancer mortality rates in 46 Chinese counties (Forman *et al.*, 1990). In this study, the prevalence of infection was measured as the percentage of the population in the county with antibodies to the bacterium (an indication that they were or had been infected) and the cumulative gastric cancer mortality rate is the rate per 1000 men and women (summed from birth to age 64). (Note that cumulative mortality is comparable to the lifetime risk that you met in Chapter 2.) Each spot on the graph represents one of the 46 counties.

Describe the data shown in Figure 3.8. What, if anything, does this tell you about the role of *H.pylori* infection in causing stomach cancer?

There is not a perfect association, but the graph indicates that counties with a higher prevalence of *H. pylori* infection also tend to have higher stomach cancer rates and, perhaps more importantly, counties with a low prevalence of *H. pylori* have low stomach cancer rates. This hints that *H. pylori* might play a role in the development of stomach cancer; however, the fact that some counties have a high *H. pylori* prevalence but a low stomach cancer rate suggests that infection alone is not enough to cause cancer. Other factors must also play a role.

This example illustrates the key characteristic of ecological studies – *they compare the prevalence of exposure and occurrence of disease in populations or groups of people, not individuals.* The points on the graph represent the population prevalence of infection (in this case, taken from special surveys of individuals in each county) and the rate of disease in the population. The focus is on whether counties or populations with a high prevalence of infection also had a high cancer rate. In general, ecological studies are attractive because they are easy to do, especially if the routine data are readily available, but they can be difficult to interpret. The populations being compared may well differ in ways other than their exposure to the factor of interest and it is possible that something else that is related to the exposure is actually responsible for the observed differences in morbidity or mortality (i.e. an apparent relation could be due to **confounding** – see Chapter 8). Another problem with this type of study is that an observed association between variables at the group level might not represent the association at the individual level. In the example above, we have no way of knowing whether the people who developed cancer were actually infected with *H. pylori*. Ascribing characteristics to members of a group that they might not possess as individuals is called an **ecological fallacy**. For these reasons, ecological studies rarely give a strong test of a causal hypothesis but, more often, they help to generate or develop hypotheses. Box 3.5 shows some other ecological studies that have been instrumental in suggesting associations between exposures and disease.

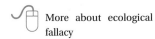 More about ecological fallacy

E-data

The massive explosion in the use of 'smart' technology has opened up a wide range of other sources of information that are increasingly being used to identify and study health problems. Mobile phones often include a global positioning system (GPS) and so can be used to track when, where and how

---

Box 3.5 Ecological studies

- In a classic study, Armstrong and Doll (1975) reported the correlation between 27 cancers and a wide range of dietary and other variables in 23 countries. Diet was strongly correlated with several types of cancer, particularly consumption of meat with cancer of the colon. Countries with low per-capita daily consumption of meat had the lowest rates of colon cancer. The findings from this study suggested that dietary factors play a role in the development of cancer and led to a burgeoning of research in this area.
- In 1979, the authors of another study reported a strong inverse association between average per-capita consumption of wine and mortality from ischaemic heart disease (high wine consumption was associated with low IHD mortality; St Leger *et al.*, 1979). Since then, more than 60 ecological, case–control and cohort studies have been conducted and most have also shown an inverse association between *moderate consumption* of wine and other alcohol and heart disease.

far people travel and we will look at a specific example of this when we consider surveillance in Chapter 12. Others have suggested monitoring terms entered into Internet search engines to identify increases in specific symptoms that might provide early warning of, for example, a flu epidemic – although 'Google Flu Trends' (www.google.org/flutrends/) has not, to date, been as accurate in its predictions as was hoped (Lazer *et al.*, 2014).

Confidentiality

We cannot end any section on health data without touching on the issue of confidentiality. Clearly, information about an individual's health is private and should not be accessible to anyone else other than their health care providers. Much of the available health data is in the form of summary statistics such as rates so that it is impossible to identify specific individuals, and this information can be made freely (or at least readily) available. To gain access to data on individuals it will almost certainly be necessary to sign a confidentiality agreement, have permission from a Human Research Ethics Committee or Institutional Review Board, and/or obtain consent from the individual patients and sometimes their physicians as well. Rapidly changing and expanding privacy legislation in many countries is adding to the challenges. While properly highlighting ethical use of data, the increasing emphasis on the principle of autonomy has created tensions between the need to protect personal information on the one hand and the desire for public good, which may require some access to individual data, on the other.

Summary

You have now seen the most common types of descriptive data and where they come from and also some examples of the many ways in which they can be used. These data are core to health planning and, as you will see in later chapters, are also essential for identifying new health problems and monitoring the effects of health interventions. You have also seen that although it cannot provide strong evidence about the causes of disease, creative use of descriptive epidemiology can generate new ideas about causality. These hypotheses then need to be tested in more formal 'analytic' studies and we will move on to discuss these in the next chapter.

Questions

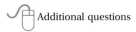
Additional questions

1. Figure 3.9 shows how mortality among males in Thailand changed between 1960 and 1970. The numbers are the differences in the number of deaths (per 10,000) between the two time points. Describe and interpret this pattern.

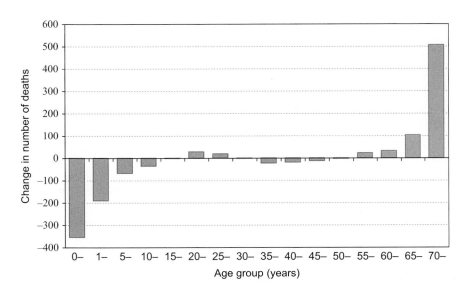

Figure 3.9 Changes in the expected age distribution of deaths (per 10,000 deaths) among males in Thailand between 1960 and 1970 (adapted from Carmichael, 2011).

2. How representative do you think a convenience sample of people surveyed at a shopping mall at 11:00 a.m. on a weekday morning would be of the local population? Would it be any different if the survey were conducted in the evening or at a weekend?

3. Why do the curves for the USA in Figures 3.6 and 3.7 look so different?

REFERENCES

 References

Armstrong, B. and Doll, R. (1975). Environmental factors and cancer incidence and mortality in different countries, with special reference to dietary practices. *International Journal of Cancer*, 15: 617–631.

ABS (Australian Bureau of Statistics). (2006). Mental health in Australia: a snapshot, 2004–05. Cat no. 4824.0.55.001. Downloaded from: http://www.abs.gov.au/AUSSTATS/abs@.nsf/mf/4824.0.55.001, accessed 20 August 2016.

Carmichael, G. A. (2011). Exploring Thailand's mortality transition with the aid of life tables. *Asia Pacific Viewpoint*, 52: 85–105.

CDC (Centres for Disease Control). (1981). Pneumocystis pneumonia – Los Angeles. *Morbidity and Mortality Weekly Review*, 30: 250–252. http://www.cdc.gov/mmwr/preview/mmwrhtml/june_5.htm

Centre for Global Health Research. (2015). Million Death Study. http://www.cghr.org/index.php/projects/million-death-study-project/, accessed 30 March 2015.

Corsi, D. J., Neuman, M., Finlay, J. E. and Subramanian, S. V. (2012). Demographic and health surveys: a profile. *International Journal of Epidemiology*, 41: 1602–1613.

De Leo, D., Dudley, M. J., Aebersold, C. J., *et al.* (2010). Achieving standardised reporting of suicide in Australia: rationale and program for change. *Medical Journal of Australia*, 192: 452–456.

Delaunay, V., Douillot, L., Diallo, A., *et al.* (2013). Profile: the Niakhar Health and Demographic Surveillance System. *International Journal of Epidemiology*, 42: 1002–1011.

Forman, D., Sitas, F., Newell, D. G., *et al.* (1990). Geographical association of *Helicobacter pylori* antibody prevalence and gastric cancer mortality in rural China. *International Journal of Cancer*, 46: 608–611.

Goldacre, M. J. (1993). Cause-specific mortality: understanding uncertain tips of the disease iceberg. *Journal of Epidemiology and Community Health*, 47: 491–496.

Gregg, N. M. (1941). Congenital cataract following German measles in the mother. *Transactions of the Ophthalmological Society of Australia*, 3: 35–46. Reprinted (1991) *Epidemiol Infect*, 107: iii–xiv. http://www.ncbi.nlm.nih.gov/pmc/articles/PMC2272051/.

Haenszel, W. and Kurihara, M. (1968). Studies of Japanese migrants. I. Mortality from cancer and other diseases among Japanese in the United States. *Journal of the National Cancer Institute*, 40: 43–68.

Jordan, W. M. and Anand, J. K. (1961). Pulmonary embolism. *Lancet*, 2: 1146.

Lazer, D. M., Kennedy, R., King, G. and Vespignani, A. (2014). The parable of Google Flu: traps in big data analysis. *Science*, 343: 1203–1205.

Maclaine, G. D., Macarthur, E. B. and Heathcote, C. R. (1992). A comparison of death certificates and autopsies in the Australian Capital Territory. *Medical Journal of Australia*, 156: 462–463, 466–468.

Mindell, J., Biddulph, J. P., Hirani, V., *et al.* (2012). Cohort profile: the health survey for England. *International Journal of Epidemiology*, 41: 1585–1593.

Porapakkham, Y., Rao, C., Pattaraarchachai, J., *et al.* (2010). Estimated causes of death in Thailand, 2005: implications for health policy. *Population Health Metrics*, 8: 1–11.

Rampatige, R., Mikkelsen, L., Hernandez, B., Riley, I. and Lopez, A. D. (2014). Systematic review of statistics on causes of deaths in hospitals: strengthening the evidence for policy-makers. *Bulletin of the World Health Organization*, 92: 807–816.

Requejo, J., Victora, C. and Bryce, J. (2014). Data Resource Profile: Countdown to 2015: maternal, newborn and child survival. *International Journal of Epidemiology*, 43: 586–596.

Sankoh, O. and Byass, P. (2012). The INDEPTH Network: filling vital gaps in global epidemiology. *International Journal of Epidemiology*, 41: 579–588.

St Leger, A. S., Cochrane, A. L. and Moore, F. (1979). Factors associated with cardiac mortality in developed countries with particular reference to the consumption of wine. *Lancet*, 1: 1017–1020.

Tunstall-Pedoe, H., Kuulasmaa, K., Mahonen, M., *et al.* for the WHO MONICA. (1999). Contribution of trends in survival and coronary event rates to changes in coronary heart disease mortality: 10-year results from 37 WHO MONICA populations. *Lancet*, 353: 1547–1557.

United Nations. (2008). *Principles and Recommendations for Population and Housing Censuses*. Revision 2. Series M No 67. New York, NY: United Nations. http://unstats.un.org/unsd/demographic/sources/census/docs/ P&R_Rev2.pdf, accessed 30 March 2015.

United Nations. (2012). *World Population Prospects: The 2012 Revision*. New York, NY: United Nations. http://esa.un.org/unpd/wpp/index.htm, accessed 6 June 2015.

WHO (World Health Organization). (2014). *Mortality Database*. Geneva: World Health Organization. http://www.who.int/healthinfo/statistics/mortality_ rawdata/en/index.html, accessed 17 November 2014.

WHO (World Health Organization). (2015). *International Classification of Diseases – 10th Edition*. Geneva: World Health Organization. http://www.who .int/classifications/icd/en/, accessed 30 March 2015.

Xu, Y., Wang, L., He, J., *et al.* for the 2010 China Noncommunicable Disease Surveillance Group. (2013). Prevalence and control of diabetes in Chinese adults. *Journal of the American Medical Association*, 310: 948–959.

RECOMMENDED FOR FURTHER READING

- A classic ecological study that stimulated the development of nutritional epidemiology:
  Armstrong, B. and Doll, R. (1975). Environmental factors and cancer incidence and mortality in different countries, with special reference to dietary practices. *International Journal of Cancer*, 15: 617–631.
- An informative evaluation of CHD control, based on a set of special incidence studies:
  Tunstall-Pedoe, H., Kuulasmaa, K., Mahonen, M., *et al.* for the WHO MONICA. (1999). Contribution of trends in survival and coronary event rates to changes in coronary heart disease mortality: 10-year results from 37 WHO MONICA populations. *Lancet*, 353: 1547–1557.

Healthy research: study designs for public health

Box 4.1 Oranges and lemons

In 1747, James Lind conducted an experiment to test six different cures for scurvy. While at sea, he identified 12 patients with scurvy whose 'cases were as similar as I could find them' and prescribed a different treatment to each pair of patients. After a few days he found that the two patients fortunate enough to have been prescribed oranges and lemons were almost fully

(continued)

Box 4.1 (*continued*)

recovered whilst no improvement was seen in the other 10, who had been subjected to various regimens including seawater, gruel, cider and various elixirs. From this, Lind inferred that inclusion of citrus fruit in the diet of sailors would not only cure, but also prevent scurvy (Lind, 1753). Limes or lime juice thus became a part of the diet on ships, earning British sailors their nickname of 'limeys'.

When we discussed what epidemiologists do in Chapter 1, we touched on some of the different types of study that we use to collect the information we need to answer questions about health. In Chapter 3 we looked at the data systems and *descriptive* studies that provide the 'bread-and-butter' information of public health; in this chapter, we will look at the *analytic* studies that are our main tools for identifying the causes of disease and evaluating health interventions. Unlike descriptive epidemiology, analytic studies involve planned comparisons between people with and without disease, or between people with and without exposures thought to cause disease. They try to answer the questions 'Why do some people develop disease?' and 'How strong is the association between exposure and outcome?'. This group of studies includes the **intervention** and **cohort studies** that you met briefly in Chapter 1, as well as **case–control studies**. Together, descriptive and analytic epidemiology provide information for all stages of health planning, from the identification of problems and their causes to the design, funding and implementation of public health solutions and the evaluation of whether they really work and are cost-effective in practice.

As we discussed in Chapter 1, people talk about many different types of epidemiology, but ultimately almost all epidemiology comes back to the same fundamental principles; the only things that differ are the health condition of interest and the factors that might influence that condition. When we discuss the various study designs in this chapter we will do so mainly in the context of looking for the 'exposures' that cause 'disease'. However, the approaches that we will discuss are generic and are equally applicable to studies:

- of treatment, prognosis and patient outcomes (e.g. survival, improved physical function, or quality of life) in clinical medicine, dentistry, nursing or any of the allied health professions;
- of the effects of our occupation or our socioeconomic and physical environment on health;
- aiming to identify factors that influence health behaviours such as smoking, alcohol consumption, or whether parents choose to have their children vaccinated;

- evaluating programs that attempt to change behaviours in order to improve health outcomes;
- evaluating the effects of changes in health practice or policy . . .

And the list could go on. Likewise, the range of exposures or study factors that might influence health – for good or bad – is incredibly broad. The 'exposure' we are interested in could be an environmental factor such as an infectious agent, radiation, or some chemical, it could be a behavioural factor like smoking or drinking habits, an intrinsic characteristic of the individual such as sex, age, skin colour, or an underlying genetic factor. Furthermore, while most of these are personal exposures that affect us at the individual level, epidemiology is expanding and *social epidemiology* encompasses the additional influences of the broader social environment. At another level, *lifecourse epidemiology* attempts to integrate exposures over an individual's lifetime. While different questions place different demands on the specifics of data collection, all can be addressed via the same suite of research designs, although different designs will be more or less appropriate in different situations.

It is important to bear in mind that the study designs we discuss have their strengths, but they also have limitations, and we will touch briefly on these as we go. We will come back to pick up on some of these limitations in more detail when we talk about *bias* and *confounding* in Chapters 7 and 8 and when we look at how to report, read and interpret the results of epidemiological studies in Chapter 9. But first let us consider if there is an ideal study that would give us a completely unbiased picture of the effect of an exposure on an outcome.

Ignoring ethical and practical issues for a minute, what do you think would be the best way to determine whether factor A caused outcome B?

The ideal study

If a laboratory scientist wanted to see whether something caused a particular effect they would set up an experiment. This would involve creating two identical test systems under identical conditions, adding the particular factor of interest to one of them and then waiting to see what happened. Any differences between the outcomes in the two systems could then be fairly conclusively attributed to the presence of that factor (save for the play of chance, as discussed in Chapter 6). Unfortunately, life is not so straightforward when we are interested in human health.

One way to assess whether a factor affects health outcomes would be to compare the outcomes in a group of people exposed to the factor of interest to those among a group who were not exposed. If the outcomes differ, the challenge is then to decide whether it really was the exposure that caused the difference. For example, if we observe that people who exercise regularly (the 'exposed' group) are less likely to have depression than those who do not exercise ('unexposed'), can we really be sure that physical activity is preventing depression?

What other reasons might explain the lower rate of depression among people who exercise?

In all likelihood, the two groups won't differ only in their exposure status (level of physical activity), but they will also differ with respect to other factors that are correlated with the exposure. For example, people who exercise may have a more healthy diet, drink less alcohol, and be less likely to be overweight or to smoke than those who do not exercise. They will also be less likely to have chronic physical conditions that make exercise difficult. So how can we be sure it is not one of these other factors that led to the different rates of depression in the two groups? To rule out this possibility (a phenomenon known as **confounding** that we will come back to in Chapter 8) we would like our 'exposed' and 'unexposed' groups to be as similar as possible to each other in every respect except the exposure of interest, i.e. they need to be what is sometimes called **exchangeable**. In this situation, any difference in outcomes can only be due to the presence of the exposure in one group. The only way to be 100% sure that a particular exposure caused a specific outcome in a given individual or group of individuals would be to wind back the clock to see whether the same people would have experienced the same outcomes if they had lived lives identical in every way to their real lives, except they were now not exposed to the potential cause. If in this hypothetical situation the individual(s) did not develop the outcome, we could say with some certainty that the exposure did indeed cause the event. This imaginary parallel world which differs only from the real world with regard to the exposure of interest is often described as **counterfactual** (because it is contrary to fact) and, as epidemiologists, much of our effort is directed to designing studies that come as close to this hypothetical ideal as possible.

In practice, the closest that we can come to this is with what is known as a **crossover trial** in which the outcomes among a group of people exposed to the factor of interest are compared to the outcomes in the *same group of people* when they were unexposed. Although people cannot be exposed and unexposed at exactly the same time, as required by the counterfactual model, we hope the periods when they are exposed and unexposed are close enough together that nothing else changes. This type of study is, however, rarely possible in practice, so before we discuss it further we will take a step backwards to consider the epidemiological equivalent of a laboratory experiment – the intervention study or *trial* – more generally.

> In this situation it is also possible that people who are depressed are less likely to exercise. This is often described as called **reverse causality** where it is the depression that causes inactivity rather than the other way around.

Intervention studies or trials

If there is good reason to believe that something might improve health then it is possible to conduct an **intervention study** where the investigator actively intervenes to change something to see what effect this has on disease occurrence. This is what James Lind did in his small, but classic study on scurvy in 1747 (Box 4.1). Such studies include *clinical trials* comparing two (or more) forms of treatment for patients with a disease, as well as *preventive trials*, in which the aim is to intervene to reduce individuals' risk of developing disease in the first place. As with experiments in other sciences, the investigator controls who is exposed and who is not: for example, who is allocated to a new treatment regimen and who receives the old treatment, or who is enrolled in a 'stop smoking' campaign and who is not. Box 4.2 hints at the range of

---

Box 4.2 Some large-scale intervention studies

- In the early 1950s, one of the largest epidemiological studies, and almost certainly the largest formal human 'experiment', was conducted in the USA. This was a field trial of polio vaccine in which over 400,000 school children were assigned to receive either the vaccine or a placebo (inactive) injection. The trial clearly demonstrated both the efficacy and the safety of the vaccine, which was then given to millions of children throughout the world (Francis *et al.*, 1955). This has led to a major drop in the incidence of polio in both industrialised countries and also many developing countries which have now been declared polio-free by WHO.
- The ISIS (International Studies of Infarct Survival) investigators recruited more than 100,000 patients around the world into a series of trials testing treatments to prevent early death after a suspected myocardial infarction (heart attack). These treatments included aspirin and streptokinase which were found to be highly effective in ISIS-2 (ISIS-2 Collaborative Group, 1988).
- In the US Physicians' Health Study (we have already met the British Doctors and the US Nurses' Health studies), 22,000 physicians were randomly allocated to take aspirin, in an attempt to prevent cardiovascular disease, and/or β-carotene, in an attempt to prevent cancer (Hennekens and Eberlein, 1985). After 12 years of follow-up, rates of cancer were very similar in the β-carotene and placebo groups, and, while aspirin was shown to lower the rates of heart attack, so few of these very healthy doctors died that the trial could not determine whether aspirin saved lives from cardiovascular disease.

(continued)

> **Box 4.2** *(continued)*
>
> • A randomised, controlled community trial involving almost 26,000 preschool children was conducted to evaluate the effectiveness of vitamin A supplementation to prevent childhood mortality in Indonesia (Sommer *et al.*, 1986). In 229 villages, children aged 1–5 years were given two doses of vitamin A while children in the 221 control villages were not given vitamin A until after the study. Mortality among children in the control villages was 50% higher than that in the villages given vitamin A.

interventions that can be studied experimentally. In each study the investigators 'intervened' to change something in the hope that this would improve the future health of the participants. The participants in the ISIS trials were already sick (patients who had had a heart attack), and the intervention (treatment) was intended to increase their chances of surviving – aspirin and streptokinase were shown to be very effective. In contrast, the children in the polio vaccine trial were healthy and it was hoped that the vaccine would prevent them from becoming ill. Similarly, it was hoped that vitamin A supplementation would reduce childhood mortality but, in this example, the intervention was given to whole villages rather than individual children.

Randomised controlled trials (RCTs)

The best way to evaluate a new treatment is to identify a group of patients with the same condition and then randomly allocate them to either receive the treatment or to a control group that does not receive the treatment. A preventive trial differs only in that it involves people who are disease-free but thought to be at risk of developing disease. **Random allocation** (also called **randomisation**) of individuals to the study groups is the only way to ensure that all of the groups are as similar as possible (i.e. *exchangeable*) at the start of the study. It is important because if one group were in some way more ill (or less healthy) than the other at the start, this might make this group appear to have worse outcomes, even if the intervention really had no effect (another example of *confounding*). While we can look for and deal with some factors that differ between study groups in our analysis, there may also be other important factors that we either do not know about or cannot measure well. *The real strength of randomisation is that, on average, it will also balance these other unknown or poorly measured factors across the groups.* It is because of this aspect of RCTs – the close similarity of the groups in all respects other than the intervention – that they are generally considered to give the best evidence of all epidemiological studies.

> There is an important distinction between '**random selection**' where we select people at random to be in our study but we do not control whether or not they are exposed (unless it is a RCT), and '**randomisation**' where we do control exposure by randomly allocating people to the exposed and non-exposed groups in an intervention study.

> **Randomisation does not always work.** Equality of the groups at baseline is highly dependent on group size. Even if participants are allocated to groups at random, if the groups are small it is unlikely that all of the factors that could affect the outcome will be evenly distributed across the groups.

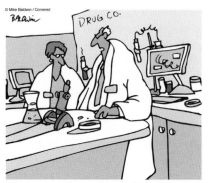

"Do a double-blind test. Give the new drug to rich patients and a placebo to the poor. No sense getting their hopes up. They couldn't afford it even if it works."

Figure 4.1 The design of a randomised controlled trial.

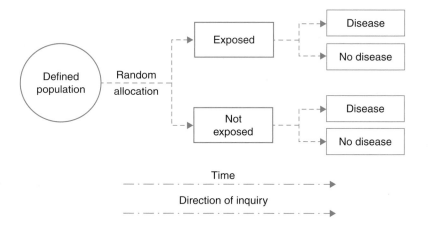

The **control** or comparison group is essential so that outcomes in the treated group can be compared with the outcomes among similar people who have not been treated. Sometimes the patients in the control group receive no treatment but, preferably, they are given a placebo (something that resembles the real treatment but is not active). And if an acceptable standard treatment is available the control group must be given this – it would be unethical to withhold it – and this is compared with the new experimental treatment. Figure 4.1 shows the design features of a simple RCT.

Ideally, both the trial investigators and the participants should be unaware of whether the participant is in the active intervention or placebo group, creating a 'double-blind' or 'masked' study. If only the patient is unaware of their allocation, it is a single-blind study. Blinding is important because knowledge of the treatment might affect both the participant's response and an observer's measurement of outcome. If the participant knows they have been given the new treatment they might feel better simply because they believe it will do them some good (a **placebo effect**) and, likewise, an observer might be more likely to report signs of improvement in someone if they know they received the active treatment. In some situations (e.g. comparing medical treatment with surgery) there may be no feasible way of blinding patients and study personnel to the differences in treatments. Minimising measurement bias in this situation may be best accomplished by bringing in an independent 'blinded' observer whose only involvement is to assess the outcome measure. Blinding of outcome measurements obviously becomes more crucial as the measurement becomes more subjective. When the outcome is objective and less dependent on interpretation, as in a biochemical parameter or death, blinding is less important.

Apart from participants and trial investigators, there are many others (e.g. health care providers, data collectors, outcome assessors, data analysts) involved in the conduct of a trial who can introduce bias through their knowledge of treatment allocation. For this reason there is a growing tendency to abandon the terms single- and double-blind in favour of a transparent reporting of the blinding status of each group involved in the trial.

The other crucial feature of an RCT is good follow-up. It is important to know what has happened to all of the participants in the study because if many people are 'lost to follow-up' such that we don't know if they experienced the health outcome of interest, then the results of the study may be biased. This is a form of *selection bias* and we will discuss it further in Chapter 7.

Crossover trials

The trials we discussed above and shown in Figure 4.1 are what are known as **parallel group trials**, in which individuals are randomly allocated to one of the two groups, which are then followed in parallel. In a **crossover** design, the participants serve as their own controls and thus, as described above, we come closer to achieving the counterfactual ideal where we observe the same people twice under conditions that are identical except with respect to the exposure of interest. For example, in a simple two-period crossover study to assess the efficacy of an intervention we would randomly assign each participant to either the intervention or the control (I or C) for a specified period of time and then the alternative for a similar period of time. Thus, approximately half of the participants would receive the interventions in the sequence I–C and the other half in the sequence C–I, reducing the impact of any factors that might change between the first and second period.

One of the biggest advantages of this design is that it removes much of the variability that is inherent when we compare different groups of people and that can never be completely eliminated by randomisation. In particular, it ensures the groups are truly exchangeable from a genetic perspective and in terms of other factors that do not change over time. As a result, crossover trials can produce statistically and clinically valid results with fewer participants than would be required with a parallel design. However, it is important to remember that while we are comparing the participants to themselves, time has moved on and so it is impossible to be completely sure that nothing else has changed. As a minimum it is likely that the weather will have changed and this may affect various aspects of behaviour. Also, not all interventions are suitable for assessment in this way. We can only use crossover trials to assess the effects of factors that have a rapid effect and where the effect wanes rapidly when the exposure is removed. If the effects of the intervention during the first period are likely to carry over into the second period then this design is clearly inappropriate, as is also true for assessing long-term benefits and harms.

n-of-1 trials

A variant of the crossover trial is the single patient trial, often called an **_n_-of-1 trial**. Here, an individual patient receives the experimental and control treatments in random order on multiple occasions, with specific outcomes being monitored throughout the trial period. Ideally both the patient and the treating doctor are blinded to the treatment being received and the trial usually ends when it becomes clear that there are (or are not) important differences between the treatments. As with the crossover trial, a strength of these studies is that by comparing the same person on and off treatment we come closer to achieving true exchangeability. Again, we have the problem that we are comparing the active treatment and control at different points in time but, by giving them multiple times in a random order, we hope to minimise any bias that might result from this. Although the results of n-of-1 trials are not generalisable to the same extent as those of typical RCTs, they do provide a good guide to individual clinical decisions.

> "**_n_**" is often used to denote the sample size in a study; an n-of-1 study is thus a study where $n = 1$ person.

Cluster randomised controlled trials

For many public health and practice/policy interventions it is impossible to intervene at an individual level so the answer is a *cluster randomised controlled trial* where groups or clusters of people are randomised together. An example is a study that evaluated a 'Comprehensive Health Assessment Program' (CHAP) to enhance interaction between adults with intellectual disability, their carers and general practitioners. To avoid *contamination* whereby participants randomised to the control arm were inadvertently exposed to the intervention via their housemates, individuals living in the same house or who saw the same GP were randomised together as a 'cluster'. In this study the clusters were of very different sizes so they were matched to another cluster of similar size and characteristics and one of each pair was allocated at random to the intervention and one to the control arm. The study showed increased detection of health problems and increased screening rates in the intervention group (Lennox *et al.*, 2007).

Community trials

Community trials are cluster trials in which the intervention is implemented at the community level. They are generally conducted when it would be impossible to offer (or evaluate) the intervention at the individual level. An example is the studies of water fluoridation and dental health conducted in various countries. When investigators wanted to study the effects of adding fluoride to the water supply on dental health it was clearly impossible to add fluoride to some people's water and not to others', so whole towns were allocated to receive fluoride in their water or not. The controlled trial of water fluoridation which gave the most striking results was carried out in the towns of Newburgh and Kingston in New York State, USA. After 10 years of fluoridation, the DMF (decayed, missing or filled teeth) score for Newburgh children aged 6–16 was 50% lower than that for children in the unfluoridated town of Kingston (Ast and Schlesinger, 1956). The assumption underlying this result was that, apart from the water, there was no other major difference between the towns that could explain the effect (i.e., there was no confounding). (Note that, although this and other studies clearly showed the benefits of low levels of fluoride on dental health, continuing controversy about the possible adverse effects of fluoride on other organs in the body, particularly the bones, has meant that universal fluoridation of water supplies has not occurred.) Because only two towns were included in this study, in practice it is little different from a non-randomised comparison (see below). Other cluster designs involve larger numbers of groups, so that the random allocation of multiple groups to intervention or no intervention gives more of the benefits of randomisation in terms of balancing out other factors across the groups (e.g. the vitamin A study, Box 4.2).

Non-randomised designs

The fact that a study is described as a trial or clinical trial does not necessarily mean that it is a randomised controlled trial. While RCTs remain the gold standard for initial evaluation of new clinical and public health interventions, the effectiveness of these interventions in practice can often only be determined from 'before and after' type comparisons in whole communities or populations. You will see examples of this throughout the book, and particularly when we discuss prevention in Chapter 14 and screening in Chapter 15. Probably the most common non-randomised design in the health setting is one that uses 'historical controls' where health outcomes following the introduction of a new treatment or preventive measure are compared to the outcomes experienced by the same population before the change in practice (also sometimes called a pre–post study). For example, in many countries, mortality rates from road traffic accidents fell dramatically after the introduction of legislation requiring drivers to wear seat belts. Similarly, patient survival rates might be compared before and after the introduction of a new surgical technique.

> **More pre–post study designs:** if measures are obtained at multiple time points before and after the intervention this may be described as an *interrupted time series*, while if multiple groups are involved it is sometimes called a *multiple baseline* design.

What is the major problem with a pre–post study of this type?

The main problem with this design is that it assumes that the only (or most important) thing that has changed is the new legislation or the type of surgery, and that may not be the case. Another variation on the cluster trial is the 'stepped wedge' design, where the intervention is sequentially introduced to all of the study groups. We will not discuss these designs further here, but see Sanson-Fisher *et al.* (2014) for further information.

Observational studies

Although the ideal way to study whether something is causally related to the occurrence of disease is through an experiment or intervention study, this would often be unethical (you cannot deliberately expose someone to something thought to be harmful) or impractical. As a result, epidemiology is rarely an experimental science. Most of the time an epidemiologist will just go out (after a lot of thoughtful planning) and measure the rate of occurrence of a disease or other health outcome, or will compare patterns of exposure and disease to identify particular exposures or risk factors associated with that disease. This is purely an *observational* role: the researcher does not intervene in any way. They leave nature to take its course, and record what happens, or what happened in the past. These are commonly described as *observational studies*.

Cohort studies

The next best thing to a randomised trial is a **cohort study** (sometimes described as a *prospective* or *longitudinal* study). Like a trial, we follow people forwards (prospectively) over time to see what happens to them and, again like a trial, the cohort might be a group of initially healthy people whom we follow to measure the occurrence of disease or a group of patients whom we follow to study their disease outcomes, i.e. their prognosis. Figure 4.2 shows the design of a typical cohort study.

> In Ancient Rome, a **cohort** was one of 10 divisions of a Roman military legion. It comprised young men of similar age from one region. In service its members were often injured or killed and they were not replaced. The cohort was then disbanded when the term of enlistment was over.

Figure 4.2 The design of a cohort study (adapted from Beaglehole *et al.*, *Basic Epidemiology*, 1993, with permission).

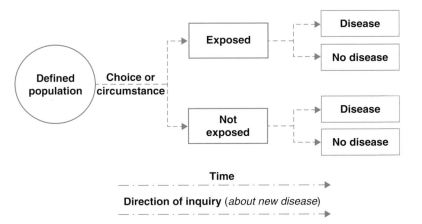

Compare Figures 4.1 and 4.2. How does a cohort study differ from an RCT?

The fundamental difference is that in a trial the investigator controls who is exposed to the factor of interest and who is not, ideally by assigning people to the different exposure groups at random, whereas in a cohort study participants are living the lives they have chosen, and the researcher has to discover and measure the exposures they have chosen for themselves.

Why is this a problem?

The challenge with this type of study is to disentangle the effects of the exposure that we are interested in from those of other personal characteristics or behaviours that are correlated with that exposure. In a randomised trial these other factors should be distributed evenly across the study groups, but this is unlikely to be the case in a cohort study where people who choose to smoke, for example, may also be more likely to drink alcohol or coffee, or to exercise less and so on, i.e. the groups are intrinsically less similar (exchangeable) than the arms of a randomised trial.

One classic example of a cohort study is the Framingham Heart Study (Dawber, 1980). It was started in 1948 at a time when heart disease had become the USA's number one killer, and the principal aim was to identify biological and environmental factors that might be contributing to the rapid rise in cardiovascular death and disability. The epidemiological approach was quite novel at the time and it was designed to discover how and why those who developed heart disease differed from those who escaped it. The town of Framingham, Massachusetts was selected by the US Public Health Service as the study site, and 5209 healthy men and women between 30 and 60 years of age were enrolled and followed over time to see who developed disease and/or died. Framingham was appealing because it had a stable population and a single medical facility, suggesting that it would be relatively easy to carry out the follow-up. The study was expanded in 1971 when 5124 children (and their spouses) of the original cohort were recruited for a second study, the Offspring Study.

Before Framingham, the notion that scientists could identify, and individuals could modify, *risk factors* (a term coined by the authors of the study) tied to heart disease, stroke and other diseases was not part of standard medical practice. With over 50 years of data collected from residents of Framingham (and the publication of more than 1000 scientific papers), the Framingham researchers have identified major risk factors associated with heart disease, stroke and other diseases and created a revolution in preventive medicine. The study identified several risk factors associated with increased risks of heart disease including cigarette smoking (1960), high cholesterol levels and high blood pressure (1967), obesity and low levels of physical activity (1967). These are so commonly accepted today, both by health professionals and by the public, that it is difficult to imagine a time when we did not know their importance.

The Framingham Study is quite small by modern standards: the European Investigation into Cancer (EPIC) established in 1995 includes more than half a million individuals from 10 European countries (Bingham and Riboli, 2004) and the Million Women Study was initiated in the UK in 1996 (The Million Women Study Collaborative Group, 1999). The Framingham study therefore needed particularly long follow-up to accumulate enough endpoints to give robust results. A crucial trade-off is that the smaller size and the setting permitted regular detailed physical examination and other 'hands-on' investigations such as the recording of electrocardiograms, giving a rich array of high-quality exposure data that cannot be gathered on a very large scale.

Of all the observational designs, cohort studies generally provide the best information concerning the causes of disease and the most direct and intuitive measurements of the risk of developing disease. The participants must be free of the outcome of interest at the start of the follow-up, which makes it easier to be confident that the exposure preceded the outcome (i.e. to rule out the possibility of *reverse causality*). However, if there is a long pre-clinical phase before a disease is diagnosed, as may be the case for many types of cancer, the apparent exposure–disease sequence can still be wrong, and for this reason many cohort studies do not count cases of disease that occur in the first few years of follow-up. The other advantage of collecting exposure data before people develop disease is that measurement of exposure is not biased by knowledge of outcome status, i.e. it avoids **recall bias**. It is important to note, however, that if a cohort study has a very long follow-up period and exposure data were only collected at baseline then people may have changed their behaviours over the intervening years. For example, smokers may quit smoking or meat eaters may become vegetarian and it is also an unfortunate fact that many of us will gain weight as we get older. Depending on when the critical period of exposure occurs, this may mean that people are wrongly classified with regard to their exposure (e.g. past smokers as current smokers). This is a problem of **misclassification**. Many cohort studies, for example the US Nurses' Health Studies (see Box 4.3), avoid this problem by re-contacting study participants every few years to collect updated exposure data. (We will discuss misclassification and recall bias further in Chapter 7.)

Selection of participants is an issue at two points of a cohort study: who is selected into the cohort at the start of the study, and who is lost from the cohort during follow-up. Who is selected into a cohort can influence the generalisability (see Chapter 9) of its findings because they may apply only to the sorts of people who agreed to take part. However, as in a trial, if many people are 'lost to follow-up' and we don't know their outcome status, then the results of the study may be biased (see Chapter 7).

Cohort studies are by nature very time-consuming and expensive. However, the benefit:cost ratio of a well-run cohort study can be high given that many

Box 4.3 Some other notable cohort studies

- The British Doctors Study cohort was established in 1951 and followed for more than 50 years, although most of the original 40,701 participants are now dead. It has been of enormous value, particularly in relation to identifying the manifold health consequences of smoking. This is despite the fact that, compared with studies today, only limited exposure data were collected on a very short postal questionnaire mailed to the doctors at 10-year intervals since 1951 (Doll and Hill, 1964; Doll *et al.*, 2004).
- The US Nurses' Health Study (www.nurseshealthstudy.org/) started in 1976 with 121,964 female nurses aged 30–55, and 5 years of funding. Since then, its focus has widened enormously from the oral contraceptive–breast cancer links for which it was first funded (Stampfer *et al.*, 1988) to cover many exposures (including diet) and a multitude of outcomes. It has now accumulated more than 30 years of follow-up and is still going strong. It is very expensive to run, but the scientific and public health yield has been exceptional. The Nurses' Health Study II began in 1989 with 117,000 nurses aged 25–42 (Rockhill *et al.*, 1998) and in 2010 they started the Nurses' Health Study III, an entirely web-based study targeting nurses aged 20–46 years in the USA and Canada.
- ALSPAC (The Avon Longitudinal Study of Parents and Children, www.bristol.ac.uk/alspac/) was started in 1990 to determine ways in which an individual's genes combine with environmental pressures to influence health and development. Comprehensive data have been collected on over 10,000 children and their parents, from early pregnancy until the present. Because the study is based in one geographical area of the UK, linkage to medical and educational records is relatively simple, and hands-on assessments of children and parents using local facilities allows good quality control (Golding *et al.*, 2001).

different outcomes can often be assessed in a single study. For example, over the last decade, the Nurses' Health Study (see Box 4.3) has been the basis for between 30 and 50 publications every year covering exposures as diverse as air pollution and shift work. A limitation is that studies established to look at many different health conditions have to collect information on a very wide range of potential risk factors and so they often cannot collect much detail on these. In principle, a long-term cohort study also has the potential to deliver the public health knowledge of most value, by showing the full array of harms and benefits associated with a given exposure. The British Doctors Study is an outstanding example of this with regard to cigarette smoking because while it, like other studies, shows that there is a potential benefit of cigarette smoking with regard to Parkinson's disease, it also clearly shows the overwhelming negative effects of smoking on many other health conditions which put control of smoking at the top of the public health agenda.

Historical cohort studies

It is sometimes possible to avoid the long follow-up period common to many cohort studies by establishing a retrospective or **historical cohort**. This requires good records of past exposure for a group of people who can then be traced to determine their current health. Until fairly recently, such studies have been most common in industry or the military where good personnel records exist, but they have also been used to study the development of disease in relation to characteristics at birth (e.g. weight and length at birth) because this information can often be obtained retrospectively from birth records. In the absence of close follow-up – the usual situation – they are generally limited to studying mortality or cancer outcomes, given the lack of universal records for other non-fatal endpoints. Some interesting and useful variations include the use of college alumni records in the USA to study the benefits of physical activity as a young adult (Paffenbarger *et al.*, 1986) and the Boyd Orr Study based on detailed dietary records collected from over 4000 British children in the 1930s (Frankel *et al.*, 1998).

Now, with the increasing opportunities for linking other health records, studies of this type are becoming more common and increasingly sophisticated.

Record linkage

As health data are increasingly stored in electronic formats, the scope for what is often described as **record** or **data linkage** is increasing exponentially. Traditionally, investigators performing cohort studies have enhanced their follow-up by 'linking' the identities of their individual cohort members to centralised cancer and death registries in order to find out about new outcomes. Some studies now also rely on record linkage to provide information about potential exposures and other health outcomes without having to rely on people's memories for accurate information. For example, the '45 and Up' cohort study is following more than 250,000 men and women aged 45 and older in the Australian state of New South Wales to look at outcomes ranging from health conditions to use of health services and quality of life. Although the investigators asked participants to complete a standard health questionnaire when they joined the study, they also asked them for consent to access their health records to allow linkage to a wide range of health databases (45 and Up Study Collaborators, 2008). In addition to cancer and death records, in Australia it is now possible to link to data from the national Pharmaceutical (drug prescriptions) and Medicare (tests and procedures) Benefits Schedules and, in some states including New South Wales, it is also possible to link data for hospital admissions, emergency presentations, midwives, notifications and mental health records. Obtaining information from these databases has the benefit of being less reliant on individual memory, and also broadens the scope of questions that the study can answer by capturing richer exposure (e.g. detailed medication use) and outcome data (e.g. health service use). Western Australia and, notably, the Scandinavian countries also have excellent systems for linking data from a wide range of health and other databases. The matches are made in a variety of ways, including using a common personal identification number as in many Scandinavian countries and the USA (social security number), or through probabilistic approaches based on a variety of personal identifiers (e.g. name, date of birth and address).

There are also studies based entirely on record linkage that are essentially the modern version of the historical cohort study. They are effectively cohort studies in which both exposure and outcome information come from electronic records. Until recently, they had been used mostly to link health services and outcomes. For example, by linking data from hospital morbidity and death records, Western Australian researchers were able to show that the presence of other medical conditions (comorbidity), but not advancing age, predicted repeat admission to hospital for adverse drug reactions (Zhang *et al.*, 2009). This information will allow better identification and monitoring of those most at risk of an adverse reaction. However, increasing computerisation of medical information is now making more conventional aetiological research possible by this means. As an example, Swedish investigators were able to use the Swedish Inpatient Register to identify a cohort of 29,187 patients hospitalised for type-1 diabetes between 1965 and 1999. They then 'linked' these names to the Swedish Cancer, Total Population, Migration and Death Registers. This told them who had been diagnosed with cancer, the type of cancer and date of diagnosis, and also who had migrated or died from some other cause and so was no longer at risk of being diagnosed with cancer in Sweden. They calculated standardised incidence ratios (SIRs) for the cohort compared with the general population and found that diabetes was associated with significantly increased risks of cancer of the stomach (SIR = 2.3), cervix (SIR = 1.6) and uterus (SIR = 2.7) (Zendehdel *et al.*, 2003).

Research based on linking health (and other) records does, however, raise a number of issues regarding confidentiality, and current privacy concerns and legislation in some countries have the potential to limit this avenue of research. The 45 and Up Study, like many other large cohort studies, asks all participants to consent to allow the investigators access to their health records when they join the study. However, it is often not possible or practical for researchers to contact all of the individuals concerned to get their permission to access their data. To solve this problem, pure record-linkage studies are conducted where the data custodians perform the linkage centrally and remove all identifying information

> **Data linkage** can also provide an opportunity for real-time monitoring of drug safety by linking prescribing data to other health databases, although currently few systems exist to do this in practice (e.g. www.mini-sentinel.org in the USA).

such as names, addresses and dates of birth before giving the linked data to the investigators for analysis. Even so, many health data custodians are still prevented by law from releasing even such 'de-identified' information without individual consent. Much effort is being expended to enable a constructive resolution of the tensions between maximising individual autonomy (by protecting against inappropriate access to personal health data) and ensuring that the public good delivered by health research is not compromised (Lawlor and Stone, 2001).

Prognostic or survival studies

As we mentioned above, cohort studies can also be used to see what happens to patients after they are diagnosed with a condition. In this case, the cohort would comprise patients with the condition of interest who were at the same point in the course of their illness, e.g. at diagnosis (often called an *inception cohort*) or after completion of their primary treatment. They would then be followed for a fixed period or until they experience the outcome of interest, which might be death, recurrence of the disease, or quality of life at a given time point. Studies of this type can identify patient characteristics that predict their outcome, for example demographic factors such as age, gender or socio-economic status; disease-specific factors such as the severity or stage of disease at diagnosis; genetic factors and the presence of other health conditions (known as comorbidities). Such characteristics are called *prognostic factors*; they may not actually *cause* the outcome, but must be associated with it strongly enough to *predict* it. Event rates tend to be high, so prognostic studies can usually be much smaller than cohort studies of risk factors.

They are also increasingly being used to investigate potentially modifiable factors such as diet and lifestyle that might affect patient outcomes. For example, an Australian study found that among women diagnosed with ovarian cancer, a cancer that typically has a high mortality rate, those who ate more vegetables survived for longer than those who ate fewer vegetables (Nagle *et al.*, 2003).

Case–cohort studies

In many cohort studies, all participants provide a wide range of information at the time of recruitment, including answers to detailed dietary questionnaires and blood and urine samples. Because of the large numbers and cost, these resources – especially the biological samples – are often not analysed in detail at the time but are stored for future use. It is then possible to use this information more efficiently by conducting either a **nested case–control study** (see below) or **case–cohort study**. In the case–cohort design a subset of participants is selected from the full cohort at baseline. Detailed exposure information can then be retrieved for this subcohort and *all* of the people in the full cohort who develop the disease of interest. This maintains the major advantage of a cohort study in that the exposure data were originally collected before the development of disease, while the much smaller scale reduces effort and cost. It also has the advantage that the subcohort can be used for comparison with multiple different case groups. However the case–cohort study requires a somewhat more sophisticated data analysis than the traditional cohort and nested case–control studies.

Nested case–control studies

As the name suggests, this is essentially a case-control study (we will discuss these further below) that is 'nested' within an existing cohort study. As in the case-cohort study, the cases are all cohort members who developed the disease of interest, but this time each case is matched to one or more non-cases selected at random from cohort members of the same gender and age *who were disease-free at the time the case was diagnosed*. As in the case-cohort study, it is assumed that the information obtained from these 'controls' represents the exposure experience of all of the non-cases in the cohort when the case was diagnosed. Nested case-control studies are simpler to analyse than case–cohort studies, but have the disadvantage that they require a separate control group to be selected for each case group.

Case–control studies

One drawback of most cohort studies is that they can only be used to study conditions that are relatively common (obviously the very large cohorts we mention above are exceptions). If we were interested in a very rare disease we would need to follow a large number of people for a very long time to identify many people with the disease. In this situation an alternative study design called a **case–control study** is often used. You have already seen how a nested case-control study can be conducted within a cohort study and the underlying principle is the same for a traditional case-control study, except that here the underlying cohort study does not actually exist. For a case-control study we first identify a notional cohort which might include everyone in a particular geographic region or even a whole country. Depending on how common the disease is, we would then try to recruit everyone in that population who develops the disease of interest or a representative sample of these people (cases), but we recruit only a small fraction of the people without the condition. These 'controls' are selected at random and, as in the nested example above, we hope that they will be representative of the wider target population. We then ask both the cases and controls about their previous exposures. Thus, instead of identifying people on the basis of their exposure status and waiting to see who develops disease, we effectively start from the end and work backwards (see Figure 4.3). For instance, if we wanted to know whether smoking was associated with lung cancer, we could compare people with lung cancer and controls without lung cancer to see if they differed in their smoking habits, exactly as Doll and Hill did back in 1950 (see Chapter 1).

> **Controls:** Some authors prefer to call the comparison group the 'reference' group and so will describe the study as a *case–reference* or *case–referent* study.

Figure 4.3 The design of a case–control study (adapted from Beaglehole *et al., Basic Epidemiology,* 1993, with permission).

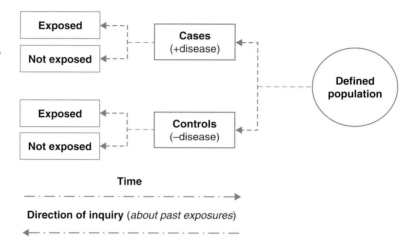

A classic case–control study was conducted in Germany in 1961 (Mellin and Katzenstein, 1962). The mothers of children born with unusual limb malformations (cases) were compared with mothers of normal children (controls) with respect to their exposures in pregnancy. Forty-one of the 46 case mothers (89%), but none of 300 control mothers, had taken thalidomide early in their pregnancy. This strongly suggested that thalidomide use early in pregnancy could be responsible for the birth defects. (It should be noted that this study was stimulated by data from an earlier case series.)

Modern case–control studies tend to be much larger; for example, the Australian Ovarian Cancer Study included more than 1500 women with ovarian cancer and a similar number of control women. It has confirmed the strong inverse associations with pregnancy and oral contraceptive pill use and risk of ovarian cancer such that women who have several children and/or who use the 'pill' for several years have about half the risk of nulliparous women or non-pill users (Jordan *et al.,* 2008). A wide range of other possible causes have also been examined within this one study and this is one of the major appeals of the case–control design. Because the focus is usually on a single health outcome, participants can be asked very detailed questions about relevant exposures; this is often not possible in a cohort study, which will usually collect less detailed information on a much wider range of exposures in order to study multiple different outcomes. Participants can be asked about many different exposures, allowing multiple factors to be evaluated within the same study. Box 4.4 gives further examples of case–control studies which have led to direct health benefits.

Ideally, case–control studies include only **incident** (new) **cases** of disease as they arise. However, some studies, especially those of very rare diseases, also include **prevalent cases**. This makes them rather like cross-sectional studies

Box 4.4 Case–control studies

- Phenacetin was introduced as an analgesic in 1887 and used extensively until it was suggested that it might be associated with kidney disease. A case-control study involving 554 adults with newly diagnosed kidney disease and 516 matched control subjects selected randomly from the same geographical area was conducted in the USA to investigate this (Sandler *et al.*, 1989). After allowing for the effects of other types of analgesic, the risk of kidney disease was five times higher among daily users of phenacetin and three times higher among daily users of paracetamol (acetaminophen, a metabolite of phenacetin) than it was among infrequent users of these drugs. There was little association between aspirin use and kidney disease. Results from this study and others confirmed the risks of phenacetin, which was withdrawn from the market.

- In a case-control study conducted in Tasmania, Australia, the parents of 58 children who had died from SIDS (sudden infant death syndrome) and of 120 control children were interviewed about the sleeping practices of their children. Children who were placed face-down had a fourfold higher risk of SIDS than children placed in other positions. This risk was increased even further if the child slept in a heated room, was tightly wrapped or had recently been ill (Ponsonby *et al.*, 1993). The results of this study and others have led to campaigns aimed at persuading parents to place babies on their backs to sleep in order to reduce rates of SIDS.

(see below), with the possible problem of determining a clear time sequence for the exposure–disease relation. (That is, a factor may appear to be related to disease risk simply because it extends the duration of disease.)

Case–control studies offer a number of advantages over follow-up studies. They are generally quicker and more economical to perform (but are still not a trivial undertaking) and, as we noted above, are good for studying rare outcomes. Case–control studies are also good for evaluating many different exposures, all of which can be asked about at the one interview as we noted above.

The central problem in the design of a case–control study is selection of the control group. *Controls should represent the population from which the cases have come such that their exposure prevalence is very similar to that of the whole population. In practice this means that appropriately selected controls should have been identified as cases if they had developed the condition of interest*. If the cases form a population-based series (e.g. if all cases from a defined geographical region are included), then the control group should be representative of that population. **Population controls** can be selected in a number of ways, including from population registers or comprehensive electoral rolls, or by sampling residential telephone numbers at random (random-digit dialling), although this latter approach is losing its appeal as the use of mobile phones increases and fewer households have landlines. Another traditional approach to identify controls, that also works when the case group does not originate from a clearly defined geographical population, was to recruit a control from the local neighbourhood of the case, for example someone living in a nearby street. This approach is time-consuming and expensive, but it is effective and is still used in many lower- and middle-income countries. A variant that has been used where telephone numbers are assigned by residential area involves matching telephone numbers with random selection of the last few digits. In the ovarian cancer study described above, the controls were selected from the national electoral roll because enrolment to vote is compulsory in Australia; this strategy would not work in countries where voting is not mandatory because electoral rolls would be much less complete. In the UK, selection of controls from the patient lists of the general practitioners (GPs) who referred the cases is often a viable alternative because most of the population is registered with a GP.

Whilst population or neighbourhood controls are ideal, practical reasons mean that **hospital controls** are still used, although not as frequently as in the past. This is usually accomplished by selecting controls from patients admitted to the same hospitals as the cases for conditions other than the one being studied (see e.g. Box 4.5). Although this is a much more efficient and economical process than selecting population controls, it is associated with an obvious major drawback. The controls are themselves ill and thus different from most healthy people in the source population from which the cases come. Indeed, their distribution of risk factors (especially personal habits such as smoking, excessive alcohol consumption, etc.) may well resemble that of the cases rather more than that of the source population, leading to biased results. However, thoughtful use of such designs can still provide good public health information and Box 4.6 shows an example of such a study that has been used for post-marketing drug surveillance (sometimes called pharmacoepidemiology).

An important issue related to the selection of both cases and controls is that they must be chosen *independently of their exposure status*. In a case–control study of oral contraceptive pill use and deep vein thrombosis, for example, whether or not a woman is using the pill should not affect her chances of being recruited as either a case or a control. Knowledge of the exposure status of individuals could lead to bias in participant recruitment called **selection bias**. Another type of bias that can occur within case–control studies arises when the

In high-income countries it is getting increasingly hard to persuade healthy people to participate in research and response rates among controls are only ~50%. Refusal to take part is often related to health and lifestyle factors so controls who do take part may not represent the wider population, introducing the potential for **selection bias** (see Chapter 7).

Bias with hospital controls: When data from 47 studies were combined, the cohort and population-based case–control studies suggested that obesity increased the risk of ovarian cancer, but the opposite was seen in the hospital-based studies (Collaborative Group, 2012), perhaps because the hospital controls were, on average, heavier than other women.

Box 4.5 Hospital controls: the pros and cons

Tertiary referral clinics may attract patients from an unpredictably wide variety of geographical and social origins. If cases are identified through these clinics it can then be a major challenge to find a group of disease-free controls who represent the same geographical and social backgrounds as the cases. For example, a colonoscopy is needed to diagnose adenoma (polyps) of the large bowel, so a colonoscopy clinic is an ideal place to identify cases for a study. If controls are selected at random from the local population there is no guarantee that they would have been picked up as cases if they had adenoma – they might have gone to a different facility. Similarly, we would miss all of those people from outside the local population who would, nonetheless, have travelled to that clinic for treatment. An alternative then is to select controls from among other patients attending the clinic who have a colonoscopy but do *not* have bowel polyps. This solution ensures that the controls will represent the geographical and social distribution of the cases, but it is important to be aware that it might also introduce other biases. For example, if there are characteristics, such as a family history of bowel cancer, that make someone more likely to be referred for colonoscopy, then these characteristics will be over-represented in the control group. This example serves to emphasise that epidemiological studies will rarely be perfect – the important thing is to do the best that is possible in a given situation and then to consider the likely effects of any bias (see Chapter 7).

information collected from the cases and controls is not comparable. This can occur if an interviewer elicits or interprets exposure information differently when the disease status of the individual is known (**interviewer bias**) or because people with disease recall their exposures or experiences more precisely than or otherwise differently from those without disease (**recall bias**). We will revisit bias and other forms of inaccuracy in data collection and discuss the potential impact of these types of error on the results of a study in Chapter 7.

There are several modern variants of the case–control study design. Two, the *nested case–control* and *case–cohort* studies which we discussed under cohort studies above, are essentially a different way of analysing cohort data. A third is the *case–crossover* study.

Case–crossover studies

The **case–crossover** design is especially suited to identifying the effects of transient exposures on the risk of an acute-onset disease. Instead of recruiting

Box 4.6 Using hospital controls for pharmacoepidemiology

Hospital controls have been used very successfully to identify harmful side effects of prescription medications in a number of settings. One of the earliest and longest-running pharmacoepidemiology research projects using this design is the Case–Control Surveillance Study run by the Slone Epidemiology Center at Boston University (www.bu.edu/slone/research/studies/ccs/), which ran for over 30 years until 2009, with over 100 publications. Its purpose was to systematically evaluate the relationship of medications to the incidence of certain illnesses and to screen for unsuspected drug–disease associations. Since 1983, the main focus of the study was on various cancers. Patients newly diagnosed with a cancer of interest and who resided in the study area (cases) were recruited from a network of hospitals. Patients from the same area with acute conditions such as appendicitis or chronic conditions such as kidney stones or gallstones diagnosed within the past year were recruited as controls. All patients were interviewed to collect a wide range of information about lifestyle and a medical and lifetime medication history. Altogether over 80,000 patients were interviewed, including over 25,000 with cancer, leading to multiple publications such as a recent report providing reassurance that use of statins to lower cholesterol levels does not increase an individual's risk of cancer (Coogan *et al.*, 2007).

a separate group of controls, each case is also their own control and their exposure in a defined period prior to the onset of disease is compared with their normal exposure frequency. This innovative design eliminates many of the problems inherent in studies that compare different groups of people and comes closest to the theoretical (but unattainable) ideal, which would be to study an exposed population and then wind back the clock and study exactly the same population again when they had not been exposed.

In the seminal case–crossover study, Maclure (1991) examined the influence of a variety of possible precipitating factors, including sexual activity, on the occurrence of myocardial infarction (MI, or heart attack). He classified cases as exposed if they had been sexually active in the two hours before their MI and then compared this with their usual frequency of sexual activity over a one-year period. He hypothesised that, if sexual activity were a risk factor for MI, then more cases would have been sexually active shortly before their MI than would be expected from their usual frequency. After interviewing 300 cases he estimated that sexual activity increased an individual's risk of MI more than twofold.

Cross-sectional studies

In Chapter 3 we discussed the surveys that many countries conduct on a fairly regular basis to measure the prevalence of different health behaviours and health conditions in their population (for example, the NHANES studies in the USA – see Box 3.3) and we showed how these can be used to look at the relationships between behaviour and health. The key factor of these surveys is that they aim to select people in such a way that they are representative of the whole population so that information collected from the study sample can be generalised directly to the whole population. Studies like this, that set out to look at the relation between an exposure and a health outcome in a 'cross-section' of the population, are called **cross-sectional studies**. As you will see, they have a number of drawbacks compared to other study designs but, because of their relatively simple design (summarised in Figure 4.4), they are often conducted as an early investigation into the possible causes of ill health.

> Longitudinal **cross-sectional studies** recruit a *different* sample of people for each survey and then study changes in the population prevalence of disease or potential risk factors for disease over time. They therefore differ from cohort studies which follow the *same* people over time.

For example, a group of researchers in India wanted to estimate the prevalence of and risk factors for suicidal behaviour in young people in Goa. They invited all 16–24-year-olds from two rural and two urban communities to be interviewed for the study and achieved a participation rate of almost 95%. Overall, 3.9% of the 3662 participants reported some form of suicidal behaviour in the previous three months. Multiple factors were associated with suicidal behaviours, including female gender, not attending school and experience of sexual and recent physical abuse (Pillai *et al.*, 2009).

This cross-sectional study was both *descriptive* in that it defined the scope of the problem (how common is suicidal behaviour) and *analytic* in that it also identified (and measured the prevalence of) a number of possible causal factors. All these data, descriptive and analytic, can be valuable for planning health and social system responses. The key feature of the study is that the young people were not recruited because they had (or had not) exhibited suicidal behaviour or because of their particular histories but solely because they were assumed to be typical of young people in Goa.

Cross-sectional studies such as this may be conducted to gather information about any aspects of health and lifestyle and, as in the example above, participants should be recruited without knowledge of either their exposure

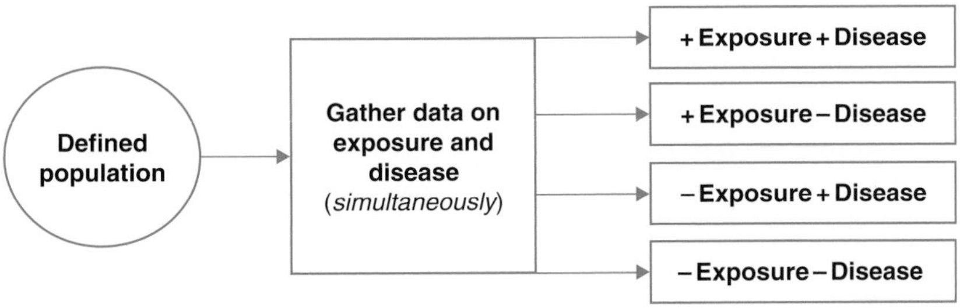

Figure 4.4 The design of a cross-sectional study.

status (presence or absence of the exposures of interest) or their disease status (presence or absence of the diseases of interest). This is essential to avoid **selection bias** – something that we will come back to discuss in Chapter 7. Information on the outcome (suicidal behaviour in the example above) and the exposures (gender, education, previous abuse, etc.) is usually obtained at the same time. For this reason, it can be difficult to identify which came first – the exposure or the outcome (disease). This problem of **reverse causality** is a major issue in cross-sectional studies – does A really cause B, or might the reverse be true such that B causes A? Does being overweight reduce your chance of developing lung cancer, or does the development of lung cancer make you lose weight so you are less likely to be overweight? Cross-sectional studies can, however, be particularly useful for examining exposures that do not change over time (for example, personal characteristics such as gender and blood group) or that occurred many years previously.

Another important thing to note about cross-sectional studies is that they evaluate *prevalent* cases of disease – those that are already present in the population at the time of the survey. As we discussed in Chapter 2, prevalence is a function both of the incidence and of the duration of a disease. People who have a disease for longer are more likely to be ill at the time of a cross-sectional study than those who are sick for a shorter time. An association between exposure and prevalence of disease can thus reflect not only a link between exposure and the occurrence of new disease, but also a link between exposure and factors that affect survival or persistence of a diseased state.

Thinking back to the study of suicidal behaviour described above:

Is there any problem with the time-directionality of the link between (i) gender, (ii) lifetime sexual abuse, and (iii) not attending school and suicidal behaviour?

Are the young adults studied likely to be typical of all young adults in Goa, India?

In this study it is unlikely that there is a problem with the time-directionality of the relationships with gender (as this does not change over time) or sexual abuse, as this was recorded over the lifetime and thus is very likely to have preceded the suicidal behaviour, which was recorded for the last 3 months only. The relation with not attending school is, however, more problematic, as it is possible that young adults with suicidal tendencies may be more likely to miss school than the other way around. In relation to the **generalisability** of the findings, the results from the study were based on young people from two rural and two urban communities. The participation rates were very high (much higher than would be achieved in most studies in developed countries now), but before generalising the results beyond the study areas we would

Box 4.7 Diagnostic studies

A study to evaluate the accuracy of a diagnostic test can be thought of as a special type of cross-sectional study in which the data are collected from diagnostic test results or physical examination rather than from interviews or questionnaires. Typically, individuals with symptoms of disease are selected randomly or consecutively from a clinic or hospital to undergo the test of interest (the *index test*). Then, independently (and blinded to the results of the index test), the same individuals undergo the best test available to diagnose the disease (the *reference test* or '*gold standard*'). The results of the two tests are then compared and the accuracy of the index test (its **sensitivity** and **specificity**) can be determined (we will discuss the mechanisms of this in Chapter 15). As in all cross-sectional studies, it is important that the people selected are representative of the target population – in this case the patients in a particular setting – in whom the test would be used in real life.

need to know that the selected communities were representative of all communities in Goa (or India).

Another type of cross-sectional study that you may come across in the clinical setting is one conducted to evaluate the performance of a diagnostic or screening test or to validate a self-reported diagnosis in a research setting: see Box 4.7.

Ecological studies

We mentioned these in Chapter 3 because they compare exposure and disease in populations rather than individuals, but they do attempt to link exposures and outcomes and so could equally well be considered analytic studies. After observing a correlation between rates of infection with the gastric bacterium *Helicobacter pylori* and gastric cancer mortality in China as shown in Figure 3.8, the investigators conducted a similar study comparing infection rates and gastric cancer incidence in 17 centres from the USA, Japan and Europe. From this they were able to estimate that mortality from gastric cancer in a population where everyone was infected with *H. pylori* would be about six times that in a population with no infection (i.e. the relative risk for the relation between *H. pyori* and death from gastric cancer was ~6; The Eurogast Study Group, 1993). It is, however, always important to remember that communities that differ in one way – for example, the prevalence of *H. pylori* infection – probably differ in other ways too. It is therefore impossible to be sure that the factor of interest is what is actually driving their different health outcomes, in this case mortality from gastric cancer.

Ecological studies can be particularly useful for evaluating changes in health policy. As an example, investigators looked at the relation between cancer survival and measures of health expenditure and adherence to standard care across Europe to serve as a baseline against which they could assess the efficacy of new European initiatives to improve cancer survival. They found a positive relation between total national expenditure on health and 5-year age-adjusted relative all-cancer survival rates, such that individuals from countries that spent more on health had better survival (Gatta *et al.*, 2013).

A word about ethics

We touched on this under record linkage above, but it would be remiss of us to end this discussion of study design without some consideration of the subject of research ethics. Before conducting any research on humans (or animals), most developed countries require the study protocol to be approved by a Human Research Ethics Committee (or Institutional Review Board, IRB, in the USA). This is to ensure that the rights of participants are fully protected in any research study – that they are fully informed of any risks and benefits associated with participation and that the benefits of the research (to the individual or, more often, to society) sufficiently outweigh the potential risks.

Current guidelines for medical research ethics can be traced back more than 50 years to the end of World War II (see Box 4.8), although some of the core concepts go back as far as Hippocrates. They are based on four moral principles:

Beneficience – do good;
Non-maleficence – do no harm, in practice this has to be balanced against the principle of beneficience – the potential benefits should outweigh the possible risks;
Respect for autonomy – respect the rights of the individual; this includes the right to privacy and the right to make informed decisions and thus the need for study participants to give their 'informed consent' before enrolling in a study;
Justice – equity, impartiality and fairness.

These principles were first codified in a practical form after the Nuremburg trials of German medical researchers at the end of World War II. The resulting 'Nuremburg Code', which underpins all subsequent codes of health research ethics, is shown in Box 4.9. However, this Code was largely ignored at the time and formal statements outlining requirements for the ethical conduct of research did not start to appear until the late 1970s after continuing reports of disquieting ethical practices such as the Tuskagee Study (see Box 4.8) and

Box 4.8 Notable events and documents in the development of modern ethical guidelines

<1945 German scientists accused of experimenting on human subjects in Nazi concentration camps during World War II; also the beginnings of large-scale research in the USA using groups such as orphans, the mentally handicapped and prisoners.

1947 The **Nuremberg Code**
A list of 10 principles of medical and research ethics developed from the Nuremberg trials in Germany at the end of World War II (see Box 4.9), but largely ignored at the time.

1964 The **Declaration of Helsinki**
Developed at a meeting of the World Medical Association in Helsinki as a statement of ethical principles to provide guidance to physicians and other participants in medical research (www.wma.net/en/20activities/10ethics/10helsinki/).

1966 **Beecher's Report**
Publication of a report citing 22 post-war studies that were ethically flawed despite being conducted at prestigious institutions and published in top journals (Beecher, 1966).

1972 Publication of a report from the **Tuskegee syphilis study** in the USA (1932–1972)
This caused outrage when it became clear that study participants had been misled and deprived of treatment (www.cdc.gov/tuskegee/timeline.htm).

1978 **The Belmont Report**
A document developed by what was then the United States Department of Health, Education, and Welfare entitled 'Ethical Principles and Guidelines for the Protection of Human Subjects of Research' (archive.org/details/belmontreporteth00unit).

the Willowbrook Study (1963–1966) where children in an institution for the mentally handicapped were deliberately infected with hepatitis virus to study the course of the infection.

Tensions continue today between the need to protect the rights of individuals (often via strict privacy laws) and the public need for good-quality information to improve health. Rigid application of privacy laws can make some forms of epidemiological research almost impossible. As discussed above, this is especially true for record linkage studies where it may be impractical or

Box 4.9 The Nuremberg code, 1947

1. The voluntary consent of the human subject is absolutely essential. This means that the person involved should have legal capacity to give consent; should be so situated as to be able to exercise free power of choice, without the intervention of any element of force, fraud, deceit, duress, over-reaching, or other ulterior form of constraint or coercion; and should have sufficient knowledge and comprehension of the elements of the subject matter involved as to enable him to make an understanding and enlightened decision. This latter element requires that before the acceptance of an affirmative decision by the experimental subject there should be made known to him the nature, duration, and purpose of the experiment; the method and means by which it is to be conducted; all inconveniences and hazards reasonable to be expected; and the effects upon his health or person which may possibly come from his participation in the experiment.

   The duty and responsibility for ascertaining the quality of the consent rests upon each individual who initiates, directs or engages in the experiment. It is a personal duty and responsibility which may not be delegated to another with impunity.

2. The experiment should be such as to yield fruitful results for the good of society, unprocurable by other methods or means of study, and not random and unnecessary in nature.

3. The experiment should be so designed and based on the results of animal experimentation and a knowledge of the natural history of the disease or other problem under study, that the anticipated results will justify the performance of the experiment.

4. The experiment should be so conducted as to avoid all unnecessary physical and mental suffering and injury.

5. No experiment should be conducted where there is an a priori reason to believe that death or disabling injury will occur; except, perhaps, in those experiments where the experimental physicians also serve as subjects.

6. The degree of risk to be taken should never exceed that determined by the humanitarian importance of the problem to be solved by the experiment.

7. Proper preparations should be made and adequate facilities provided to protect the experimental subject against even remote possibilities of injury, disability, or death.

(continued)

Box 4.9 (*continued*)

8. The experiment should be conducted only by scientifically qualified persons. The highest degree of skill and care should be required through all stages of the experiment of those who conduct or engage in the experiment.

9. During the course of the experiment the human subject should be at liberty to bring the experiment to an end if he has reached the physical or mental state where continuation of the experiment seems to him to be impossible.

10. During the course of the experiment the scientist in charge must be prepared to terminate the experiment at any stage, if he has probable cause to believe, in the exercise of the good faith, superior skill and careful judgment required of him that a continuation of the experiment is likely to result in injury, disability, or death to the experimental subject.

From *Trials of War Criminals before the Nuremberg Military Tribunals under Control Council Law No. 10, Vol. 2, pp. 181–182*. Washington, DC: US Government Printing Office, 1949.

> **Research ethics:** the US National Institute of Health (NIH) has a free online ethics tutorial (https://phrp.nihtraining.com). Although primarily for NIH grant holders, most of the content is generic and applicable to all.

even impossible to obtain consent from individuals to access their information. The costs of complying with human research guidelines can also drive up the costs of research with studies often needing to obtain approval from, and report back to multiple different ethics committees. However, as the historical examples cited above emphasise, we cannot ignore the need for real autonomy in relation to participation in research.

Summary

Before starting any study it is important to be very clear about the question you want to answer because different study designs can answer different questions (we will come back to this issue in Chapter 9). Randomised trials like those described at the start of the chapter are theoretically the ideal way to look for associations between exposure and a disease or health outcome because they are the best way to ensure that the groups we are comparing are exchangeable in all ways except the exposure of interest. They do, however, have to be designed, run and reported rigorously to realise this potential in terms of providing convincing evidence about causality.

Unfortunately, they are often inappropriate (for ethical reasons), not feasible or unaffordable. Furthermore, because they are often conducted in highly selected groups of volunteers, it can be challenging to generalise their findings and we will come back to this problem in Chapter 11. The non-experimental study designs, particularly cohort and case–control studies, are therefore of central importance in public health and, as you will see when we discuss causation in Chapter 10, other designs such as ecological studies can also provide valuable information. The fundamental importance of descriptive studies in monitoring the health of a population and for identifying emerging health problems should already be apparent, and you will see further examples of their essential role in evaluating the effects of population interventions when we discuss prevention in Chapter 14 and screening in Chapter 15. Each design thus has an important role to play and different designs will be more or less appropriate in different situations. It is also essential to recognise the strengths and limitations of each; we will consider these further in Chapters 7 and 8 when we look at some of the sources of bias in epidemiological studies.

Table 4.1 Comparing the strengths and weaknesses of different study designs.

	Ecological	Cross-sectional	Case–control	Cohort	Randomised controlled trial	Nested case–control
Investigation of rare disease or outcome						
Investigation of a rare exposure						
Testing multiple effects of an exposure						
Study of multiple exposures						
Establishing temporality[a]						
Give a direct measure of incidence						
Explore exposures from early life						
Explore exposures which change over time						
Time required						
Costs						
Ethical Problems						

[a] i.e. that the exposure came before the outcome.

Questions

1. Complete Table 4.1 to show the relative strengths and limitations of the main study designs, scoring each one on a scale from 1 = Poor (e.g. not good to investigate a rare disease or very expensive) to 5 = Excellent (e.g. very good to investigate a rare exposure or very quick to do).
2. Possible designs for the Salk polio vaccine trial described in Box 4.2 might include giving the vaccine to second-grade children in one region and comparing the rate of polio in this group to the rate in:
   - Second-grade children in another region where the vaccine was not used
   - Second-grade children the year before the vaccine was introduced
   - First- and third-grade children in the same region and year as the vaccinated group.

   What are the strengths and limitations of each of these designs and which do you think would be preferable and why?
3. Look back to the section about ethics and identify which of the four fundamental moral principles apply to each of the 10 statements in the Nuremburg Code.

Additional questions

REFERENCES

References

45 and Up Study Collaborators. (2008). Cohort profile: the 45 and Up Study. *International Journal of Epidemiology*, 37: 941–947. See also http://www.45andup.org.au

Ast, D. B. and Schlesinger, E. R. (1956). The conclusion of a ten-year study of water fluoridation. *American Journal of Public Health*, 46: 265–271.

Beaglehole, R., Bonita, R. and Kjellström, T. (1993). *Basic Epidemiology*. Geneva: World Health Organization.

Beecher, H. K. (1966). Ethics and clinical research. *New England Journal of Medicine*: 274: 1354–1360. Reprinted in *Bulletin of the World Health Organization*, 2001, 79: 367–372.

Bingham, S. and Riboli, E. (2004). Diet and cancer – the European Prospective Investigation into Cancer and Nutrition. *Nature Reviews Cancer*, 4: 206–215. See also http://epic.iarc.fr

Collaborative Group on Epidemiological Studies of Ovarian Cancer. (2012). Ovarian cancer and body size: individual participant meta-analysis including 25,157 women with ovarian cancer from 47 epidemiological studies. *PLoS Medicine*, 9(4): e1001200.

Coogan, P. F., Rosenberg, L. and Strom, B. L. (2007). Statin use and the risk of 10 cancers. *Epidemiology*, 18: 213–219.

Dawber, T. R. (1980). *The Framingham Study. The Epidemiology of Atherosclerotic Disease*. Harvard, MA: Harvard University Press. See also http://www.framinghamheartstudy.org

Doll, R. and Hill, A. B. (1964). Mortality in relation to smoking: ten years' observations of British doctors. *British Medical Journal*, 1: 1399–1410, 1460–1467.

Doll, R., Peto, R., Boreham, J. and Sutherland, I. (2004). Mortality in relation to smoking: 50 years' observations on male British doctors. *British Medical Journal*, 328: 1519.

Francis Jr, T., Korns, R. F., Voight, R. B., *et al.* (1955). An evaluation of the 1954 poliomyelitis vaccine trials: summary report. *American Journal of Public Health*, 45: 1–65.

Frankel, S., Gunnell, D. J., Peters, T. J., Maynard, M. and Davey Smith, G. (1998). Childhood energy intake and adult mortality from cancer: the Boyd Orr cohort study. *British Medical Journal*, 316: 499–504.

Gatta, G., Trama, A. and Capocaccia, R. (2013). Variations in cancer survival and patterns of care across Europe: roles of wealth and health-care organization. *Journal of the National Cancer Institute Monographs*, 46: 79–87.

Golding, J., Pembrey, M., Jones, R. and the ALSPAC Study Team. (2001). ALSPAC – the Avon Longitudinal Study of Parents and Children. I. Study methodology. *Paediatric and Perinatal Epidemiology*, 15: 74–87.

Hennekens, C. H. and Eberlein, K. (1985). A randomised trial of aspirin and β-carotene among U.S. physicians. *Preventive Medicine*, 14: 165–168.

ISIS-2 Collaborative Group. (1988). Randomised trial of intravenous streptokinase, oral aspirin, both or neither among 17187 cases of suspected acute myocardial infarction: ISIS-2. *Lancet*, 2: 349–360.

Jordan, S. J., Green, A. C., Whiteman, D. C., *et al.* (2008). Serous ovarian, fallopian tube and primary peritoneal cancers: a comparative epidemiological analysis. *International Journal of Cancer*, 122: 1598–1603. See also http://www.aocstudy.org/

Lawlor, D. A. and Stone, T. (2001). Public health and data protection: an inevitable collision or potential for a meeting of minds? *International Journal of Epidemiology*, 30: 1221–1225.

Lind, J. (1753). *A Treatise of the Scurvy. A Bicentenary Volume.* Edinburgh: Sands, Murray and Cochran.

Lennox, N., Bain, C., Rey-Conde, T., *et al.* (2007). Effects of a comprehensive health assessment programme for Australian adults with intellectual disability: a cluster randomized trial. *International Journal of Epidemiology*, 36: 139–146.

Maclure, M. (1991). The case–crossover design: a method for studying transient effects on the risk of acute events. *American Journal of Epidemiology*, 133: 144–153.

Mellin, G. W. and Katzenstein, M. (1962). The saga of thalidomide: neuropathy to embryopathy, with case reports of congenital anomalies. *New England Journal of Medicine*, 267: 1184–1193, 1238–1244.

Nagle, C. M., Purdie, D. M., Webb, P. M., *et al.* (2003). Dietary influences on survival following ovarian cancer. *International Journal of Cancer*, 106: 264–269.

Paffenbarger Jr, R. S., Hyde, R. T., Wing, A. L. and Hsieh, C. C. (1986). Physical activity, all-cause mortality, and longevity of college alumni. *New England Journal of Medicine*, 314: 605–613.

Pillai, A., Andrews, T. and Patel, V. (2009). Violence, psychological distress and the risk of suicidal behaviour in young people in India. *International Journal of Epidemiology*, 38: 459–469.

Ponsonby, A. L., Dwyer, T., Gibbons, L. E., Cochrane, J. A. and Wang, Y-G. (1993). Factors potentiating the risk of sudden death syndrome associated with the prone position. *New England Journal of Medicine*, 329: 377–382.

Rockhill, B., Willett, W. C., Hunter, D. J., *et al.* (1998). Physical activity and breast cancer risk in a cohort of young women. *Journal of the National Cancer Institute*, 90: 1155–1160.

Sandler, D. P., Smith, J. C., Weinberg, C. R., *et al.* (1989). Analgesic use and chronic renal disease. *New England Journal of Medicine*, 320: 1238–1243.

Sanson-Fisher, R. W., D'Este, C. A., Carey, M. L., Noble, N. and Paul, C. L. (2014). Evaluation of systems-oriented public health interventions: alternative research designs. *Annual Reviews in Public Health*, 35: 9–27.

Sommer, A., Tarwotjo, I., Djunaedi, E., *et al.* (1986). Impact of vitamin A supplementation on childhood mortality. A randomised controlled community trial. *The Lancet*, 327: 1169–1173.

Stampfer, M. J., Willett, W. C., Colditz, G. A., Speizer, F. E. and Hennekens, C. H. (1988). A prospective study of past use of oral contraceptive agents and risk of cardiovascular diseases. *New England Journal of Medicine*, 319: 1313–1317.

The Eurogast Study Group. (1993). An international association between *Helicobacter pylori* infection and gastric cancer. *Lancet*, 341: 1359–1362.

The Million Women Study Collaborative Group. (1999). The Million Women Study: design and characteristics of the study population. *Breast Cancer Research*, 1: 73–80. See also http://www.millionwomenstudy.org

Zendehdel, K., Nyrén O., Östenson, C.-G., *et al.* (2003). Cancer incidence in patients with type 1 diabetes: a population-based cohort study in Sweden. *Journal of the National Cancer Institute*, 95: 1797–1800.

Zhang, M., Holman, C. D. J., Price, S. D., *et al.* (2009). Comorbidity and repeat admission to hospital for adverse drug reactions in older adults: retrospective cohort study. *British Medical Journal*, 338: 155–158.

RECOMMENDED FOR FURTHER READING

- 10-and 50-year follow-up reports from the British Doctors Study:
  Doll, R. and Hill, A. B. (1964). Mortality in relation to smoking: ten years' observations of British doctors. *British Medical Journal*, 1: 1399–1410, 1460–1467.

Doll, R., Peto, R., Boreham, J. and Sutherland, I. (2004). Mortality in relation to smoking: 50 years' observations on male British doctors. *British Medical Journal*, 328: 1519.

• Report from the seminal polio vaccine trial:

Francis Jr, T., Korns, R. F., Voight, R. B., *et al.* (1955). An evaluation of the 1954 poliomyelitis vaccine trials: summary report. *American Journal of Public Health*, 45: 1–65.

• A review of alternative study designs for public health research:

Sanson-Fisher, R. W., D'Este, C. A., Carey, M. L., Noble, N. and Paul, C. L. (2014). Evaluation of systems-oriented public health interventions: alternative research designs. *Annual Reviews in Public Health*, 35: 9–27.

Why? Linking exposure and disease

Description Chapters 2–3	Association Chapter 5: Measures of association	Alternative explanations Chapters 6–8	Integration & interpretation Chapters 9–11	Practical applications Chapters 12–15

Box 5.1 Who does all the housework?

His view: Australian men do **three times more** housework today than they
did 40 years ago . . .

Her view: Australian men spend 5 minutes a day on laundry now
compared to 1.6 minutes 40 years ago – an **extra 3½ minutes a day** . . .

(Maushart, 2003.)

As you saw in Chapter 1, one of the main uses of epidemiology is to identify the causes of disease, and this is of fundamental importance in all areas of public health – if we can work out what is causing ill health then we can work to prevent it. In Chapter 2 we looked at the ways in which we can measure the occurrence of disease and touched on some ways in which we can compare different populations. However, while measuring the occurrence of a disease in a population can tell us about the health of that population, it does not directly shed much light on the underlying causes of the disease. To identify the aspects of people or their environment (exposures) that might lead to the onset of disease, we need to *compare* disease occurrence in groups with and without the exposures of interest. In Chapter 4 we looked at some of the study designs that we can use to do this; now we will look more closely at the measures we use to quantify the associations between 'exposures', or potential causes of disease, and the disease itself. By quantifying the association between an exposure and disease we can start to make judgements as to whether the exposure might actually cause the disease (we will discuss causality in more detail in Chapter 10). If we believe that it is causing disease, we can then identify the importance of that exposure in terms of its overall effect on the health of a community.

In this chapter we will look at the ways in which we calculate, use and interpret these 'measures of association', so-called because they describe the association between an exposure and a health outcome. An understanding of these measures will help you to interpret reports regarding the causes of ill health and the effects of particular exposures or interventions on the burden of illness in a community. Note that, while we will discuss the measures in the context of an 'exposure' and 'disease', they can be used to assess the association between any measure of health status and any potential 'cause'.

You will often see **measures of association** referred to as 'effect' measures. Although this name suggests a cause and effect relationship (i.e. that the exposure *causes* the outcome to occur), we are actually only measuring *associations* and these may or may not be causal (see Chapter 10).

Exchangeability:
Throughout this chapter we assume that the groups we are comparing are comparable in all ways except with regard to the exposure of interest – i.e. that they are *exchangeable*. We will discuss some of the issues we face when they are not exchangeable when we discuss *bias* and *confounding* in Chapters 7 and 8.

Looking for associations

We all know that smoking is a cause of lung cancer, but might it also increase the risk of stroke? To answer this question we could compare the incidence of stroke in a group of women who smoke with that in a group of non-smokers.

Table 5.1 displays data from a cohort study in which the investigators followed a large group of women for several years (person-years of observation). They classified the women as never smokers, ex-smokers and current smokers, recorded how many women had a stroke during the follow-up period and calculated the **incidence rate** of stroke in each group.

Table 5.1 Stroke incidence rates in female nurses, by smoking category.

Smoking category	No. of cases of stroke	Person-years of observation	Incidence rate per 100,000 person-years
Never smoked	70	395,594	17.7
Ex-smoker	65	232,712	27.9
Current smoker	139	280,141	49.6
Total	274	908,447	95.2

(Colditz *et al.*, 1988)

How many **times as likely** was
  (i) a current smoker to have a stroke than a never smoker, and
  (ii) an ex-smoker to have a stroke than a never smoker?

Compared with non-smokers, how many **extra** strokes were there per 100,000 person-years in
  (i) ex-smokers, and
  (ii) current smokers?

The answers to these questions reflect the two main ways in which we can compare smokers and non-smokers. First, ex-smokers were *1.6 times* (27.9 ÷ 17.7) and current smokers were *2.8 times* (49.6 ÷ 17.7) as likely to have a stroke as never smokers during the follow-up period. An alternative way to look at the data would be to say that, all other things being equal, if the smokers had never smoked we would have expected them to have the same rate of stroke as the never smokers, i.e. 17.7/100,000 person-years. This means that, compared with never smokers, there were an *extra 10.2 strokes per 100,000 person-years* (27.9 – 17.7) in ex-smokers and an *extra 31.9 strokes per 100,000 person-years* (49.6 – 17.7) in current smokers.

  What we calculated above were, first, the **rate ratio** and, second, the **rate difference** for the association between smoking and stroke. These measures give us two different ways of quantifying the relation between an exposure and a disease. The rate ratio tells us how many times higher the rate of disease is in one group than in another group (e.g. current smokers are almost three times as likely to have a stroke as never smokers). This gives an indication of the *strength* of the association and can help us to decide whether smoking could be a cause of stroke. The rate difference tells us how much extra disease occurred in one group compared with another group (e.g. there were an extra 32 strokes per 100,000 person-years among current smokers compared with non-smokers). If we believe that smoking is a cause of stroke then this extra disease can be attributed to the fact that the women are smokers and, theoretically, it would not have occurred if they had never smoked. This information gives some sense of the potential value of a preventive intervention, in this case a programme aimed at stopping women from taking up smoking. (Of course, if such an intervention were successful it would reduce the incidence of many diseases, not just stroke.)

It is important to remember that ratio and difference measures give us very different perspectives on a given situation. Look back to Box 5.1 at the start of the chapter. Men would probably prefer to look at the **ratio** or **relative** measure: they do three times more housework now than 40 years ago. In contrast, women would focus on the **difference** or **absolute** measure: men may do three times more laundry now than 40 years ago, but they still do an average of only 5 minutes (3.5 minutes extra) per day.

Ratio measures (relative risk)

The cholera was therefore *14 times as fatal* at this period amongst persons having the impure water of the Southwark and Vauxhall Company, as amongst those having the purer water from Thames Ditton (Snow, 1855) (from Box 1.7).

People who ate cold chicken at the youth camp were *almost four times as likely* to become ill as people who did not eat cold chicken (from Table 1.2).

Ratio or relative measures tell us how many times as likely it is that someone who is exposed to something will develop a certain disease or experience a particular health outcome compared (or *relative*) to someone who is not exposed. *They do not tell us anything about the actual amount of disease occurring in either group.* They provide information about the *strength* of the association between the exposure and the outcome and, as you will see in Chapter 10, a strong association is more suggestive that the exposure is actually causing the outcome. In the example above, the rate ratio for stroke and current smoking was 2.8. This is a fairly strong association and would add weight to an argument that smoking was actually causing strokes, although it is not as compelling as the much stronger relation between smoking and lung cancer, for which the rate ratio for current smoking is somewhere between 10 and 15.

As the example shows, ratio measures are very easy to calculate – you simply divide the frequency of disease (or of any health outcome) in the group that is exposed to the factor of interest by the frequency in the group that is not exposed to it. This can be done using either of the measures of disease incidence that you met in Chapter 2. If you divide two incidence rates you end up with a **rate ratio** (as for the stroke example above); if you divide two incidence proportions or risks then it is a **risk ratio**. It is also possible to divide two measures of prevalence to calculate a **prevalence ratio**. Note that you must always divide two measures of the same type – you cannot usefully divide an incidence rate by an incidence proportion.

Rate ratios

As you saw above, a rate ratio is calculated by simply dividing the incidence rate of disease in a group of people exposed to the factor of interest (often denoted by a subscript 'e') by the incidence rate in a group of people who are not exposed to the same factor (denoted by a subscript 'o'):

$$\text{Rate Ratio} = \frac{\text{Incidence Rate in exposed}}{\text{Incidence Rate in unexposed}} = \frac{IR_e}{IR_o} \quad (5.1)$$

This factor could be a potential cause of disease, it could be a characteristic of a person, such as their age or where they live, or it could be something that influences behaviour. Equally, it could be a preventive measure or, in the clinical context, a drug or other treatment that we hope will reduce the incidence of disease.

Risk ratios

Similarly, the risk ratio (also called the **relative risk**) is calculated by dividing the incidence proportion or risk of disease in an exposed group by the incidence proportion in an unexposed group:

$$\text{Risk Ratio} = \frac{\text{Incidence Proportion in exposed}}{\text{Incidence Proportion in unexposed}} = \frac{IP_e}{IP_o} \quad (5.2)$$

For example, In Chapter 2 we considered a randomised trial to evaluate whether taking aspirin would reduce the risk of blood clots in people with infective endocarditis. Look back at Table 2.3 on page 47 and calculate the risk ratio for the association between aspirin and blood clots.

In this trial, the risk ratio was 28.3% ÷ 20.0% = 1.4; those who took aspirin were 1.4 times as likely to develop blood clots as those who did not take aspirin. A risk ratio of 1.0 would mean that there was no difference between the groups, so those taking aspirin were 40% *more likely* to develop blood clots than those not taking aspirin (in the context of clinical epidemiology this may be described as the **relative risk increase** or RRI). If aspirin had reduced the risk of blood clots then we would have expected to see a risk ratio of less than 1.0. Clearly this intervention did not work the way the investigators had hoped it would.

Table 5.2 The results of a study evaluating the effects of calling patients on influenza immunisation rates.

| | Outcome | | |
Exposure	Immunised	Not immunised	% immunised
Received a call	328	332	50
No call	288	370	44
Total	616	702	47

(Hull *et al.*, 2002)

This approach can be used much more widely than in the search for the causes of disease. As an example, a trial was conducted in three general practices in the UK to find out whether telephoning patients to offer them an appointment for immunisation against influenza would increase immunisation uptake rates (Hull *et al.*, 2002). In this study, attending for immunisation was the outcome of interest and receiving a telephone call was the exposure. A total of 1318 patients aged 65–74 years were randomly assigned to two groups. Patients in one group ($n = 660$) received a telephone call from the receptionist at their general practice inviting them to make an appointment for immunisation (the intervention or exposed group). Patients in the other group ($n = 658$) were not called (the control or unexposed group). The investigators then waited to see who turned up for immunisation. They found that 328 of the patients who received a phone call attended, as did 288 of those who did not receive a call.

The easiest way to look at these data is in the form of a '2 × 2 table'. These tables are usually set out so that the two columns show the numbers of people with and without the outcome of interest while the rows show the numbers in the exposed and unexposed groups (Table 5.2).

What percentage of patients attended for immunisation (the incidence proportion) in each of the two groups?

How many times as likely were patients to attend if they had received a personal call to make an appointment than if they had not been telephoned?

In the intervention group 50% of patients were immunised, compared with 44% of those in the control group (despite the intervention the immunisation rates were still below the government target of 60%). This means that patients who received an invitation were 1.14 times (50% ÷ 44%) as likely to attend for immunisation. This measure is still a relative risk because it has the same structure – the incidence proportion (or risk) of a particular health outcome in one group is divided by the incidence proportion in a second group. In this case the word 'risk' seems less appropriate, but the term relative risk is still regularly used.

Prevalence ratios

As you saw when we discussed prevalence surveys in Chapter 3 and cross-sectional studies in the previous chapter, it is also possible to use measures of prevalence instead of incidence to compare the burden of disease in two groups and in this situation you end up with a prevalence ratio:

$$\text{Prevalence Ratio} \quad = \quad \frac{\text{Prevalence in exposed}}{\text{Prevalence in unexposed}} \quad = \quad \frac{P_e}{P_o} \qquad (5.3)$$

As we discussed in Chapter 2, measures of prevalence are harder to interpret than measures of incidence and for this reason prevalence ratios are used much less frequently than rate and risk ratios.

A note about relative risks

We noted above that the term **relative risk** is synonymous with **risk ratio**. In practice, it is also commonly used to describe a **rate ratio**, because both the rate ratio and the risk ratio compare the amount of disease in one group *relative* to that in another. If a disease is rare (incidence proportion or risk less than 1%), then the rate ratio and risk ratio will be almost identical; if it is not so rare then the risk ratio will be closer to 1.0 than the rate ratio although, in practice, there is little difference as long as the incidence proportion is less than about 10%. The three terms rate ratio, risk ratio and relative risk are also commonly and conveniently abbreviated as RR. When we use the term relative risk it will refer to both the rate ratio and the risk ratio.

It is also worth noting that, although relative risks are also used in the context of clinical trials, several other related measures are also used in the field of clinical epidemiology (Box 5.2).

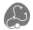

> ## Box 5.2 Relative risks in clinical epidemiology
>
> In 1998, Botti *et al.* reported a trial of the use of pressure bandages for patients undergoing coronary angiography. Some of their results are shown in Table 5.3.
>
> The relative risk of bleeding among those given pressure bandages compared with those without is $3.5 \div 6.7 = 0.52$. This tells us that those
>
> (*continued*)

Box 5.2 (*continued*)

given pressure bandages were about half as likely to develop bleeding as those who were not given bandages. The results of treatment trials are sometimes also reported as a **relative risk reduction (RRR)**. This is the amount by which the treatment has reduced the relative risk and it is calculated by subtracting the relative risk from 1.0. It may then be expressed as a percentage by multiplying by 100:

$$\text{Relative risk reduction}\,(\text{RRR}) = 1.0 - \text{RR}$$
So the RRR $= 1.0 - 0.52 = 0.48$ or 48%. $\qquad(5.4)$

Alternatively, it can be calculated directly from the incidence proportion or, using the terminology of clinical epidemiology (see Box 2.4 on page 43), the *event rates* among the experimental (EER) and control (CER) groups:

$$\text{Relative risk reduction (RRR)} = (\text{CER} - \text{EER}) \div \text{CER}$$
In this case the RRR $= (6.7 - 3.5) \div 6.7 = 0.48$. $\qquad(5.5)$

In other words, use of the pressure bandages has reduced the risk of bleeding among patients undergoing coronary angiography by 48%. Obviously, the greater the RRR the better the intervention.

For studies with a positive association (RR > 1.0) the results are turned around to give what is logically called the **relative risk increase (RRI)**. In the aspirin study discussed previously, aspirin increased the risk of bleeding by 40% (RR = 1.4).

Note that you will see associations described in this way in all fields of epidemiology, e.g. 'The risk of disease was 20% lower among those who exercised more'. It is a simple, informative mode of description that just happens to have been given a separate name in the area of clinical epidemiology.

Table 5.3 Use of pressure bandages in patients undergoing coronary angiography.

Pressure bandages	Total	Number with bleeding	Incidence proportion or event rate
Yes	519	18	$\text{EER}^a = 3.5\%$
No	556	37	$\text{CER}^b = 6.7\%$
Total	1075	55	5.0%

[a] EER, experimental event rate or incidence proportion in the treatment group
[b] CER, control event rate or incidence proportion in the comparison group
(Botti *et al.*, 1998.)

Standardised incidence and mortality ratios

We discussed these measures in Chapter 2 (pages 56–58) because of the links between direct and indirect standardisation, but they also deserve a mention here because they compare the rate of disease (or death) in two populations and so, in effect, are also measures of relative risk.

Difference measures (attributable risk)

As we noted above, the relative risk tells us nothing about the actual amount of disease that is occurring. If the incidence proportions or risks of disease in exposed and unexposed groups were 0.5% and 0.1%, respectively, the relative risk would be 5.0. Similarly, if the risks were 50% and 10%, the relative risk would also be 5.0. The major difference between these two situations is obvious: the actual amount of disease that is occurring is vastly different – in fact, in the second example it is 100 times greater. This vital public health information cannot be obtained from the relative risk.

The approach to measuring the excess amount of disease occurring among those exposed to a potential risk factor is just as intuitive, and the measures are as simple to calculate as the relative risk. As you saw in the smoking and stroke example at the start of the chapter, we can calculate the *extra* amount of disease that is occurring in the exposed group by simply subtracting the incidence in the unexposed group (IR_o, CI_o or **background risk**) from the incidence in the exposed group (IR_e, CI_e). This can again be done using either of the measures of disease incidence (incidence rate or incidence proportion) that you met in Chapter 2. If you are subtracting two incidence rates (as in the stroke example) you end up with a **rate difference**, whereas if you are subtracting two incidence proportions or risks (as in the immunisation example) you have a **risk difference**. These measures are also sometimes described as the **excess rate** and **excess risk** as they measure the extra disease that only occurs in the presence of the exposure. If we think that it is reasonable to assume that the excess disease can be *attributed* to the exposure, i.e. the exposure is causing the disease, then both of these measures can also be described as the **attributable risk** (in the same way that *relative risk* is used to describe both rate ratios and risk ratios).

Rate differences

Consider the smoking and stroke example again (Table 5.1). Compared with never smokers, there were an extra 10.2 strokes (27.9 – 17.7) per 100,000 person-years in ex-smokers and an extra 31.9 strokes (49.6 – 17.7) per 100,000 person-years in current smokers. These differences are illustrated

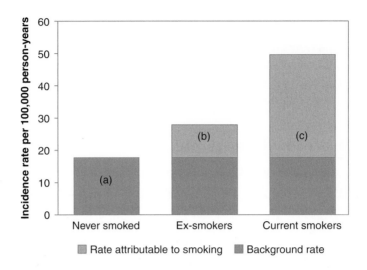

in Figure 5.1. The left-hand bar (a) shows the incidence rate of stroke in non-smokers. This is often called the *reference* or **background rate** because it reflects the natural occurrence of the disease in an unexposed population. We expect this to operate on all members of the population regardless of their smoking status, and this is shown for the ex- and current smokers. This lets us visualise directly the extra burden of stroke added by past and present smoking habits. Thus the second bar shows the extra incidence of stroke in ex-smokers (b) that is presumably due to the fact that the women had smoked in the past. Similarly, the third bar shows the far greater added rate of stroke in current smokers (c) that is attributable to their smoking. This extra disease is simply the difference between the rate in the exposed group (smokers) and the rate in the unexposed group (non-smokers). The total rate of disease in exposed individuals is therefore the sum of the background rate (due to other causes) and the additional rate due to the exposure in question.

If the groups differ only in their smoking habit *and if we believe that smoking is actually causing strokes to occur* then we can say that the extra disease in the smokers is attributable to their smoking – if they had not smoked then it would not have occurred. This **rate difference** is also called the **attributable risk** (AR) because it measures the actual amount of disease that can be attributed to a particular exposure:

Rate difference or attributable risk

$$= \text{Incidence rate in exposed} - \text{Incidence rate in unexposed}$$
$$= IR_e - IR_o \tag{5.6}$$

Risk differences

Look back to the example of immunisation against influenza in Table 5.2.

What percentage of patients in the intervention group would have been expected to attend for immunisation even if they hadn't received a phone call (background 'risk')?

What extra percentage of patients presumably attended only because they had received a call (i.e. how many attendances could be attributed to the phone call)?

We would have expected 44% of patients in the intervention group to go for immunisation even if the practice receptionists had not called to offer them an appointment. We can therefore say that an extra 6% of patients (50% – 44%) in the intervention group presumably went for immunisation only because they had received a call, i.e. their immunisation can be attributed to this. Here we have calculated a risk difference (as opposed to a rate difference) because we are subtracting incidences proportions (or risks):

Risk difference or attributable risk

= Incidence proportion in exposed – Incidence proportion in unexposed

= $IP_e - IP_o$

$$(5.7)$$

> Again we are assuming the two groups are *exchangeable* and that if the intervention group had not been invited to go for immunisation their rate of attendance would have been the same as that in the control group.

Attributable fractions (AFs)

In addition to the attributable risk, it may also be informative to consider the *proportion* of cases in the exposed group that would not have occurred in the absence of the exposure. This measure is often called the **attributable fraction** or **attributable proportion**, although you will also come across it described as the **attributable risk percent**. To calculate the attributable fraction you simply divide the attributable risk by the incidence in the exposed group:

$$\text{Attributable Fraction (AF)} = \frac{\text{Attributable Risk}}{\text{Incidence in exposed}}$$

$$\text{or} \quad = \frac{\text{Incidence in exposed} - \text{Incidence in unexposed}}{\text{Incidence in exposed}}$$

Again, this can be done using either the incidence rate or the incidence proportion:

$$\text{Attributable Fraction (AF)} = \frac{AR}{IR_e} \quad \text{or} \quad \frac{AR}{IP_e} \qquad (5.8)$$

$$= \frac{IR_e - IR_o}{IR_e} \quad \text{or} \quad \frac{IP_e - IP_o}{IP_e} \qquad (5.9)$$

Consider the smoking and stroke example again. The rate of stroke among current smokers was $49.6/10^5$ person-years and the rate difference or attributable risk was $31.9/10^5$ person-years. The attributable fraction is therefore 0.64 or 64%, i.e. of all the strokes occurring *among current smokers*, about two-thirds could be attributed to the fact that the women smoked:

$$\text{Attributable Fraction (AF)} = \frac{49.6 - 17.7}{49.6} = 0.64 = 64\%$$

Interpretation of the attributable risk

The attributable risk tells us how much extra disease actually occurred in the *exposed* group. If the exposed and unexposed groups are *exchangeable* in all ways except their exposure status, then this extra disease presumably occurred as a result of the exposure. By implication, we can then say that, *if the association is causal*, this is the amount of disease that we could prevent in a comparable group of people in the future *if* we could prevent them from being exposed. This measure is, therefore, of direct use to health planning and policy setting. Note that in the field of clinical epidemiology, what we have called the *attributable risk* is often called the **absolute risk reduction (ARR)** or **absolute risk increase (ARI)** depending on whether the event rate is reduced or increased in the treatment group (see Box 5.3). The ARR and ARI are identical to the attributable risks used elsewhere in epidemiology and are calculated in exactly the same way – the only difference is in the names.

In practice, of course, it is often impossible to remove or prevent an exposure altogether. Someone who smokes cannot go back to being a never-smoker, but they can become an ex-smoker. This means that current smokers who stop smoking will not realise the full benefit predicted by the standard attributable risk (which would compare smokers with the unexposed group, in this case never smokers). Rather, the best we could achieve with a 100% effective 'stop smoking' campaign would be to reduce the rate of stroke among smokers to the level seen among ex-smokers, a rate difference given by:

$$\text{IR}_{current} - \text{IR}_{ex} = 49.6 - 27.9 = 21.7 \text{ strokes/100,000 person-years}$$

Population attributable risks (PARs)

The attributable risk tells us about the amount of extra disease occurring in the exposed group because of the exposure. An alternative way to look at the burden due to an exposure is to consider *how much disease in the whole community* can be attributed to the exposure. To do this we need to compare the incidence of disease in the whole population or community (some of whom will be exposed and some unexposed) with the amount of disease in an unexposed group (the amount that we would expect if no one had been

Box 5.3 Attributable risks in clinical epidemiology

In the trial of the use of pressure bandages for patients undergoing coronary angiography (Table 5.3) the attributable risk or **absolute risk reduction** (ARR) of bleeding would be

$$ARR = CER - EER = 6.7 - 3.5 = 3.2\% \tag{5.10}$$

In other words, the use of pressure bandages prevented bleeding in 3.2% of patients.

　　Another quite useful way of looking at these data is in terms of the **number needed to treat (NNT)**. The NNT is the number of patients who would have to be given the experimental therapy in order to prevent one adverse event (death, complication) from occurring. It is calculated by simply dividing 1.0 by the ARR:

$$NNT = 1 \div ARR \tag{5.11}$$

In the study of pressure bandages the ARR was 3.2% or 0.032, so

$$NNT = 1 \div 0.032 = 31.3$$

This means that about 32 patients undergoing coronary angiography would need to be given pressure bandages in order to prevent one case of bleeding. (Note that the NNT should always be *rounded up* to the nearest whole number because you cannot treat part of a person.) This gives a good intuitive feel for the treatment benefit, and can aid communication with patients.

exposed). In the smoking and stroke example in Table 5.1 we know that the overall incidence rate of stroke among the women was $30.2/10^5$ person-years.

What would this rate have been if no one had smoked?

How much of the incidence of stroke in the total population is due to the fact that some women smoke or are ex-smokers?

What fraction of the overall rate of stroke in the total population is due to smoking?

　　If none of the women had smoked and if smokers and non-smokers are comparable in all other respects, the overall rate of stroke in the population would be the same as the rate in never smokers ($17.7/10^5$ person-years). This means that, in the whole population, there are an extra 12.5 cases (30.2 – 17.7) per 100,000 person-years that can be attributed to the fact that *some* of the

Figure 5.2 Attributable and
population attributable risks: the
results of a study of smoking and
stroke (*drawn from*: Colditz *et al.*,
1988).

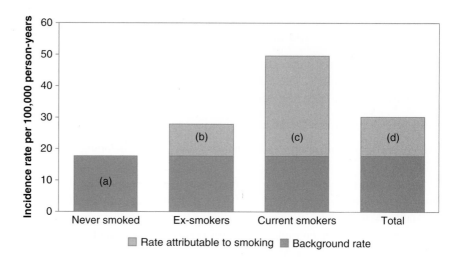

Figure 5.2 Attributable and population attributable risks: the results of a study of smoking and stroke (*drawn from*: Colditz *et al.*, 1988).

women in the population smoke or are ex-smokers. This is the ***population attributable risk* (PAR)** and is depicted (d) in the fourth bar in Figure 5.2.

There are two ways to calculate the PAR. One way, analogous to the calculation of attributable risk (Equations (5.6) and (5.7)), is to subtract the incidence in the unexposed group (IR_o, IP_o) from the incidence in the *whole population* (IR_T, IP_T). As for the attributable risk, this can be done using either incidence rates or incidence proportions:

PAR = Incidence rate in population − Incidence rate in unexposed

$$= IR_T - IR_o \text{ or } IP_T - IP_o \tag{5.12}$$

Clearly, the PAR will depend not only on the attributable risk among the exposed, but also on the prevalence of the exposure in the population. An alternative way to calculate the PAR is therefore to multiply the attributable risk by the prevalence of exposure in the population (P_e):

$$PAR = AR \times P_e \tag{5.13}$$

Note that, while this formula is straightforward to use when there are only two levels of exposure, it is trickier when there are more than two levels, as in the stroke and smoking example. In this situation it is much easier to use Equation (5.12) because the overall incidence rate in the population (IR_T) combines the effects of both past and current smoking in a single measure.

Population attributable fractions (PAFs)

As with the attributable risk and attributable fraction, we can also calculate the **population attributable fraction** (or **population attributable risk percent**), which indicates the proportion of all the strokes that occurred in the population that could have been avoided if no-one had smoked. The formula to calculate the PAF is analogous to that used for the attributable fraction but with the incidence in the total population used instead of the incidence in the exposed group:

$$\text{Population Attributable Fraction} = \frac{\text{Population Attributable Risk}}{\text{Incidence in total population}} \times 100$$

Population Attributable Fraction

$$= \frac{\text{Incidence in total population-Incidence in unexposed}}{\text{Incidence in total population}} \times 100$$

Again, this can be done using either incidence rates or incidence proportions:

$$\text{Population Attributable Fraction} = \frac{PAR}{IR_T} \quad or \quad \frac{PAR}{IP_T} \qquad (5.14)$$

$$\text{Population Attributable Fraction} = \frac{IR_T - IR_o}{IR_T} \quad or \quad \frac{IP_T - IP_o}{IP_T} \qquad (5.15)$$

So, in the stroke example, approximately 41% (12.5 ÷ 30.2 = 0.41) of strokes in the whole population could be attributed to smoking and, in theory, would not have occurred *if no-one had ever smoked*.

Interpretation of the population attributable risk

The PAR is exactly analogous to the attributable risk (AR) but, while the attributable risk tells us how much disease in the *exposed* group can be attributed to the exposure, the population attributable risk tells us how much disease in the *whole population* can be attributed to the exposure. The population attributable risk and population attributable fraction are functions both of the *incidence of disease* due to an exposure and of the *prevalence of the exposure*. An exposure may be associated with a very high attributable risk of a disease such that those exposed have a very high chance of developing it, but if the exposure is rare then this high risk will only affect a small proportion of the population. It will therefore have little impact in a whole community (a low PAR). The population attributable risk is the best way to measure the burden of disease in a whole community that can be attributed to a particular exposure.

As we have noted above for the AR, there is no intervention that we could implement to change a woman who is a current smoker into a never smoker; the most we could do would be to persuade her to stop smoking. If we could do this we could estimate the incidence rate of strokes in the whole group as 23.4 per 100,000 person-years (based on the new mix of never smokers and

PAF: Strictly speaking, the formulae for the PAF that we have described are only valid when there is no 'confounding' of the exposure of interest (Rockhill *et al.*, 1998), but we show them here to illustrate the underlying concepts. Equation (5.19) shows an alternative formula for the PAF that can be used in the presence of confounding. We will discuss confounding in Chapter 8.

ex-smokers[1]). This means that, if we could have persuaded all current smokers to give up smoking, we could potentially have prevented 6.8 strokes per 100,000 person-years (PAR = 30.2 – 23.4) or 22.5% of all strokes in the population (PAF = 6.8 ÷ 30.2).

In practice, however, even this is an overly simplistic view. It is very hard to persuade people to stop smoking (or to give up most unhealthy behaviours for that matter) and a more realistic goal might be to look at the health benefits that would follow if we could halve smoking rates. We will come back to this issue and will meet the PAR again when we consider disease prevention in Chapter 14. When thinking about the possibilities for intervention and prevention of disease we should also bear in mind that changing someone's smoking habit will reduce not just their risk of stroke but also their risk of many other diseases, so the public health benefits of a 'stop smoking' campaign are not limited to stroke reduction. While the overall benefits of stopping smoking are clear-cut, it is less obvious where an intervention reduces risk of one disease but increases that of another. For example, moderate alcohol consumption can reduce the risk of heart disease, but it can also increase the risk of breast cancer. These benefits and risks have to be weighed up and no-one would recommend that women should drink more alcohol to prevent heart disease.

At the global level, population attributable risks and population attributable fractions are used to calculate the impacts of various exposures on world health (see e.g. Lim *et al.*, 2012). For example, it has been estimated that in the year 2008 almost six million premature deaths around the world were attributable to tobacco use and second-hand smoke (WHO, 2011). You saw another example of this in Table 2.11 on page 69 although it looked somewhat different, because instead of looking at the *incidence* of disease attributable to an exposure, the burden of disease was measured in disability adjusted life years or DALYs. The concept is the same though. Note the variation in the relative importance of some causes depending on the affluence and thus the prevalence of exposure in the population.

A word of caution regarding attributable risks

As you have seen, attributable risks are easy to calculate. However, it is important to remember that, to be meaningful, we need accurate information regarding the rates of disease among people who are exposed and unexposed to the factor of

---

[1] If all current smokers became ex-smokers at the start of the study their stroke rate would have been 27.9/10^5 person-years so ~78 strokes would have occurred in their 280,141 person-years of follow-up. This gives a total of 213 strokes (70 + 65 + 78) in 908,447 person years or 23.4/10^5 person-years in the whole population. *Note: this assumes the full benefit is seen immediately after stopping.*

interest, and the association between exposure and outcome must be causal. It is also important to remember that while the RR of disease associated with exposure may be similar across different populations, the PAR also depends on the prevalence of the exposure in the population (see Equation (5.13)). The PAR in one population will therefore be very different from that in another population with a different prevalence of exposure. Finally, there are possibly more terms used to describe attributable risks than any other measure in epidemiology. People use different names for the same thing and, what is even more confusing, the same name for different things. This emphasises the importance of never taking things at face value – always take time to check what are being presented. The key distinction is whether people are talking about only the exposed group (what we call the attributable risk, attributable fraction or, in clinical epidemiology, the absolute risk reduction) or the whole population (what we call the population attributable risk or population attributable fraction). It is also important to distinguish between absolute differences (what we have called attributable risks) and percentage differences (attributable fractions).

Relative risk versus attributable risk: an example

In the British Doctors Study (discussed in Chapter 1) mortality rates were calculated for deaths both from lung cancer and from coronary heart disease (CHD). These rates, together with the relative risks, attributable risks and attributable fractions, are shown in Table 5.4.

Is the association with smoking stronger for lung cancer or CHD?

If everyone stopped smoking, would we prevent more cases of lung cancer or CHD?

In these data there is a very strong *relative* association between smoking and lung cancer (RR = 14), but only a modest link between cigarettes and CHD

Table 5.4 Lung cancer and CHD mortality rates in the British Doctors Study.

Disease	Smoking status	Mortality rate per 10^5 person-years	Relative risk	Attributable risk per 10^5 person-years	Attributable fraction (%)
Lung cancer	Yes	140	14.0	130	93
	No	10			
Coronary heart disease	Yes	669	1.6	256	38
	No	413			

(Doll and Peto, 1976)

Table 5.5 A comparison of relative and attributable risks.

Measure	Strengths	Uses
Relative risk (RR)	Evaluates the *strength* of an association between exposure and disease	To help identify causes of disease
Attributable risk (AR)	Measures the burden of disease attributable to exposure in the *exposed* group	To assess the magnitude of a public health problem associated with an exposure *among those exposed*
Population attributable risk (PAR)	Measures the burden of disease attributable to exposure in the *population*	To assess the magnitude of a public health problem associated with an exposure *in the whole population*
Attributable fraction (AF)	Identifies the specific exposures that cause most disease *in those who are exposed*	To identify potential targets for prevention
Population attributable fraction (PAF)	Identifies the specific exposures that cause most disease *in a population*	To identify potential targets for prevention

(RR = 1.6). On its own, this offers powerful support to a belief in smoking as a cause of lung cancer, but leaves quite a few doubts as to whether it has a causal role in the development of CHD (see also Chapter 10). Given that smoking does cause CHD as well as lung cancer (and there is plenty of other evidence to support this), the *attributable fraction* supports the view that smoking is a more important cause of lung cancer than it is of CHD: among smokers 93% of lung cancers but only 38% of CHD can be attributed to smoking. In contrast, the *attributable risks* show that the *public health impact* of smoking is twice as great for CHD mortality as for lung cancer deaths: there are almost 260 additional deaths from CHD in smokers for every 100,000 person-years compared with only 130 from lung cancer. If we look more closely at the actual rates of disease, we see that the background rate of CHD (the rate in non-smokers) is very high, so a large rate difference does not look so impressive when we calculate the RR. In contrast, the background rate of lung cancer is very low, so a much smaller rate difference leads to a very high RR. This example shows very clearly the striking difference in what these measures describe and the different implications of a large relative risk (or attributable faction) versus a large attributable risk. Table 5.5 summarises some of these differences and the uses of the different measures.

Case–control studies

All of the above measures relate to situations in which we can measure the incidence of disease. This information usually comes from a **cohort study** in which we identify groups of exposed and unexposed individuals who do not have the disease of interest and then follow them over time to see how many develop

Table 5.6 A case–control study of oral contraceptive (OC) use and ovarian cancer.

	Cases	Controls	Total
Used OC pill	413	1160	1573
Did not use OC pill	206	322	528
Total	619	1482	2101

(Jordan *et al.*, 2008)

the disease. As you saw in the previous chapter, in a **case–control study** we usually select only a sample of all possible people without disease as controls. This often means that we can no longer calculate disease incidence, so we need different methods to calculate measures of association in a case-control study.

In the early 2000s a case-control study of ovarian cancer was conducted in Australia. It included the majority of women newly diagnosed with ovarian cancer across the whole of Australia between 2003 and 2005. The controls were a sample of women who did not have ovarian cancer and who were chosen at random from the national electoral roll to give a similar age and state distribution as the cases (we will discuss this process where we 'match' cases and controls further in Chapter 8). The investigators found that 413 of the 619 women with ovarian cancer and 1160 of the 1482 controls had previously used the oral contraceptive (OC) pill (Jordan *et al.*, 2008), as shown in Table 5.6.

> **Estimating incidence in a case–control study:** If the sampling fraction of controls (i.e. the proportion of the total population that participate as controls) is known then it is possible to estimate the incidence of disease in a case–control study, but this is rarely done in practice.

What percentage of the OC users have ovarian cancer? Does this reflect the likely incidence of ovarian cancer in OC users?

In this case-control study 26% (413 ÷ 1573) of the OC users have ovarian cancer. It is tempting to interpret this as meaning that the incidence of ovarian cancer among oral contraceptive users was 26% but, even if you don't know anything about ovarian cancer, this should ring some warning bells! The OC pill would never be prescribed if almost half of the women who used it developed cancer. The numerator (the number of women with cancer) is fine because most of the women with cancer were included, but the denominator (the total population) is wrong because only a tiny proportion of all the women without ovarian cancer have been included. This means that, in a case-control study, we cannot calculate the usual measures of disease incidence directly, and so cannot calculate relative risks in the same way.

Relative risk in case–control studies

In a case-control study we calculate another measure of association known as the **odds ratio** (OR). This involves calculating the *odds* that a case had used OCs in exactly the same way as odds are calculated in horse racing. Among the

Table 5.7 Calculation of the odds ratio in a case–control study.

	Cases	Controls	Total
Exposed	a	b	$a + b$
Unexposed	c	d	$c + d$
Total	$a + c$	$b + d$	$a + b + c + d$

cases, 413 women had used the OC pill and 206 had not, so the 'odds' of a case having used the pill are '413 to 206' or $413 \div 206 = 2.00$.

What are the odds that a control had used the OC pill?

Among the controls, 1160 women had used the pill and 322 had not. The odds that a control had used the pill are therefore $1160 \div 322 = 3.60$. We can then calculate the **odds ratio** by dividing the odds that a case had used the pill (i.e. was exposed) by the odds that a control had used the pill. In this example:

Odds ratio (OR) = $2.00 \div 3.60 = 0.56$

An alternative and simple way to calculate the odds ratio that is often used in practice is as follows. Your data must be arranged in a standard way as shown in Table 5.7 (note that this is the same as the way in which the data are shown in Table 5.6).

The odds that a case used the OC pill = $a \div c$

The odds that a control used the OC pill = $b \div d$

Therefore the ratio of these odds = $(a \div c) \div (b \div d)$

or

$$\text{Odds Ratio} = \frac{a \times d}{b \times c} \tag{5.16}$$

So, for the ovarian cancer data, the OR associated with OC use is

$$\text{Odds Ratio} = \frac{413 \times 322}{1160 \times 206} = 0.56$$

In other words, the odds of a case having used the OC pill is almost half the odds that a control had used the pill. As you will see below, we can interpret this as meaning that a woman who uses the OC pill is almost half as likely to get ovarian cancer as a woman who has not used the pill. But be warned, it is not always possible to interpret an odds ratio in this way – especially if the disease of interest is quite common.

Interpreting odds ratios

How we interpret an odds ratio depends to a large extent on how the control group was recruited for that particular study, as in different situations the odds ratio can be a good estimate of either the risk (incidence proportion) ratio or the incidence rate ratio (see Box 5.4). In many studies the controls are recruited using what is called *density sampling* and in this situation the odds ratio is a good estimate of the rate ratio. For density sampling, the controls for the study must be identified during the period when the cases were occurring, *not* at the beginning or end of the study. In practice this does not make a lot of difference if the disease is rare, but if the disease is common it means that it is possible for someone to be recruited as a control early in a study and then to be recruited again as a case if they later develop the disease of interest. Although ovarian cancer is a rare disease, one woman participated as a control in a case–control study similar to the one described above but was diagnosed with ovarian cancer a year later. She then participated in the study a second time as a case. This is not only valid but essential for true density sampling.

Box 5.4 Rate ratios, risk ratios and odds ratios

Each of the three measures of association is a valid measure in its own right, but the relationship among them varies in different situations and depends on how the controls were selected for the study (see Rodrigues and Kirkwood, 1990).

- If they were selected at the *start* of the case-recruitment period and so included anyone who was disease-free at that point in time (regardless of whether they went on to develop disease) then

Odds ratio ≈ Risk ratio

so an OR of 3.0 can be interpreted as meaning that the *risk* of disease in those who were exposed was three times that among those who were not exposed.

- If they were selected at the *same* time as cases were being recruited (i.e. density sampling), as is usually the case in practice, then

Odds ratio ≈ Rate ratio

so an OR of 3.0 can be interpreted as meaning that the *rate* of disease in those who were exposed was three times that among those who were not exposed.

- If they were selected to include only people who were still disease-free at the end of the study then the odds ratio will still provide information about the strength of the association but, if the disease is not rare, it might not be a good estimate of the relative risk. That is, if an OR = 3.0 it tells us that the association is strong but it does *not* necessarily mean that those who were exposed were precisely three times as likely to develop disease compared to those who were not exposed.

In practice, however, if a disease is rare – and for the purposes of epidemiology many diseases are rare – then all three measures, the rate ratio, risk ratio and odds ratio, will be approximately equal and all can be interpreted as a relative risk. This is often described as the '**rare disease assumption**' (see Appendix 6 for the mathematical derivation of why this is true for the risk ratio and odds ratio).

Odds ratios in cross-sectional studies

In a cross-sectional study we compare the *prevalence* of disease in different exposure groups and the logical measure to use to do this is the **prevalence ratio** (PR). However, prevalence ratios are not as easy to work with as odds ratios and, as a result, you will find that the results of cross-sectional studies are often presented as odds ratios, sometimes called prevalence odds ratios (POR). As for the odds ratio (see above), the POR will also be a good estimate of the prevalence ratio in a cross-sectional study *if the outcome is rare*. However, in many cross-sectional studies the outcome is *not* rare and in this situation the POR will be more extreme (further from the null value of 1.0) than the prevalence ratio. In other words, if the PR is 2.0 the POR will be > 2.0; likewise, if the PR is 0.8 the POR will be < 0.8. This means that when the outcome is not rare, a POR of 2.0 suggests there is an association between the exposure and outcome, but it *cannot* be interpreted as meaning the outcome was twice as common in the exposed group compared to the unexposed group.

Attributable risk in case–control studies

Because we cannot usually calculate the actual incidence of disease in exposed and unexposed subjects in a case–control study, we cannot calculate the attributable risk of disease associated with the exposure. We can, however, estimate the attributable fraction using the following formula (see Box 5.5 for an explanation of where this formula comes from):

$$\text{Attributable Fraction (AF)} = \frac{(OR - 1)}{OR} \times 100 \tag{5.17}$$

We can also estimate the population attributable fraction, as follows:

$$\text{Population Attributable Fraction (PAF)} = \frac{P_e(OR - 1)}{P_e(OR - 1) + 1} \times 100 \tag{5.18}$$

where P_e is the prevalence of exposure in the population, estimated by measuring the prevalence in the *control* group.

Or, alternatively,

> ## Box 5.5 Deriving the formula for AF in a case–control study
>
> From Equation (5.9) $AF = \dfrac{IR_e - IR_o}{IR_e}$
>
> If we then divide each component of this formula* by the incidence of disease in the unexposed group (IR_o) we get:
>
> $$AF = \frac{(IR_e \div IR_o) - (IR_o \div IR_o)}{(IR_{e-} \div IR_o)}$$
>
> But $IR_e \div IR_o$ = the relative risk (Equation (5.1)) and $IR_o \div IR_o = 1$ so we have: $AF = \dfrac{RR - 1}{RR}$
>
> Or, in a case–control study where we use the OR to estimate the RR:
>
> $AF = \dfrac{OR - 1}{OR}$
>
> * *This is legitimate as long as we divide both the top and bottom of the equation by the same thing as this does not change the answer.*

Population attributable fraction = $P_{e(\text{cases})} \times AF$

$$= P_{e(cases)} \frac{(OR - 1)}{OR} \times 100 \qquad (5.19)$$

where $P_{e(\text{cases})}$ is the prevalence of exposure among the *cases*. This version of the equation is perhaps more intuitive than Equation (5.18) because while the AF tells us the proportion of cases in the exposed group that can be attributed to the exposure, when we calculate the PAF we also have to allow for the cases that were not exposed. For example, if 80% of exposed cases were attributable to an exposure but only half of the cases were exposed ($P_{e(\text{cases})} = 0.5$) then in the whole population only 40% of cases (80% × 0.5) would have been attributable to the exposure. Another advantage of Equation (5.19) is that it can also be used in the presence of confounding by using the OR that has been 'adjusted' for the confounders (see Chapter 8).

These measures are the only way of assessing the potential public health importance of an exposure from a case–control study. (Note that these formulae can also be used for follow-up studies by substituting the RR for the OR.)

Another example comes from a study of the effectiveness of bicycle helmets for preventing head injury in children (Thomas *et al.*, 1994). The cases were 98 children who presented to the local children's hospital with bicycle-related head injuries and the controls were 266 children treated for other bicycle-related injuries. In total, 207 children, 67 of the cases and 140 controls, were not wearing a helmet at the time of the accident. (Note that we will consider *not wearing a helmet* as the exposure in this example.)

Table 5.8 A case–control study of bicycle helmets and head injury.

	Cases	Controls	Total
No helmet (exposed)	67	140	207
Wearing a helmet (unexposed)	31	126	157
Total	98	266	364

(Thomas *et al.*, 1994.)

What is the OR for the association between not wearing a helmet and head injury?

What percentage of head injuries occurring among the children not wearing a helmet could be attributed to the fact that they were not wearing a helmet (AF)?

What proportion of the control children were not wearing a helmet (P_e)?

What percentage of all bicycle-related head injuries in children could be attributed to not wearing a helmet (PAF)?

Table 5.8 shows the results of the study laid out in a standard 2 × 2 table. The odds ratio for the association between not wearing a bicycle helmet and head injury is

$$OR = \frac{a \times d}{b \times c} = \frac{67 \times 126}{140 \times 31} = 1.95$$

This indicates that children who do not wear helmets are almost twice as likely to sustain a head injury in a bicycle accident as children who do wear helmets.

The attributable fraction tells us the proportion of head injuries among those not wearing a helmet that could be attributed to the fact that they were not wearing a helmet:

$$AF = \frac{(OR - 1)}{OR} \times 100 = \frac{1.95 - 1}{1.95} \times 100 = 49\%$$

This tells us that 49% of head injuries *among children not wearing helmets* could be attributed to the fact they were not helmeted and were therefore potentially preventable if they had been wearing a helmet.

Out of the 266 controls, 140 or 53% were not wearing a helmet. We can use this information to calculate the population attributable fraction to estimate the proportion of all head injuries that could be attributed to the fact that some children were not wearing a helmet:

$$\text{PAF} = \frac{P_e(OR-1)}{P_e(OR-1)+1} \times 100 = \frac{0.53 \times 0.95}{(0.53 \times 0.95)+1} \times 100 = \frac{0.5035}{1.5035} \times 100 = 33\%$$

The results suggest that, in the study population, almost one-third of all child head injuries incurred while cycling could be prevented if all children wore bicycle helmets. (Note that it is important not to round off the numbers during calculations like this because this may make the answer inaccurate. Rounding should be used only for communication of the final answer.)

Looking for associations when the measures are continuous

In everything we have discussed above we have looked at what are called *dichotomous* outcomes – outcomes where people either experience the outcome of interest or they do not. We have also looked only at dichotomous (exposed vs. unexposed) or *categorical* exposures, such as the comparisons of never, former and current smokers. However, there are of course many health measures that cannot be captured by a simple yes/no outcome. For example, we might be interested in factors that affect blood pressure, body mass index, blood glucose levels, etc., or we might be interested in how these *continuous* measures – so-called because they can take any value (within a plausible range) – affect disease. In these situations it is sometimes appropriate to dichotomise or categorise the outcome, e.g. to look at the proportion of people whose blood pressure is above a certain level versus those whose blood pressure is below this level. However, if we do this we lose a lot of information because we are not differentiating between someone whose blood pressure is only just above the cut point and someone whose blood pressure is very high. The best methods for analysing continuous variables of this type depend on the type of data. They can be found in any good biostatistics textbook and we will not consider them here.

Summary

Box 5.6 gives an example that summarises the calculation and interpretation of the various measures of association that you have just met. It is based on *incidence rates* of type-2 diabetes but the formulae also apply to *incidence proportion* or risk data – simply substitute IP for IR. In a case–control study it is not usually possible to calculate the AR or PAR, but we can use the odds ratio (Equation (5.16)) in place of the RR to calculate the AF and PAF. After working through this example and the questions at the end of the chapter you should feel comfortable calculating and interpreting any of the common measures of association that you come across in the health literature.

Box 5.6 An example – obesity and type-2 diabetes

Imagine that 30% of the population in a particular community is over-weight, 82.5% of diabetics are overweight and the rate of type-2 diabetes is
- $330/10^5$ person-years in the obese (IR_e),
- $30/10^5$ person-years in the non-obese (IR_o) and
- $120/10^5$ person-years in the whole population (IR_T).

Then we can calculate the following.

(1) The **rate ratio** or **relative risk** (RR) using Equation (5.1):

$$RR = \frac{IR_e}{IR_o} = \frac{330}{30} = 11.0$$

The **relative risk** tells us that the rate of type-2 diabetes is 11 times as high among people who are obese than among non-obese people.

(2) The **rate difference** or **attributable risk** (AR) using Equation (5.6):

$$AR = IR_e - IR_o = 330 - 30 = 300 \text{ per } 10^5 \text{ person-years}$$

The **attributable risk** tells us that, if obesity is a cause of type-2 diabetes, then, *among obese people*, 300 cases per 10^5 person-years can be attributed to their obesity.

(3) The **attributable fraction** (AF) using Equation (5.9):

$$AF = \frac{(IR_e - IR_o)}{IR_e} \times 100 = \frac{(330 - 30)}{330} \times 100 = 91\%$$

or Equation (5.17) (using the RR instead of the OR):

$$AF = \frac{(RR - 1)}{RR} \times 100 = \frac{(11 - 1)}{11} \times 100 = 91\%$$

The **attributable fraction** tells us that more than 90% of type-2 diabetes in obese people would not occur if they were not overweight.

(4) The **population attributable risk** (PAR) using Equation (5.12):

$$PAR = IR_T - IR_o = 120 - 30 = 90/10^5 \text{ person-years}$$

or using Equation (5.13):

$$PAR = AR \times P_e = 300 \times 0.3 = 90/10^5 \text{ person-years}$$

where P_e = prevalence of exposure in the population = 30% or 0.3.
The **population attributable risk** tells us that, in the **whole population**, 90 cases of type-2 diabetes per 10^5 person-years can be attributed to obesity.

(continued)

Box 5.6 (*continued*)

(5) The **population attributable fraction** (PAF) using Equation (5.14):

$$PAF = \frac{PAR}{IR_T} \times 100 = (90 \div 120) \times 100 = 75\%$$

or Equation (5.18) (using the RR instead of OR):

$$PAF = \frac{P_e(RR-1)}{P_e(RR-1)+1} \times 100 = \frac{0.3 \times (11-1)}{(0.3 \times (11-1))+1} \times 100 = \frac{3}{4} \times 100 = 75\%$$

or Equation (5.19):

$$PAF = P_{e(cases)} \frac{(RR-1)}{RR} \times 100 = 0.825 \times \frac{(11\text{-}1)}{11} = 0.825 \times 0.91 \times 100 = 75\%$$

The **population attributable fraction** tells us that 75% of all cases of type-2 diabetes would not occur if no one was grossly overweight.

  Note: the estimates of PAF are all identical because we have assumed that there is no confounding (see Chapter 8*). In the presence of confounding, Equation (5.19) should be used with the adjusted estimate of the relative risk.*

Questions

1. In an industry employing 10,000 people, 2500 were employed in areas where they were exposed to pesticides, while the remaining 7500 were not exposed. At the beginning of the study, all employees were free of disease. The entire population of 10,000 was followed for 10 years to determine whether exposure to pesticides increased the risk of developing a particular disease. For this disease, the findings were as given in Table 5.9. 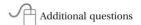 Additional questions
   (a) Calculate the incidence proportion for the disease in
       (i) the exposed workers,
       (ii) the unexposed workers, and
       (iii) all workers combined.
   (b) Calculate the relative risk of this disease in those exposed to pesticides. What does this tell us?
   (c) How much disease in the exposed workers could be due to their pesticide exposure (attributable risk)?
   (d) Calculate the population attributable fraction. What does this tell us?
2. The Family Planning Association in Oxford, England studied 17,000 women who had been enrolled in a cohort study between 1968 and 1974 to look at the association between oral contraceptive (OC) use and venous thromboembolism (Vessey *et al.*, 1989). For current users of OCs, person-time

Table 5.9 The results of a hypothetical study of the effects of pesticide exposure.

	Developed disease	Did not develop disease	Total
Exposed to pesticides	40	2,460	2,500
Not exposed	60	7,440	7,500
Total	100	9,900	10,000

was counted from the time a woman began using OCs. For never or past users, it was counted from the time a woman enrolled in the study. Woman-years were counted until venous thromboembolism occurred, the woman was lost-to-follow-up, or the end of the study.

(a) The incidence rate of venous thromboembolism was 53 per 100,000 woman-years among current OC users and 6 per 100,000 woman-years among never or past users. Calculate the relative risk of venous thromboembolism for current users compared with never or past users.

(b) The incidence rate of thromboembolism was 62 per 100,000 among users of OCs containing higher dosages of oestrogen and 39 per 100,000 among users of lower-dose OCs. Calculate the relative risk of venous thromboembolism for

(i) low-dose users compared with never or past users, and

(ii) high-dose users compared with never or past users.

(c) What can you conclude about the risk of thromboembolism for users of OCs containing different doses of oestrogen?

3. Doll and Hill first evaluated the proposition that smoking was a risk factor for lung cancer in a case–control study (Doll and Hill, 1950). They found that, of 649 men with lung cancer (cases), 647 had smoked at some time, compared with 622 of the 649 men without lung cancer (controls).

(a) Draw up a clearly labelled and appropriate 2 × 2 table to show these data.

(b) How many times as likely was a smoker to develop lung cancer than a non-smoker?

(c) Calculate the proportion of lung cancers attributable to smoking among (i) *smokers* and (ii) the *whole population*.

(d) What are these measures called and how does their interpretation differ?

4. The association between decreased duration of sleep and incidence of coronary heart disease (CHD) was studied among women enrolled in the Nurses' Health Study (Ayas *et al.*, 2003). Among women who reported sleeping for 7 or 8 hours per night, there were 541 incident cases of CHD during 451,393 person-years of follow-up. Among those who slept for

6 hours per night there were 267 cases in 175,629 person-years, and among those sleeping 5 or fewer hours per night there were 67 cases during 30,115 person-years of follow-up.

(a) Calculate the incidence rate of CHD among
    (i) women who reported sleeping 7–8 hours per night,
    (ii) women who reported sleeping for 6 hours per night,
    (iii) women who slept 5 or less hours per night, and
    (iv) all women.

(b) How strong is the association between sleep duration and the incidence of CHD?

(c) What percentage of CHD cases could theoretically be prevented if all women slept for 7–8 hours per night?

REFERENCES

Ayas, N. T., White, D. P., Manson, J. E., *et al.* (2003). A prospective study of sleep duration and coronary heart disease in women. *Archives of Internal Medicine*, 163: 205–209. References

Botti, M., Williamson, B., Steen, K., McTaggart, J. and Reid, E. (1998). The effect of pressure bandaging on complications and comfort in patients undergoing coronary angiography: a multicentre randomized trial. *Heart and Lung*, 27: 360–373.

Colditz, G. A., Bonita, R., Stampfer, M. J., *et al.* (1988). Cigarette smoking and risk of stroke in middle-aged women. *New England Journal of Medicine*, 318: 937–941.

Doll, R. and Hill, A. B. (1950). Smoking and carcinoma of the lung. *British Medical Journal*, 2: 739–748.

Doll, R. and Peto, R. (1976). Mortality in relation to smoking: 20 years' observations on male British doctors. *British Medical Journal*, 2: 1525–1536.

Hull, S., Hagdrup, N., Hart, B., Griffiths, C. and Hennessy, E. (2002). Boosting uptake of influenza immunisation in a randomised controlled trial of telephone appointing in general practice. *British Journal of General Practice*, 52: 712–716.

Jordan, S. J., Green, A. C., Whiteman, D. C., *et al.* (2008). Serous ovarian, fallopian tube and primary peritoneal cancers: a comparative epidemiological analysis. *International Journal of Cancer*, 122: 1598–1603.

Lim, S. S., Vos, T., Flaxman, A. D., *et al.* (2012). A comparative risk assessment of burden of disease and injury attributable to 67 risk factors and risk factor clusters in 21 regions, 1990–2010: a systematic analysis for the Global Burden of Disease Study 2010. *The Lancet*, 380: 2224–2260.

Maushart, S. (2003). Domesticator: rise of the machines. *The Weekend Australian Magazine*, August, 16–17.

Rockhill, B., Newman, B. and Weinberg, C. (1998). Use and mis-use of population attributable fractions. *American Journal of Public Health*, 88: 15–19; correction in *American Journal of Public Health*, 98: 2119.

Rodrigues, L. and Kirkwood, E. R. (1990). Case–control designs in the study of common diseases: updates on the demise of the rare disease assumption and the choice of sampling scheme for controls. *International Journal of Epidemiology*, 19: 205–213.

Snow, J. (1855). *On the Mode of Communication of Cholera*, 2nd edn. London: Churchill. (http://www.ph.ucla.edu/epi/snow.html).

Thomas, S., Acton, C., Nixon, J. *et al.* (1994). Effectiveness of bicycle helmets in preventing head injury in children: case–control study. *British Medical Journal*, 308: 173–176.

Vessey, M. P., Villard-Mackintosh, L., McPherson, K. and Yeates, D. (1989). Mortality among oral contraceptive users: 20 year follow up of women in a cohort study. *British Medical Journal*, 299: 1487–1491.

WHO (World Health Organization). (2011). *Global Status Report On Non-communicable Diseases 2010*. Geneva: World Health Organization.

RECOMMENDED FOR FURTHER READING

- More about the use of population attributable fractions:
  Rockhill, B., Newman, B. and Weinberg, C. (1998). Use and mis-use of population attributable fractions. *American Journal of Public Health*, 88: 15–19; correction in *American Journal of Public Health*, 98: 2119.
- A discussion of the relationship between the odds ratio estimated in a case-control study and risk and rate ratios:
  Rodrigues, L. and Kirkwood, E. R. (1990). Case–control designs in the study of common diseases: updates on the demise of the rare disease assumption and the choice of sampling scheme for controls. *International Journal of Epidemiology*, 19: 205–213.
- Snow's classic account of his work investigating cholera:
  Snow, J. (1855). *On the Mode of Communication of Cholera*, 2nd edn. London: Churchill. (http://www.ph.ucla.edu/epi/snow.html).

Heads or tails: the role of chance

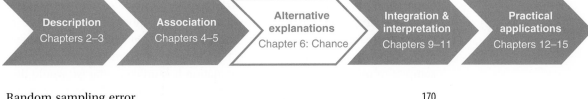

If the results of a study reveal an interesting association between some exposure and a health outcome, there is a natural tendency to assume that it is real. (Note that we are considering whether two things are *associated*. This does not necessarily imply that one *cause*s the other to occur. We will discuss approaches to determining causality further in Chapter 10.) However, before we can even contemplate this possibility we have to try to rule out other possible explanations for the results. There are three main 'alternative explanations' that we have to consider whenever we analyse epidemiological data or read the reports of others, no matter what the study design: namely, could the results be due to

- chance,
- bias or error, or
- confounding?

We will discuss the first of these, **chance**, in this chapter and will cover **bias** and **confounding** in Chapters 7 and 8, respectively.

Random sampling error

When we conduct a study or survey it is rarely possible to include the whole of a population[1] so we usually have to rely on a *sample* of that population and trust that this sample will give us an answer that holds true for the general population. If we select the sample of people wisely so they are truly representative of the target population (the population that we want to study) and, importantly, if most of those selected agree to participate, then we will not introduce any **selection bias** into the study (we touched on the issue of selection bias in Box 3.2, and will discuss it further in Chapter 7). However, even in the absence of any selection bias, if we were to study several different samples of people from the same population it is unlikely that we would find exactly the same answer each time, and unlikely that any of the answers would be exactly the same as the true population value. This is because each sample we take will include slightly different people and their characteristics will tend to vary from those in other samples – just by chance. This is known as **random sampling error**.

Imagine that you were interested in the health effects of obesity and wanted to know the average body mass index (BMI) of 10-year-old children in your community. If you weighed and measured just one or two children you would not obtain a very good estimate of the average BMI of all children – but the more children you studied, the better your estimate would be. The same is true if we are looking for the association between an 'exposure' and 'outcome', for example the relation between BMI and age. If we only survey a small group of 10-year-olds and another small group of 12-year-olds we might find that, just by chance, the 10-year olds are bigger than the 12-year olds, but the larger our study, the better or more *precise* our estimate of the true association between age and body-size will be. In general, if we select a small sample of a population then our results are more likely to differ from the true population values than if we had selected a larger sample. The best way to reduce sampling error is thus to increase the size of the study sample as far as is practical. Of course, there is always a trade-off between study size and cost. There are ways in which we can calculate how many people we should include in a study to reduce sampling error to an acceptable level. This is known as the **power** of the study and we will come back to consider this further after we have looked at some ways to assess the amount of random sampling error in a study.

When we conduct a study to evaluate the relationship between an exposure and disease we may see an association or we may not. We then have to use the information from the sample of people in the study to infer

---

[1] Notable exceptions are the population censuses that we discussed in Chapter 3.

STUDY RESULTS (Known)	TRUTH (Unknown)	
	No association	Association
No association	Correct	Type II error (probability = β)
Association	Type-I error (probability = α)	Correct (probability = $1-\beta$) = Power

Figure 6.1 Possible outcomes of an epidemiological study.

whether the exposure and outcome are truly related in the wider population. There are four possible outcomes for any study, as shown in Figure 6.1.

If there is really no association between the outcome and exposure then we hope that our study will find just that. Conversely, if the exposure and outcome are truly associated in the population then we want our study to show this association. What we want to minimise are the situations where our study shows an apparent relationship between exposure and outcome when the truth is that there is none (often called a 'type I' or alpha error), or our study says there is no association when, in truth, there is (a 'type II' or beta error). Unfortunately, in practice we can never know for sure whether we are right or wrong, but we strive to limit this uncertainty by maximising study power (see below) to restrict the role of chance. (We will consider strategies to minimise other types of error in the next two chapters.)

Statistical significance: could an apparent association have arisen by chance?

One way to assess whether an association might have arisen by chance is to carry out what is known as a **hypothesis test**. This works on a similar principle to many justice systems where someone is presumed innocent until there is sufficient evidence to suggest they are guilty. Here we assume that there is really no association, the 'null' hypothesis, unless this is so unlikely to be true that we feel we can reject it in favour of the 'alternative' hypothesis that there is a real association. To do this we calculate the probability that we would have seen an association as strong as (or stronger than) the observed association *if there were really no difference between the groups* (i.e. if the null hypothesis were true). The results of these statistical tests take the form of a **p-value** (or probability value) and they give us some idea of how likely it is that the groups are truly different and the association is real, or whether the results might just be due to random sampling error or chance (in other words,

The **null hypothesis** (H_0) and **alternative hypothesis** (H_1) for a study looking at the relation between drinking coffee and migraine might be:

H_0: there is no association between drinking coffee and migraine (i.e. RR = 1.0)

H_1: there is an association between drinking coffee and migraine (RR $\neq$ 1.0).

a type I error, α). For example, if a survey of children shows that girls have a higher average BMI than boys, is this likely to be a true difference or could it just be chance that the girls in the study sample happened to have a higher BMI than the boys?

Imagine that the average BMI of the girls in a survey was 2 units higher than the average BMI of the boys and that statistical testing gave a p-value of 0.01 associated with this difference. We can say from this that, if the average BMIs of boys and girls were in fact the same (i.e. the null hypothesis is true), then we would have only a 0.01 or 1% probability of seeing an apparent difference of 2 units (or more) purely by chance. This is a very low probability, it would occur only 1 in 100 times, thus it seems *unlikely* to be a chance finding, although it still could be. Conventionally, results are considered to be *statistically significant*, i.e. unlikely to have arisen by chance, if the p-value is less than 0.05 ($p < 0.05$); in other words, if the probability that the result would have arisen by chance is less than 5% (i.e. the probability that we are making a type I error, α, is less than 0.05). Using this criterion, we would, therefore, reject the null hypothesis and conclude that the 2-unit difference in BMI between boys and girls was unlikely to have arisen by chance and that, all else being equal, girls probably do have a higher BMI than boys.

Imagine a study which found that, compared with people who exercised regularly, those who did not exercise were three times as likely to have a heart attack (RR = 3.0) and that the p-value for this association was 0.005.

What would the relative risk be if the risk of having a heart attack were the *same* for people who exercised and those who did not?

How often would we expect to see a relative risk as big as 3.0 if there were really no association?

Is it likely that a study would give a relative risk of 3.0 ($p = 0.005$) if there were really no association between exercise and heart attack?

If the risk of having a heart attack were the same regardless of how much a person exercised, i.e. there was *no* association between exercising and having a heart attack, then the relative risk would be 1.0. In the example above the study found a relative risk of 3.0, $p = 0.005$. The small p-value suggests that it is very unlikely that the study would have given a relative risk as big as 3.0 if the true relative risk were 1.0. (With a p-value of 0.005, we would expect this to happen only about 5 in 1000 or 1 in 200 times.) The observed association between heart attack and exercise is therefore unlikely to have arisen by chance.

Confidence intervals

A hypothesis test is a qualitative assessment of whether or not an observed association is likely to have arisen simply because, by chance, the people who ended up in the study differed in some way from the population norm. A more quantitative way to assess the likely effects of this random sampling error on our estimates is to calculate what is a called a **confidence interval** around the result. This is in effect an explicit admission that the result of a study,[2] often referred to as the 'point' or 'effect' estimate, is probably not exactly right, but that the real answer is likely to lie somewhere within a given range – the confidence interval. A narrow confidence interval therefore indicates *good precision* or little random sampling error and, conversely, a wide confidence interval indicates *poor precision*. The most commonly used confidence intervals are 95% intervals (95% CI) and they are often described slightly inaccurately as meaning that we can be '95% confident' that the real value is within the range covered by the confidence interval. What the confidence interval really means is that if we were to repeat the study many times with different samples of people, then 95% of the 95% confidence intervals we calculated would include the true value. *Note that this also means that 5% of the time (or 1 in 20 times) the 95% CI would not include the true value and we will never know which times these are.* Other percentages can be used, such as 90%, which gives a narrower confidence interval but less certainty that it will contain the true value (we will be wrong about 1 time in 10); and 99%, which will be more likely to contain the true value (we will only be wrong about 1 time in 100) but will give a wider interval.

To consider a practical example, imagine two studies that have evaluated the association between exposure to air pollution and asthma.

Study 1 finds a relative risk of 1.5 with a 95% confidence interval (CI) of 1.2–1.9.

What does this tell us about the association between air pollution and asthma?

This is a fairly precise estimate. It tells us that people who are exposed to air pollution are about one and a half times *as* likely (or 50% *more* likely) to develop asthma than those who are not exposed. It tells us that the risk might be as much as 1.9 times, but also that it might be as little as 1.2 times as high (i.e. a 20% increase) in those who are exposed. It also tells us that the relative risk is unlikely to be more than 1.9 or less than 1.2 (but it still could be outside these values).

---

[2] This would typically be an OR or RR, but it could also be a single measure of prevalence or a rate.

Study 2 finds a relative risk of 2.5 (95% CI 0.9–6.9).

What is the most likely value for the relative risk of asthma in people exposed to air pollution in the second study?

Is it possible that the result could have arisen by chance and there is really no association (i.e. the 'true' population relative risk is 1.0)?

Which of the two studies would give you most concern that air pollution was associated with asthma?

In the second study, the most likely value for the relative risk is 2.5 and the true relative risk could be as high as 6.9. However, the confidence interval is very wide, indicating poor precision, and it also includes the value 1.0 (remembering that an RR of 1.0 suggests no effect), so it is possible that there is really no association and the result of 2.5 arose by chance. Both results suggest a possible effect of air pollution in inducing asthma. Assuming there is no bias, the first study implies that there is a real association between air pollution and asthma but the effect is not very great. The second study suggests the relative effect might be larger and thus more important clinically, but because of the wide CI we are left with some uncertainty as to how 'true' that value really is. We should certainly not ignore the result just because chance is one possible explanation for our findings; after all, the real value is just as likely to be close to 6.0 (a very strong association), as it is to be close to 1.0 (no effect). However, we should be cautious, and acknowledge the possibility that it could merely reflect the play of chance. In practice, if we had to make a judgement about the public health effects of air pollution we would want to consider the results of *both* studies together to increase the precision of our estimate. We will look at ways to do this in more detail in Chapter 11. For now, it is important to remember that narrow confidence intervals (indicating good precision) are always more informative than wide confidence intervals (indicating poor precision).

> See Appendix 7 for some of the most useful formulae for calculating **confidence intervals**.

The relationship between *p*-values and confidence intervals

> The **null value** is the value a measure takes when there is *no association*, e.g. the rate of disease in two groups is the same. For a relative risk (e.g. RR, OR) the null value is 1.0; for an absolute risk the null value is 0.

If a 95% CI does *not* contain the 'no-effect' or 'null' value then the *p*-value from a statistical test would be < 0.05. Conversely, if the 95% CI *does* include the null value then $p \geq 0.05$. This means that if both ends of a CI around a relative risk are greater than 1.0 (example (a) in Figure 6.2), it suggests that the positive association between the exposure and outcome is unlikely to be due to chance; similarly if both ends of the CI are less than 1.0, it suggests an inverse association that is unlikely to be due to chance (d). However if the CI includes the null value, i.e. the lower bound is less

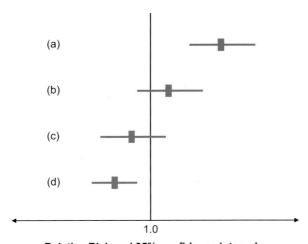

Figure 6.2 Relative risks and confidence intervals from four hypothetical studies.

(a)

(b)

(c)

(d)

1.0

Relative Risk and 95% confidence interval

than 1.0 and the upper bound is greater than 1.0 as shown in examples (b) and (c), then we cannot rule out the possibility that the true relative risk is really 1.0 and thus that there is really no association between the exposure and outcome. In the hypothetical asthma studies above, the 95% CI for study 1 does not include the null value so the corresponding p-value would be less than 0.05 and the result would be termed 'statistically significant'. The result of study 2, on the other hand, would not be statistically significant because the 95% CI includes the value 1.0 so the p-value would be ≥ 0.05.

Power: could we have missed a true association?

In addition to considering whether an observed association might have arisen by chance, if we do not see an association we should consider whether we could have *missed* a true relation by chance. Is it possible that an exposure is linked to an outcome but the study was just too small to detect this reliably (a type II error, β)? Or, returning to the legal analogy, that the person really was guilty but that we had insufficient evidence to convict them? Consider again the hypothetical study above that reported a relative risk of 3.0 ($p = 0.005$) for the association between a lack of regular exercise and heart attack. What if the study had been smaller and the p-value was only 0.1? In this situation $p \geq 0.05$ so it is possible that the observed RR of 3.0 has arisen by chance and there is truly no association between lack of exercise and risk of heart attack; but it is also possible that there really is a meaningful association but the study was just too small to detect this with any certainty.

As shown in Figure 6.1, the probability of making a type II error, i.e. saying there is no association when one truly exists, is often denoted β. The **power** of a study, i.e. the probability that it will show an association if it exists, is therefore $1 - \beta$.

Public domain software for sample size and power calculations

DES is a synthetic oestrogen that was used between 1940 and 1970 to prevent spontaneous abortion and premature delivery.

To avoid such a situation it is important to ensure that a study is big enough or, in other words, that it has enough *power* to detect a true association with sufficient precision. The power of a study is the probability that it will detect an association of a particular size if it truly exists in the general population. Imagine that an exposure truly causes a twofold increase in the risk of disease (of course, we can never know this in practice). If a study has 80% power to detect a relative risk of 2.0 between the exposure and outcome then we can say that 80% of the time, or four times out of five, that study would determine that the exposure and outcome were related. It also means that there is a 20% or one in five chance that we would miss the association. There is no hard and fast rule as to how much power a study should have but, in general, most people would probably want a minimum of 80% power and many would aim for 90%.

If we are looking to measure the strength of association between an exposure and an outcome, power or sample size calculations involve some knowledge, first, of the smallest difference that we want to be able to detect and, second, of the prevalence of the exposure and/or incidence of the outcome in the population. They also require a decision as to how precisely we wish to measure the effect, i.e. how much sampling error we are prepared to accept in our result. If we are looking for a large effect and the exposure and/or disease are quite common then we do not need a large study to show this. For example, in 1971 a tiny case–control study ($n = 40$) showed that young women who had been exposed in utero to diethylstilboestrol (DES) had an increased risk of developing a rare type of vaginal cancer (clear cell adenocarcinoma) (Herbst *et al.*, 1971). In this situation, the frequency of DES use among the mothers of the cases was so high (7 out of 8) and the difference was so large (none of 32 control mothers had used DES) that the investigators needed to study only those 40 women to show that there was a clear association. Unfortunately, in modern epidemiology we are often looking for much smaller effects and our studies have to be much larger than this to detect them with certainty. Table 6.1 shows how the prevalence of exposure and the size of the association affect the number of people you need to study to have 80% power to be able to detect the association ($\alpha = 0.05$).

A major problem in epidemiology is that, for financial or other practical reasons, researchers often cannot conduct as large a study as they would like. However, if they compromise and conduct a small study that shows an association between the exposure and outcome but this is not statistically significant (i.e. poor precision), it is difficult to interpret the results. Is there really an association, i.e. the estimated effect is close to the truth, but the study was just too small to detect this with any certainty? Or was the observed

Table 6.1 Number of cases required for a case–control study to detect a statistically significant association with varying levels of exposure prevalence.[a]

Prevalence of exposure in controls (%)	Odds ratio			
	1.2	1.5	2.0	2.5
1	43,685	7,960	2,395	1,244
5	9,172	1,686	513	269
10	4,885	908	280	149
20	2,799	532	169	92
30	2,172	422	138	77

[a] Number of cases required (assuming 1 control per case), to achieve 80% power at $\alpha = 0.05$.

association just due to chance and the 'truth' is that there is no association? The smaller the effect, the more important it is that we can estimate it precisely in order to distinguish between a real association and chance. This is a major problem in the context of genetic studies when the associations with disease are likely to be weak (RR < 1.2). This makes it very hard to identify which, if any, observed associations are real and, as a result, genetic association studies have to be very large (tens of thousands of cases) in order to give sufficient precision.

The question is also particularly important in the context of clinical trials when we need to know whether small improvements seen for a new treatment really do represent a benefit that should be passed on to patients (see Box 6.1).

This raises an important ethical issue that most human research and ethics committees would now consider before giving a study approval to proceed. Is the study big enough to detect the effects the investigators are looking for? If the answer is no then it has to be questioned whether the study should be allowed to go ahead.

Interpreting *p*-values and confidence intervals

Significance testing is very common and it is easy to get fixated on *p*-values and to implicitly believe an association is real if $p < 0.05$ and to assume it is not real (i.e. it is due to chance) if $p \geq 0.05$. However, it is important to note that the conventional distinction between $p < 0.05$ (statistically significant) and $p \geq 0.05$ (not statistically significant) is purely arbitrary. It is also important to remember that even if $p < 0.05$ this does not guarantee the association is real. Similarly, just because $p > 0.05$ it does not necessarily mean that there

The level of 0.05 for assessing **statistical significance** came from R.A. Fisher who concluded 'we shall not often be astray if we draw a conventional line at 0.05 . . .' (Fisher, 1950).

> ### Box 6.1 RCTs failed to show a benefit of streptokinase
>
> Between 1959 and 1988, 33 randomised clinical trials were conducted to test whether intravenous streptokinase reduced the risk of death after heart attack. Most of the studies ($n = 25$) found that mortality was lower among the groups given streptokinase, but many were small and so their results were not 'statistically significant' (i.e. $p \geq 0.05$). As a result the benefits of streptokinase were not fully appreciated. In 1992, however, a group combined the results of all the individual streptokinase studies using a technique called **meta-analysis** (we will discuss this further in Chapter 11). This showed that streptokinase was associated with more than a 20% reduction in mortality after heart attack and, because of the large sample size, a total of 36,974 patients when all the studies were combined, this effect was now highly statistically significant ($p < 0.001$) (Lau *et al.*, 1992). Importantly, they also found that if the results of just the first eight studies, involving a total of only 2432 patients, had been combined, the 20% reduction in mortality among those given streptokinase would have been apparent back in 1973. The problem was that individually most of the early studies were simply not big enough to detect this effect with sufficient certainty. As a consequence, their results were rarely statistically significant and so were dismissed. If some of them had been bigger (or if more emphasis had been placed on the size of the reduction in mortality and less on statistical significance) the beneficial effects of streptokinase would have been discovered much sooner and thousands of lives could probably have been saved.

is no association; it just means that we do not have enough evidence to conclude that there is an association – a subtle but important distinction. You will often read statements in the literature along the lines of 'there was no association between X and Y (OR = 1.9, $p > 0.05$)', but all this can really tell us is that there is insufficient evidence to conclude that there is an association. It may well be that Y really is twice as common among people exposed to X but this study was just too small (i.e. it had insufficient power) to detect an effect of this magnitude with any certainty.

Hypothesis tests and p-values are tools that can be used to help assess the results of a study, but they should not be used blindly to decide whether or not an association exists (see Box 6.2). They are aids to judgement, not absolute arbiters. It is also important to remember that although when you use a significance level (α) of 0.05 there is only a 1-in-20 chance that you will

Box 6.2 Why you should not rely only on *p*-values

The convention of describing a result as 'statistically significant' if $p < 0.05$ is now so strongly ingrained that some people tend to believe a result if $p < 0.05$ but not if $p > 0.05$. For example, a relative risk of 2.5 ($p = 0.049$) would, by convention, be called 'statistically significant' because 0.049 is less than 0.05. In contrast, a relative risk of 2.5 ($p = 0.051$) would not be classed as statistically significant because 0.051 is greater than 0.05. However, the relative risk is the same in both cases and $p = 0.049$ is so similar to $p = 0.051$ that it is illogical to believe the first result but not the second. *P*-values are also highly dependent on the size of the study – the bigger the study the smaller the *p*-value (for the same effect size). Imagine a study with 80 cases and 80 controls that found an odds ratio of 1.7 with a *p*-value of 0.11. By convention this result would not be statistically significant and we would say that the association could have arisen by chance. If the same study had been twice as big (160 cases and 160 controls) we would have found the same odds ratio (1.7) but now the *p*-value would have been 0.02, so we would have concluded that the association *was* statistically significant. These problems associated with the blind dependence on *p*-values have led to suggestions from some epidemiologists that *p*-values should not be used at all for assessing associations. (For further discussion of this issue see Sterne and Smith, 2001).

reject the null hypothesis in error, i.e. you will conclude there is an association when really there is none, the chance that this will happen increases as you do more tests. For example, if you do 20 tests then you would expect to see 1 statistically significant result by chance; if you do 100 tests you would expect to see about 5 significant results by chance alone. This problem of 'multiple testing' (see Box 6.3) is not uncommon. In dietary studies, for example, people may look at dozens of different food items and genetic studies now often include hundreds of thousands or millions of genetic variants.

For these reasons, the epidemiological and wider health literature has seen a shift away from using *p*-values in recent years towards reporting confidence intervals because of the additional information they provide and to reduce the dependence on '$p < 0.05$' which, as you have seen, can be misleading or mean that important results are missed. A *p*-value simply gives an indication of whether an observed association could be 'due to chance' and there might really be no effect (i.e. the true RR or OR is 1.0). It effectively focuses on the

Box 6.3 The problem of multiple testing

The more hypotheses that we test, the more likely it is that some apparently statistically significant results will arise by chance. For this reason, statisticians often recommend 'correcting' for this problem of multiple testing. A simple form of this is to reduce the α-level at which a result is considered to be statistically significant based on the number of tests performed. For example, if 20 separate tests are conducted within a single study then the p-value at which a result is considered statistically significant would be reduced from 0.05 to $0.05 \div 20 = 0.0025$. The net result is that fewer results, those with the strongest associations, will be deemed statistically significant and, hopefully, these are also the results that are less likely to be due to chance. However many epidemiologists have pointed out the illogicality of such an arbitrary rule (for example, should an epidemiologist adjust their results based on the number of statistical tests performed that day or for the number of tests they have ever done? (Rothman, 1990)) and prefer to take a more common-sense approach. One notable exception is in the context of modern genetic studies, which may evaluate tens or hundreds of thousands of genetic markers at the same time. In this situation, increased stringency is essential to minimise the thousands of spurious results that will arise simply by chance if we accept a significance level of 5% (5% of 100,000 genes is ~5000 significant results by chance!). Results from the new 'genome-wide association studies' (GWAS) which may look at 1 million or more genetic variants in relation to disease are usually not considered statistically significant unless p is less than about 5×10^{-8} (0.00000005).

end of the confidence interval that is closest to the null (does this or does it not include the null value?) and ignores the other end completely. In contrast, the width of a confidence interval gives an indication of the precision of the estimate and the two bounds tell us both how weak the association might be and also how strong it might be. It is also important to remember that the real answer is most likely to be somewhere near the point estimate in the middle of a confidence interval. It is much less likely to be near the ends of the interval and even less likely to be outside it completely. Thus if an OR = 2.5 with a 95% CI from 0.9 to 6.9, then the real effect is much more likely to be close to 2.5 than it is to be close to 1.0; furthermore, it is just as likely to be close to 6.0 or 7.0 as it is to be as low as 1.0 (see Figure 6.3).

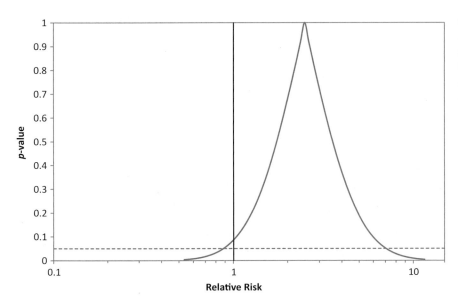

Figure 6.3 A typical *p*-value function (OR = 2.5; 95% CI = 0.9–6.9) showing the true effect is much more likely to be near the middle of the confidence interval than towards the ends.

Statistical versus clinical significance

Randomised controlled trials evaluating the drug finasteride for treatment of lower urinary tract symptoms in men have shown that there is a *statistically* significant improvement in symptom score (a measure of the symptoms experienced), from 2.5 to 2.8, in men treated with finasteride (Hirst and Ward, 2000). However, for men to experience a subjective change in quality of life, their symptom score has to change by at least three points. An increase of 0.3 points, although a 12% improvement, is therefore not *clinically* significant. This underscores the need to also consider how meaningful the result of a study is in practical terms; that is, we should assess a result in terms of its social, preventive, biological or clinical significance.

This is illustrated in Figure 6.4, which shows the results of four hypothetical intervention studies. In study (a) the result is both practically important and statistically significant because the point estimate falls beyond the '*minimum practically important difference*' line and the confidence interval does not include the value 1.0 (in fact, even the lower bound is above the minimum important difference line). The tightness of the confidence interval around the RR also gives reassurance of its precision. In study (b) the result is again practically important but not statistically significant, as the confidence interval is wide and does include 1.0. The width of the confidence interval suggests that the study was small, leaving imprecision and some uncertainty about the role of chance. The finding could be important but we really need more data for a confident judgement. In contrast, the results shown for (c) are statistically

Figure 6.4 Statistical and clinical significance: point estimates and confidence intervals from four hypothetical studies.

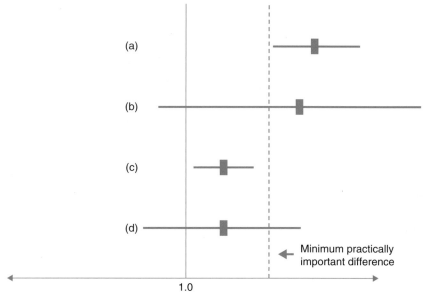

significant but not important, as in the finasteride example above. The narrow confidence interval tells us that our estimate is fairly precise (i.e. there are plenty of data). Finally, the results of study (d) are neither statistically significant nor practically important. This study provides little useful evidence about the benefit of the intervention – the very wide confidence interval that spans well across the null shows that this is a very poor test of the original hypothesis.

In summary, *statistical significance* is evident on looking at the *p*-values from appropriate statistical tests and from the confidence intervals around the point estimates; and the extra information the latter give as to the *precision* of an effect estimate is valuable. In health research where we are looking to improve outcomes through preventive, clinical or other interventions, we may have a fair idea of how big an effect needs to be for it to be *clinically or practically significant*. This might be a certain percentage improvement (i.e. a relative effect) or an absolute increase (as in the finasteride example above) and this might also have to be weighed against any adverse effects of the therapy. In observational (aetiological) epidemiology, however, there is no clear rule as to how big an effect should be for it to be meaningful. A relative risk greater than 2.0 would probably be considered fairly strong and thus, by implication, *practically significant*. An RR less than this would not, however, be dismissed immediately because, as you saw in the example of smoking and coronary heart disease in Table 5.4, a modest *relative risk* may still lead to a high *absolute* or *attributable risk*.

Summary

In any study there will always be an element of chance as to who is studied and who is not – this type of random error is called *sampling error*. As you have seen, statistical methods have been developed to assess the amount of sampling error that is likely to be present in any particular study and these are commonly presented in the form of confidence intervals and *p*-values from hypothesis tests. Epidemiologists usually prefer to use confidence intervals because these convey more information than a single *p*-value. Nonetheless, it remains easy to be seduced by statistics, so it is important to be able to interpret the results of a study practically, regardless of what the investigator might claim. Just because a result is 'statistically significant' does not mean that it could not have arisen by chance or that it is meaningful at a clinical or practical level. Conversely, just because a non-null result is not statistically significant it does not mean there is no association – just that the study did not have sufficient power to reliably measure an association of that magnitude. There is a difference between 'no association' and a possible association that is not statistically significant (see Figure 6.4). It is, however, important to reiterate that all of the preceding discussion of random sampling error assumes that any differences between the study population and the wider target population are random. If the study participants were not selected carefully and are not representative of the wider population (i.e. they differ from the target population in a *systematic* way) then we will introduce *selection bias* into the study. This is a completely separate issue and we will discuss it in more detail in the next chapter.

Questions

1. The authors of a study report a RR of 1.8 (95% CI 1.6–2.0) for the association between alcohol intake and cancer. The authors of a second study report an OR of 1.8 (95% CI 0.7–3.5) for the association between caffeine intake and the same cancer. What do the results of these studies tell us (i) about the studies and (ii) about risk factors for the cancer?

2. What is the best way to reduce sampling error in a study?
   (a) Select people from the population at random.
   (b) Increase the size of the study.
   (c) Calculate a 95% confidence interval for the results.
   (d) Use a more reliable instrument to measure exposure.

3. A randomised, placebo-controlled trial was conducted in Indonesia to study the effects of vitamin A for treating children with measles. The investigators reported a confidence interval for the relative risk of 0.26 to 0.94. Which of the following statements are true?

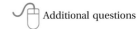 Additional questions

(a) Because the confidence interval does not include zero we can say the result is statistically significant.

(b) Because the confidence interval does not include zero we can say the result is not statistically significant.

(c) Because the confidence interval does not include the value 1.0 we can say the result is statistically significant.

(d) Because the confidence interval does not include the value 1.0 we can say the result is clinically significant.

4. What is the difference between statistical significance and clinical significance?

REFERENCES

 References

Fisher, R. A. (1950). *Statistical Methods for Research Workers*. London: Oliver and Boyd.

Herbst, A. L., Ulfelder, H. and Poskanzer, D. C. (1971). Adenocarcinoma of the vagina. Association of maternal stilbestrol therapy with tumor appearance in young women. *New England Journal of Medicine*, 284: 878–881.

Hirst, G. H. L. and Ward, J. E. (2000). Clinical practice guidelines: reality bites. *Medical Journal of Australia*, 172: 287–291.

Lau, J., Antman, E. M., Jimenez-Silva, J., *et al.* (1992). Cumulative meta-analysis of therapeutic trials for myocardial infarction. *New England Journal of Medicine*, 327: 248–254.

Rothman, K. J. (1990). No adjustments are needed for multiple comparisons. *Epidemiology*, 1: 43–46.

Sterne, J. A. and Smith, G. D. (2001). Sifting the evidence – what's wrong with significance tests? *Physical Therapy*, 81: 1464–1469.

RECOMMENDED FOR FURTHER READING

- A classic and very readable discussion of why adjustment is not needed for multiple comparisons:

    Rothman, K. J. (1990). No adjustments are needed for multiple comparisons. *Epidemiology*, 1: 43–46.

- A discussion of the uses and abuses of *p*-values and the concept of statistical significance:

    Sterne, J. A. and Smith, G. D. (2001). Sifting the evidence – what's wrong with significance tests? *Physical Therapy*, 81: 1464–1469.

All that glitters is not gold: the problem of error

Description	Association	Alternative explanations	Integration & interpretation	Practical applications
Chapters 2–3	Chapters 4–5	Chapter 7: Error	Chapters 9–11	Chapters 12–15

Box 7.1 Bigger isn't always better!

In the run-up to the 1936 presidential election in America, the *Literary Digest* conducted a poll of more than two million voters and confidently predicted that the Republican candidate, Alf Landon, would win. On the day it was the Democrat candidate, Franklin D. Roosevelt, who won a landslide victory. The *Digest* had correctly predicted the winner of the previous five elections, so what went wrong in 1936?

The *Digest* sent polling papers to households listed in telephone directories and car registration records. In 1936, however, telephone and car ownership were more common among more affluent households and these were the people who were also more likely to vote Republican. The generally less-affluent Democrat voters were thus under-represented in the sample of voters polled. In contrast, a young George Gallup conducted a much smaller poll of a few thousand representative voters and correctly predicted the Roosevelt win. As a result of this fiasco the *Digest* folded but Gallup polls are still conducted today.

We saw in Chapter 6 that larger studies are less likely to get the wrong results due to chance (or random sampling error) than smaller studies; however, the example in Box 7.1 shows that a large sample size is not sufficient to ensure we get the right results. The enormous presidential poll conducted by the *Literary Digest* didn't get the right answer because it included the 'wrong' people, i.e. they were not representative of everybody in the voting population. Furthermore, in epidemiology we frequently rely on records that have been collected for some other purpose, and we have already discussed some of the problems inherent in this in Chapter 3. Even when the data we use have been collected specifically for our research they are unlikely to be completely free of error. We often have to rely on people's memories, but how accurate are they? And biological measurements such as blood pressure and weight are often subject to natural variation as well as being affected by the performance of the measurement system that we use.

People live complicated lives and, unlike laboratory scientists who can control all aspects of their experiments, epidemiologists have to work with that complexity. As a result, no epidemiological study will ever be perfect. Even an apparently straightforward survey of, say, alcohol consumption in a community can be fraught with problems. Who should be included in the survey? How do you measure alcohol consumption reliably? All we can do when we conduct a study is aim to *minimise* error as far as possible, and then *assess the practical effects* of any unavoidable error. A critical aspect of epidemiology is, therefore, the ability to recognise potential sources of error and, more importantly, to assess the likely effects of any error, both in your own work and in the work of others. In this chapter we will point out some of the most common sources of such error in epidemiological studies and how these can best be avoided. We also want to emphasise from the outset that some degree of error is inevitable, but this need not invalidate the results of a study.

Sources of error in epidemiological studies

In an epidemiological study we usually want to measure the proportion of people with a particular characteristic or identify the association between an exposure and an outcome. To do this we have to recruit individuals into the study, measure their exposure and/or outcome status and then, if appropriate, calculate a measure of association between the exposure and outcome. We also want the results we obtain to be as close to the truth as possible. (Note that, although we will discuss error in the context of exposure and disease, when we talk about an exposure we mean anything from a gene to a particular behaviour, and the outcome need not be a disease but could be any health-related state.)

As you will discover, there are dozens of different names that have been given to the kinds of error that can occur in epidemiological studies. Fortunately, in practice, all types of error can be classified into one of two main areas: they relate either to the **selection** of participants for study or comparison, or to the **measurement** of exposure and/or outcome. These errors can in turn be either **random** or **systematic**. Random error or poor precision is the divergence, by chance alone, of a measurement from the true value. Systematic error occurs when measurements differ from the truth in a non-random way.

We will now discuss the main types of both selection and measurement error in more detail and will also consider the effects that they may have on the results of a study. Remember that in practice it is impossible to eliminate all error and the most important thing is therefore to consider the likely practical effects of any remaining error.

Selection bias

Depending on how we select subjects for our study, and how many we select, we can introduce both random and systematic sampling errors into our study. As you saw in the previous chapter, even if the people selected for a study are generally representative of the population that we wish to learn about (the target population), we may still get the wrong result just because of *random* sampling error, i.e. by chance, and this is especially likely when we take only a small sample. In contrast, the example in Box 7.1 shows how the results of even a large study can be biased if the sample of people selected for the study *systematically* differ from the population that we wish to learn about in some way.

Selection bias occurs when there is a systematic difference between the people who are included in a study and those who are not, or when study and comparison groups are selected inappropriately or using different criteria. Unlike random sampling error, we cannot reduce selection bias by simply increasing the size of the study sample – the problem persists no matter how large the sample.

The issue of selection bias is a major problem in simple descriptive studies such as prevalence surveys. If the sample of people included in the survey is not representative of the wider population the results of the survey can be very wrong, as the *Literary Digest* found in their biased opinion poll which under-represented the views of poorer Americans. In analytic studies, selection bias can add to the differences between groups being compared, thereby moving them further from the ideal of complete exchangeability that we discussed in Chapter 4. This will potentially lead to biased measures of association (OR, RR, AR or PAR). It is a particular concern in case–control studies because the participants are recruited as two separate groups and it can be difficult to ensure that the final control group makes an appropriate comparison group for the cases.

A similar problem can arise in cohort studies when the exposed and unexposed groups are recruited separately, for example when the exposed group comprises workers in a particular occupation or military group and a separate unexposed group has to be identified for comparison. However, in many cohort studies, such as the Framingham and Nurses' Health studies that we discussed in Chapter 4, we recruit a single group of participants and then classify them according to their exposure. In this situation the question of how individuals were recruited is usually less important in terms of the validity of the study results (what is often called **internal validity**). However, it can influence the **generalisability** or external validity of the findings because they may apply only to the sorts of people who took part. In some situations, however, selection bias (at the point of recruitment) can also bias the effect estimates from a cohort study. As an example, consider a cohort study examining the effect of children's socioeconomic status (SES) on their risk of injury. If the families of lowest SES are more likely to refuse to participate, then this group may be under-represented in the total cohort. In this situation, measurement of the risk of injury within the low SES group and comparisons with those of higher SES should still be accurate; the low SES group will just be smaller than it might have been had more low SES families participated. If, however, those families of lower SES who refuse to take part are also those whose children are at highest risk of injury, i.e. if participation is associated with both the exposure (SES) *and* the outcome (injury), then the study will underestimate the true amount of injury in this group. It will then also underestimate the effect of low SES on injury risk because the really high-risk children in that group were not included.

As for cohort studies, selection bias at recruitment and exposure assignment is not usually a major issue for internal validity in clinical trials, although it can occur if the allocation process is predictable and the decision whether or not to enter a person into the trial is influenced by the expected treatment assignment. For example, if alternate patients are assigned to receive active drug or placebo, a physician may decide not to enter sicker patients into the trial if he or she thought they were not going to be given the active drug. This selection bias *will* affect the internal validity of the study and is another reason why the allocation process should be truly random and ideally neither the investigators nor the participant should know what group the participant is in (see Chapter 4).

For both cohort and intervention studies the more important issue is to avoid or minimise 'loss to follow-up' because selection bias can arise if those who *remain* in a study are different from those who do not, i.e. the issue is selection *out* of the study population rather than selection *in*.

Some specific sources of selection bias

Some common ways in which selection bias can arise include the following.

Volunteers

It is well known that people who volunteer to participate in surveys and studies (i.e. they spontaneously offer their involvement rather than being selected in a formal sampling scheme) are different from those who do not volunteer. In particular, volunteers are often more health-conscious and, as a result, volunteer groups will often contain a lower proportion of, say, smokers than the general population. Advertisements calling for volunteers for a survey or study may also attract people who have a personal interest in the topic area. The prevalence of various diseases or behaviours in a volunteer group may thus be very different from that in the underlying population because of this self-selection into the study. This means that volunteer groups are completely unsuitable for surveys conducted to measure the prevalence of either health behaviours or diseases in the population and they are also likely to introduce bias into studies looking for associations between exposures and health outcomes. For this reason, epidemiological research rarely uses groups of haphazardly recruited volunteers and, if it does, it is advisable to pay close attention to whether this may have biased the results in some way.

Imagine a survey about a sensitive area such as sexual behaviour where participants were recruited via advertisements in women's magazines. How representative do you think the results would be of all women?

There are two potential problems with this type of recruitment. First, different magazines target different types of women so it is likely that the readers of one particular magazine will not be representative of all women. It is also likely that the women who choose to respond to a survey of this type will differ markedly from those who do not respond; for example, they may well be more confident and out-going and thus more likely to engage in less conventional sexual behaviours (Maslow and Sakoda, 1952). This exact issue plagued Kinsey who conducted some of the earliest work on sexual behaviour in the mid-1900s (Kinsey, 1948). He reported high levels of unconventional sexual behaviours in his study groups, but was roundly criticised for using samples of volunteers, prisoners and male prostitutes, thus raising concerns about the reliability of his results. Although Kinsey attempted to address these criticisms, the concerns remained and his results still cause controversy today.

Low response rates

What might be thought of as a type of volunteer bias, and one that again is a particular problem in surveys and case–control studies, is the problem of low response rates. People who have a particular disease are often highly motivated to take part in research into that disease. Controls, however, have no such motivation to participate and investigators are finding it increasingly hard to persuade healthy people to take part in research with the result that control participation rates are now often around 50%. Even if potential controls for a study are selected at random, if a large proportion do not agree to take part then the remaining group may no longer be a true random sample of the population and the results may be biased. Box 7.2 shows an example from a study looking at passive smoking and heart attack where the authors assessed and reported the likely extent of error in their estimates of smoking rates in the control group. This degree of thoroughness is commendable but, unfortunately, rarely seen due to logistical constraints. Note also how this information can be used to make a tentative practical assessment of the likely bias this error may have introduced into the estimate of the effect of passive smoking on heart disease.

Box 7.2 Differences between responders and non-responders

In a case–control study of the effects of passive smoking on the risk of heart attack or coronary death, the investigators put a lot of effort into trying to achieve a high response rate from controls. Potential controls were initially invited to attend a study centre where they would have blood collected and physical measurements taken as well as completing a risk factor question- naire. Participants who did not respond to this invitation were sent a shorter questionnaire to complete at home and some people who still did not respond were then visited and interviewed at their homes. There were thus three types of people among the control group: the willing volunteers who replied to the initial invitation, the slightly less willing who replied to the shorter home questionnaire and the even more reluctant who agreed to take part only when visited by an interviewer. The investigators then com- pared the prevalence of smoking in these three groups (Table 7.1).

The harder it was to persuade someone to take part in the study, the more likely they were to be a current smoker, especially for women. This suggests that those who refused completely probably had even higher smoking rates. The measured prevalence of smoking in the control group is therefore likely to be an underestimate of the true level of smoking in the whole population. Using the study data, the calculated odds ratio for the association between smoking and heart disease in men was 2.3. However, if the true proportion of current smokers in the population was actually 3% higher and the proportion of non-smokers 3% lower than in the study controls, then the true odds ratio would have been lower, about 1.8. The study would thus have overestimated the strength of the association.

Table 7.1 Prevalence of smoking increases with increasing reluctance to take part in a study.

Ease of recruitment	Never smoker (%)	Ex-smokers (%)	Current smokers (%)
Men (age 35–69 years)			
Full participation (willing)	35	40	24
Short questionnaire (less willing)	30	42	28
Home interview (reluctant)	29	42	29
Women (age 35–69 years)			
Full participation (willing)	67	19	14
Short questionnaire (less willing)	66	13	21
Home interview (reluctant)	53	16	31

(Dobson *et al.*, 1991)

Loss to follow-up

In a case–control study the main concern with subject selection is with regard to who is included in the study. For both cohort and intervention studies the more important issue is to avoid or minimise selective losses from the cohort or study group. This can be a particular problem if more people are 'lost to follow-up' in one exposure group than another (i.e. loss is associated with exposure) and if loss is also related to the outcome of interest. For example, imagine a randomised clinical trial comparing a new drug with the current standard treatment. If the sickest people in the intervention group withdrew from the trial, the people remaining in the intervention group would be healthier than those in the standard treatment group and the new drug would appear to be more beneficial than it really was. The opposite situation would occur if those who were doing well were *less* likely to return for assessments and thus were more likely to be lost to follow-up. In a cohort study, participants with socially stigmatised behaviours (which these days can include smoking cigarettes) may be both less easy to follow-up and more likely to develop the health conditions being studied.

Ascertainment or detection bias

This can occur if an individual's chance of being diagnosed as having a particular disease is related to whether they have been 'exposed' to the factor of interest. An example of this type of bias was seen in early studies of the association between oral contraceptive (OC) use and thromboembolism (a condition in which a blood clot develops in the legs and subsequently breaks off and moves to another part of the body, often the lungs). Doctors who were aware of the potential for this risk were more likely to hospitalise women with symptoms suspicious of thromboembolism if they were taking OCs. Early case–control studies, which were hospital-based, then overestimated the risk of thromboembolism associated with OC use. This was because the cases were more likely to be on OCs simply because of the way in which they were selected to be sent to hospital, because in the minds of their doctors this partly determined their diagnosis.

The healthy-worker effect

This is a well-documented type of selection bias that can occur in occupational studies. People who are working have to be healthy enough to do their job, so they tend to be more robust than the general population, which necessarily includes those who are disabled or seriously ill and hence unable to work. As a result, if occupational groups are compared with the general population – which is not uncommon in cohort studies of occupational hazards – they will almost always appear to be healthier overall. Comparisons

Box 7.3 Veterans' health

There is concern that men and women who saw active service in conflicts such as the Vietnam War have worse health than those who did not. Studies that have compared mortality rates among Vietnam veterans with those in the general population are hampered by the fact that the veterans had to pass a stringent medical examination at the time of their enlistment and so, at that time, were much more healthy than the average person. An analysis of mortality rates among male Australian Vietnam veterans found that, up until 1979, mortality among the veterans was actually 18% lower than in the general population (Table 7.2). It is highly unlikely that service in Vietnam would reduce a man's subsequent risk of death, so this inverse association is likely to be due entirely to the healthy-worker (or in this case, healthy-warrior) effect. It is impossible to say how large this effect might be and to assess whether it could actually be masking an underlying increase in mortality in the veterans.

However, in the years from 1980 to 2001, overall mortality among the veterans was similar to that in the general population and cancer mortality was more than 20% higher among the veterans. With the increasing time interval since enlistment, the healthy-worker effect will have been wearing off for most causes and it now appears that the veterans do have higher rates of cancer death compared with the general population. The question of veterans' health is now a major issue in many countries.

Table 7.2 Standardised mortality ratios (SMRs) and 95% confidence intervals (CIs) for selected causes of death among male Australian Vietnam veterans.

Cause of death and time period		SMR	(95% CI)
All causes:	1963–1979	0.82	(0.77–0.87)
	1980–1990	0.95	(0.90–0.99)
	1991–2001	0.99	(0.96–1.02)
Lung cancer:	1963–1979	0.59	(0.32–0.90)
	1980–1990	1.25	(1.05–1.45)
	1991–2001	1.21	(1.08–1.33)

(Wilson *et al.*, 2005)

within a workplace can also be flawed because different types of job often attract different types of people as well as requiring different levels of fitness. Imagine a study of the effects of heavy physical work on the occurrence of heart disease in which the investigators compared a group of manual labourers with a group of people of similar SES who had desk jobs. In this situation, people who had heart disease might be incapable of doing a manual job and therefore more likely to hold a desk job. The frequency of heart disease would thus appear to be higher in those with desk jobs, falsely suggesting that heavy work was protective against heart disease. Similar problems can arise in other groups where members are selected on the basis of physical capability, e.g. the armed forces (see Box 7.3).

Control of selection bias

The question of selection bias has to be considered and then potential bias eliminated or minimised in the design and conduct of a study. Any error introduced here that leads to inappropriate comparisons cannot easily be removed in the data analysis although, as shown in the example in Box 7.2, it is sometimes possible to estimate the effects of any such bias; we will discuss this further below.

In any study, it is important to have a clear definition of the population group that you want to study (the target population). This need not be everybody, but could be a specific subgroup of the whole population, and study participants should then be selected to represent this group. In a descriptive study it is essential to ensure that the study population really is representative of the target population or any measures of disease (incidence or prevalence) may be biased. In a case–control study the critical issues are defining the case group clearly and selecting an appropriate control group. Ideally all cases from the defined population would be included, but if only a sample is used they should be truly representative of all cases arising in the population. The controls should also be selected to be representative of the same population. (We discussed options for control selection in Chapter 4.) It is then important to ensure high participation rates among both cases and controls.

A good study will also have clearly defined *eligibility criteria* to determine whether specific individuals are included. For example, in a study of myocardial infarction, specific criteria developed by the World Health Organization might be used to define a case or, in a study of cancer, only those patients with histologically confirmed cancer might be eligible. Additional eligibility criteria might require people to fall within a certain age range (e.g. children are usually excluded from studies of adult diseases), reside in a defined area or be admitted to specific hospitals. Box 7.4 gives typical eligibility and exclusion criteria, here for a case–control study of ovarian cancer.

Note that the eligibility criteria describe the target population, i.e. all women who are *eligible* to take part in the study. For practical reasons some eligible women might later be *excluded* from the study. It is important to note that if large numbers of women are excluded, regardless of how good the reasons for

Box 7.4 Eligibility and exclusion criteria for a case–control study

Eligibility criteria for cases for a study of ovarian cancer could be as follows:

- A *histologically confirmed diagnosis*: the cancer must be confirmed by a pathologist.
- *Incident*: the woman must have no previous history of ovarian cancer.
- *Primary* ovarian cancer: the cancer must originate in the ovary; metastases (cancers that have spread from another anatomical site) would thus be excluded.
- *Age 18–79*: studies often exclude children for practical reasons and in this case ovarian cancer is very rare in children. Older adults are also commonly excluded, particularly if exposure information is to be collected by questionnaire or interview because the problems of recall increase with age.
- *Resident in a specific geographical area*: women who just happen to be diagnosed with ovarian cancer while visiting that region will be excluded.

Comparable eligibility criteria for the *controls* might then be the following:

- Women aged 18–79.
- Resident in the same specific geographical area.
- No previous history of ovarian cancer.
- No history of bilateral oophorectomy (i.e. they must have at least one ovary and so be at risk of developing ovarian cancer).

Exclusion criteria might include the following:

- Women who are unable to give informed consent (for example, they have dementia).
- Women who are too sick to participate (this decision might be made by the treating doctor).
- Women who do not speak English (if the main study documents are all in English it might not be financially viable to translate them into other languages).

this, then the resulting study sample might no longer be representative of the whole population. For example, the exclusion of very sick women might mean that cases of advanced cancer are under-represented in the study group. If advanced cancers differ somehow from early cancers in terms of their aetiology then this might affect the overall results. In experiments testing new treatments, older and sicker patients are often excluded, making it more likely that adverse drug effects will be missed, only to appear once the wider population is exposed to the drug.

Exclusion criteria in trials: In 1999 rofecoxib (Vioxx) was introduced as a new anti-inflammatory drug for management of osteoarthritis. It was withdrawn in 2004 because users had elevated risks of cardiovascular disease. One reason the adverse effects were not picked up sooner was that many of the early trials only enrolled people at low risk of cardiovascular disease (Krumholz *et al.*, 2007).

In a cohort study or trial, one of the most important criteria for a high-quality study is to ensure complete follow-up of all participants because, as you have seen, the more people who are 'lost to follow-up' with unknown health status, the more likely it is that the results will be biased. It is therefore important to have measures to maximise retention of people within the study and, if possible, to follow-up those who drop out of the study. Data linkage, which we discussed in Chapter 3, can be helpful here because if the outcome of interest is likely to be captured in routine health records it may be possible to obtain this information for all of the people in the study even if they have dropped out of the study or can no longer be contacted individually. For example, studies with cancer incidence or mortality as an outcome can often use population-based cancer or death registers to obtain this information.

Assessing the likely effects of selection bias on the results of a study

In practice, participation rates in studies are rarely 100%, so it is important to assess the likely extent of any bias and the potential impact, if any, of this on the results of the study. In descriptive studies the most important consideration is whether the observed level of something in the study sample is likely to be higher or lower than that in the wider population. In analytic studies the question is usually whether an observed association is entirely due to error, or would it still exist (and perhaps be even stronger) if the error could be eliminated? Conversely, if a study shows no association, could this be because a real effect has been masked because of the way the subjects were selected (bias) or because the study was just not big enough to show a clear association (chance)? Figure 7.1 summarises the issues regarding selection bias in analytic research and also the effects of random sampling error or chance that we discussed in the previous chapter. Unfortunately, while we can quantify the effects of random sampling error or chance, questions as to the possible presence and effects of any selection bias are often more difficult to answer – if people did not agree to take part in a study then there is usually very limited information about them. Any such consideration can, therefore, only be based on informed guesswork, and the results of any case–control study with low participation rates (particularly among controls) or of a cohort study or trial with high loss to follow-up are likely to be viewed with suspicion because of the possibility that some unaccounted-for selection bias could explain the results.

It is, however, important to note that even if selection bias exists, it does not necessarily invalidate an observed association between exposure and outcome. Problems occur when the probability that someone takes part in, or is lost from, a study is related to both the exposure *and* the outcome of interest and, specifically, if the exposure–outcome association differs among participants compared to non-participants (Carter *et al.*, 2012). Selection bias is

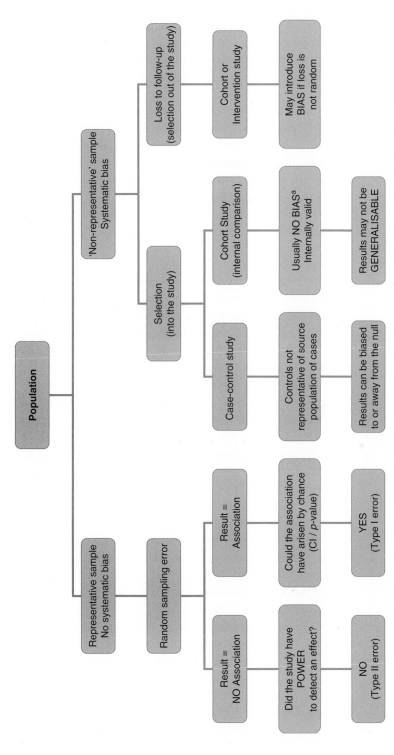

Figure 7.1 Random and systematic selection error and their consequences for effect estimation.

[a]The same cannot be said for cohorts with an external comparison group where factors like the healthy worker effect can introduce bias at this stage

particularly problematic in case–control studies because participation rates often differ greatly between cases, who have an interest in helping research into a condition that affects them, and controls who do not. As a result, the probability someone takes part in a case–control study is almost always associated with the outcome, so if it also differs by exposure status it may cause bias as in the example in Box 7.2, where people were less likely to participate as controls if they were smokers. Selection bias can also be an issue in cohort studies because loss to follow-up may be related to both the exposure and the outcome. For example, if, in a trial, those who are sicker (the outcome) and those taking the new drug (the exposure) are more likely to drop out of the study (due to ill health and treatment side effects, respectively), the results might over-state the effectiveness of the treatment being tested.

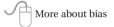 More about bias

External comparisons

Although it might not be possible to obtain information about the non-responders in a study, we may have some knowledge of the wider target population, allowing us to check for differences between it and the actual study population. For example, many countries have cancer registries, so in a case–control study of cancer we might be able to find some basic information such as the age and stage (extent of disease) distribution of all cancer patients diagnosed in a particular region at the time of the study. By comparing this information with that of the cases who took part in the study we can see whether the people who did not take part differ in some way from those who did, e.g. they might tend to be older and sicker. Similarly, it may be possible to extract information about possible risk factors such as smoking and alcohol consumption from a national health survey. If so, we can then compare, say, the smoking habits of the study population with those of the general population. If there are fewer smokers among the controls in a case–control study than in the general population, then the study may have overestimated the strength of the association between smoking and disease. For example, a recent study observed an odds ratio of 1.6 (95% CI 1.2–2.2) for the association between current smoking and risk of one type of ovarian cancer, but it was found that the proportion of current smokers in the control group was lower than would be expected from national statistics (13% vs. 19%) (Pandeya et al., 2009). By imputing (estimating) smoking status for the non-participating controls based on the assumption that the total control group should have had a similar prevalence of smoking to the general population, it was estimated that the true odds ratio would have been approximately 1.1 (95% CI 0.8–1.4). Thus, non-participation very likely biased the odds ratio upwards, making it seem as if smoking was associated with this type of ovarian cancer when, in all probability, there is really no association.

Sensitivity analysis

Even without such external data it is still possible to estimate the influence of bias on the results of a study by conducting what is known as a 'sensitivity analysis' (see Box 7.5). For example, if there is loss to follow-up in a cohort study or clinical trial, then imagine the worst-case scenario, i.e. that everyone lost from one group developed the outcome of interest and nobody lost from the other group did. How would that have affected the results of the study? What if the loss had been the other way around, or if only half of the people lost had developed disease? How bad would the loss have to have been to explain the whole association? If there is still an association after such

---

Box 7.5 The worst-case scenario

Imagine a study that compared a new anti-arrhythmic drug (drug A) with an older drug (drug B) for the prevention of sudden death. The results of this hypothetical study are given in Table 7.3.

From these results, drug A appears to reduce the risk of sudden death by about half (RR = 4.2 ÷ 8.6 = 0.49) compared with drug B. However, what if we find that some patients were lost to follow-up: 32 from group A and 16 from group B. The worst-case scenario (if we are hoping to find evidence in favour of drug A) would be if all the patients lost from group A had actually died from an arrhythmia while all those lost from group B were alive and feeling so well that they had decided not to return for follow-up. We can then recalculate the mortality for drug A on the basis of this scenario (the mortality for drug B will not change):

Mortality in group A if the 32 patients lost to follow-up died due to an arrhythmia = (36 + 32) ÷ 860 = 7.9 per 100 people

Drug A is still found to give a benefit compared with drug B, although the reduction in risk of mortality is now less than 10%. In practice it is highly unlikely that all participants lost to follow-up from group A had met an untimely arrhythmia-related death whereas none of those taking drug B had. The true reduction in risk for drug A is therefore likely to be greater than 10% and in this situation we might be happy to conclude that, even in the presence of the loss to follow-up, drug A was more useful than drug B.

Table 7.3 Results of a hypothetical study comparing two anti-arrhythmic drugs.

Drugs	Number of patients randomised	Number of sudden deaths	Mortality per 100 people
Drug A	860	36	4.2
Drug B	842	72	8.6

worst-case assumptions then the observed result cannot be an artefact due entirely to selection bias. (Note that this does not imply that the association is real, it could still be due to chance which we discussed in Chapter 6, measurement error which we discuss below or confounding (see Chapter 8).)

Quantitative bias analysis

There are ways to estimate the likely effects of selection bias (or measurement bias, see below) on the results of a study and to estimate what the results would have been in the absence of this bias. This *quantitative bias analysis* used to require the skills of an experienced statistician; however, there is now a range of more accessible tools and approaches that can be used to assess how bias might have affected an observed association (Lash *et al.*, 2009, 2014).

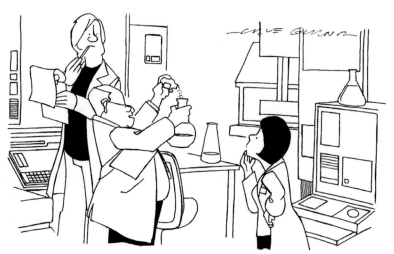

More about bias

From www.CartoonStock.com

Measurement or information error

We will now turn our attention to possible sources and effects of error in the information we collect from or about people. Few measures of exposure will be perfect and there may also be errors in the measurement of outcome, leading to **misclassification** of participants with respect to their exposure status and/or outcome (disease); i.e. someone may be labelled as 'exposed' (or as a 'case') when they were actually 'unexposed' (or a 'non-case'). This can then lead to bias in the results of the study. Some error can and will creep in whenever we measure or collect information from or about study participants and, as in the process of subject selection, this error (and any resulting misclassification) can be either random or systematic.

"...then we add a smidgin of this - that's less than a dollop, but more than a pinch... "

Random error

If you were to weigh yourself several times on the same set of scales, how similar would the results be? If there is little variation between the results we say that the measuring device is **precise**. If there is a lot of variation between the results then the precision is poor or, conversely, we have a lot of **random error**. Some measuring instruments will be better than others and although we would not expect to obtain exactly the same result every time, we would hope that if were measuring the same thing the results would all be close. If, for example, we measured someone's systolic blood pressure and the reading was 140 millimetres of mercury (mmHg), then, ideally, if we measured it again and again the results would all be close to this value – perhaps ranging from 137 to 143 mmHg. This would indicate that the measuring device was quite *precise*, i.e. it always gives approximately the same answer when measuring the same thing. But note that it tells us nothing about the **accuracy** of the measurement, i.e. whether the person's systolic blood pressure really is 140 mmHg.

Many biological parameters, including blood pressure, vary on a day-to-day, hour-to-hour and even minute-to-minute basis. Assuming that we always measure blood pressure under standard conditions and our participant has not, for example, just run up a flight of stairs, then any variation should again be largely random. Depending on when we take our measurements, we will obtain different readings that will vary around the patient's usual blood pressure. We will overestimate some people's blood pressure and we will underestimate it for others.

We can reduce random error and thus increase the precision of our measurements by taking repeated measurements on one subject, preferably on different occasions, and using the average value in the study. The more measurements we take, the more precise our answer will be. Note that this is analogous to our discussion of *precision* in the context of random sampling error or chance in the previous chapter.

Systematic error

Given that a measuring instrument was not 100% precise, we would expect some results to be a bit too high and some a bit too low, but we would still hope that the *average* results would be close to the true value. In other words, we want the device to be *accurate*. Consider the measurement of blood pressure again. If we use a sphygmomanometer that has not been calibrated for a year it might consistently read 10 mmHg too high. The person with a blood pressure of 140 mmHg would now appear to have a blood pressure of 150 mmHg. The precision of the measurements may be unchanged but, if we

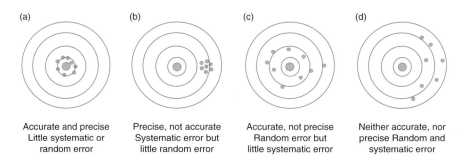

(a) Accurate and precise Little systematic or random error

(b) Precise, not accurate Systematic error but little random error

(c) Accurate, not precise Random error but little systematic error

(d) Neither accurate, nor precise Random and systematic error

were to make several measurements on each person and average them, we would find that the average value was always 10 mmHg too high. In this situation our measurements might be precise but they are not accurate because we are systematically recording everybody's blood pressure as 10 mmHg greater than it should be. We have, therefore, introduced **systematic error** or **bias** into our measurements. Unlike random error, systematic error cannot be reduced by taking repeated measurements.

We can summarise the effects of systematic and random error, or their inverse accuracy and precision, by analogy with target shooting (Figure 7.2). If someone is a good shot and they are using a gun with the sights properly aligned, their shots will tend to cluster closely around the bull's-eye in the centre (situation (a)). The shots are therefore both accurate (close to the centre) and precise (close to each other). However, if the sights on the gun are not aligned correctly, it will not be so accurate and the shooter might always hit a spot to the right of the centre (situation (b)). The results are still precise because they are tightly clustered around this point, but they are no longer accurate because they are consistently falling too far to the right. We have introduced a *systematic error*. If a less experienced shooter were to use the first gun then their shots would be more spread out, but they should still land around the bull's-eye (situation (c)). In this situation we have good accuracy because, on average, the shots are centred around the bull's-eye, but the shots are very spread out so we have more *random error* and thus less precision. Finally, an inexperienced shooter with a faulty gun would both miss the centre of the target and cover a wide area (situation (d)). In this situation we have neither accuracy nor precision. This visualisation shows how we can conceptualise the separate effects of accuracy and precision, i.e. systematic and random error.

The effects of measurement error

The effects of both biological variation and measurement error mean that measurements will never be perfect – even if there is no systematic error there will always be some degree of random error. If something is measured on a continuous scale (for example, weight in kilograms or height in centimetres) then random error alone will not lead to any bias in estimates of the *average* weight or height of the study population. This is because, although the weight of some people will be overestimated and the weight of others underestimated, if these errors are truly random, the overestimates and underestimates should cancel each other out when we calculate the average weight. However, problems arise in the presence of systematic error. If people systematically underestimate their weight then their average weight will be an underestimate of the true average for the population.

If instead of measuring something on a continuous scale we want to classify people into groups, for example normal and overweight, then both systematic *and* random errors will lead to **misclassification** of people into the wrong groups. Some normal-weight people will be wrongly labelled as overweight and vice versa. As you will see below, this misclassification will introduce bias into measures of association such as odds ratios and relative risks.

In addition to the degree of error in the measurement, a second important consideration when assessing the likely effects of measurement error is whether the errors and any subsequent misclassification are likely to be *the same* or *different* in the various study groups. In a case–control study we are usually concerned about whether errors in *exposure* measurement are the same for cases and controls. In a cohort study or a clinical trial we are often more concerned about whether the *outcome* measurement may have differed between the exposed and unexposed groups, although exposure measurement can also be an issue.

Non-differential misclassification

When measurement error and any resulting misclassification occur equally in all groups being compared, they are described as being *non-differential* (because they are the same or 'not different' in the various groups). For example, **non-differential error** occurs when the amount and type of error in exposure measurement is the same for cases and controls in a case–control study, or error in measurement of outcome is the same for the exposed and unexposed groups in a cohort study.

Imagine a case–control study in which everything is measured perfectly, with no error. The results of this hypothetical study are shown in Table 7.4 and the true odds ratio for the association between exposure and outcome is 1.80.

As we have noted above, the instrument used to measure exposure (this could be a biological test, a measuring device or a questionnaire) will, in practice, almost always have some degree of random error that results in non-differential misclassification. Imagine that 10% of all people who are exposed are misclassified as unexposed and 10% of all unexposed people are

Table 7.4 The 'true' results of a hypothetical case–control study with no measurement error.

	Cases	Controls	Total
Exposed	300	250	550
Unexposed	100	150	250
Total	400	400	800

$$OR = \frac{300 \times 150}{100 \times 250}$$
$$= 1.80$$

10% **misclassification** is the same as saying that the instrument has 90% **sensitivity** and **specificity**; it correctly identifies 90% of those who are exposed (sensitivity) and 90% of those who are unexposed (specificity). We will discuss sensitivity and specificity in more detail in Chapter 15.

Table 7.5 The effect of non-differential random measurement error: 10% of all cases and controls are misclassified with regard to their exposure status.

	Cases	Controls	Total
Exposed	300 – 30 + 10 = 280	250 – 25 + 15 = 240	520
Unexposed	100 – 10 + 30 = 120	150 – 15 + 25 = 160	280
Total	400	400	800

$$OR = \frac{280 \times 160}{120 \times 240}$$
$$= 1.56$$

misclassified as exposed. The key point here is that the misclassification is *non-differential*, namely it affects everyone in the study to the same degree. In this situation 10% or 30 of the 300 exposed cases and 25 of the 250 exposed controls will be misclassified as unexposed. In addition, 10% or 10 of the 100 unexposed cases and 15 of the 150 unexposed controls will be misclassified as exposed. This means that, instead of obtaining the true picture shown in Table 7.4, our results would look like Table 7.5.

With 20% **misclassification** instead of 10%, the odds ratio would have been

$$\frac{260 \times 170}{140 \times 230} = 1.37$$

With 30% misclassification it would have been only

$$\frac{240 \times 180}{160 \times 220} = 1.23$$

Because we have randomly misclassified some of the cases and controls with regard to their exposure, we have obtained an odds ratio of only 1.56 instead of the true odds ratio of 1.80. This makes the association seem weaker than it really is; i.e. the effect estimate, in this case an odds ratio, is biased towards the null. Note that complex exposures such as diet are particularly hard to measure and levels of misclassification are likely to be much greater than 10%. In this situation any measures of relative risk would be biased even closer towards 1.0 and real effects can disappear completely.

As we discussed above, non-differential misclassification due to random measurement error is a fact of life; it is also possible to have non-differential misclassification due to systematic measurement error if the systematic error occurs equally in all study groups. For example, 'food frequency questionnaires' ask people to report how often, on average, they eat each of a list of individual food items. When confronted with a list of 10 or 20 different vegetables people will often overestimate the total number of servings of vegetables they eat each day. If we then classify them according to whether or not they ate the recommended number of servings of vegetables per day, we would systematically misclassify some people with low vegetable intake into the high intake group and this might happen equally for cases and controls. If, for example, in the study shown in Table 7.4, 20% of all unexposed people, both cases and controls, were systematically misclassified as exposed then we would obtain an odds ratio of 1.71 which would again underestimate the true value of 1.80. Note that while these examples have all considered the effects of non-differential exposure misclassification on a case–control study, exactly the same effects occur in a cohort study (see question 5 at the end of the chapter for an example of this), or if the outcome is equally poorly measured in the unexposed and exposed groups in a cohort study or trial.

To summarise, *in the presence of non-differential misclassification of exposure (or outcome), either random or systematic, estimates of the association between exposure and outcome will usually be underestimates of the true effect.*[1] In other words, the odds ratio or relative risk will almost always be biased towards the null and the true effect will therefore be further from the null than the observed effect. This means that if a study gives a relative risk of 2.0 (or 0.8) but there is likely to be non-differential misclassification, then the true association is likely to be even stronger than that observed (i.e. > 2.0 or < 0.8). *However, non-differential misclassification can also make it harder to detect a real association.* If a relative risk is close to 1.0 this could indicate that there is really no association, or it could be a consequence of misclassification that has made a stronger effect look weaker than it really is. Also, although this is the norm, it is important to note that in some situations non-differential misclassification can bias estimates away from the null. This can happen simply by chance but is more common when we classify exposure into more than two groups (see Box 7.6 for an example).

Differential misclassification

When the measurement error and resulting misclassification occur to a greater extent in one group than another they are described as being **differential**. The effects of differential misclassification are generally harder to predict than those of non-differential misclassification.

In contrast to random error which, as discussed above, is commonly non-differential because it is usually an inherent property of the exposure being measured or the measuring device and thus affects everyone in the study, *systematic error* is often differential. It is a particular problem in standard case–control studies in which cases already have the disease of interest when the exposure information is collected or measured and so they might recall their exposure differently from controls; this type of error is known as **recall bias**.

---

[1] All else being equal; the results may still of course be influenced by other types of error.

Box 7.6 When non-differential misclassification does not bias towards the null

If an exposure has more than one level, then misclassification between two of the groups will make those two groups look more similar than they really are. In a case–control study of smoking and respiratory disease, for example, participants might be classified as non-smokers, light smokers or heavy smokers. The distinction between smoker and non-smoker is likely to be fairly clear (and for simplicity we will assume that it is perfect), but there will inevitably be some misclassification between the light and heavy smoking groups. If the non-smokers form the reference group, the misclassification will make the odds ratios for light and heavy smokers more similar than they should be. The effect of this will be to bias the odds ratios for the highest group (heavy smokers) towards the null again, but the odds ratio for the *middle group* (light smokers) will now be biased away from the null (Table 7.6). Overall, however, the net result is that the association is weakened.

Table 7.6 Non-differential misclassification can bias away from the null when there are more than two exposure groups.

	Cases	Controls	Odds ratio
Truth			
Non-smokers	150	200	1.0
Light smokers	120	125	1.3
Heavy smokers	130	75	2.3
20% of light smokers misclassified as heavy smokers and vice versa			
Non-smokers	150	200	1.0
Light smokers	122	115	1.4
Heavy smokers	128	85	2.0

For example, the cases in a case–control study of respiratory disease might systematically overestimate the amount of passive smoking they had been exposed to because they thought that this might have caused their disease. The controls, however, would have no such reason to overestimate their exposure. This might make it look as if passive smoking was associated with respiratory disease even if there was really no difference between the cases and controls.

Imagine that, in the hypothetical study shown in Table 7.4, cases overestimated their exposure and, as a result, 20% of unexposed cases were systematically misclassified as exposed, but controls were not affected.

How many of (a) the 100 unexposed cases and (b) the 150 unexposed controls would have been misclassified as exposed?

So, in total, how many (a) cases and (b) controls would have been classified as exposed and how many as unexposed?

What would the odds ratio have been?

Is this an underestimate or an overestimate of the true odds ratio?

In this situation, 20% or 20 of the 100 unexposed cases but none of the unexposed controls would be misclassified as exposed and, instead of the true picture shown in Table 7.4, we would obtain results that looked like Table 7.7 giving an odds ratio of 2.4.

We have now overestimated the true odds ratio of 1.80, making the association seem stronger than it really is. If the systematic misclassification had gone the other way and exposed cases had been misclassified as unexposed, or unexposed controls had been misclassified as exposed, then the bias would have gone in the opposite direction and we would have underestimated the effect.

Random error is less likely to be differential unless, for example, we used different measuring devices with differing levels of precision in the different study groups; however, if present, it too can make an association look either weaker or stronger than it really is (see question 6 at the end of the chapter for an example). *The best way to avoid differential random error and any consequential misclassification is thus to ensure that exactly the same instruments and methods are used in all of the different study groups.*

To summarise, if there is either systematic or random misclassification of exposure or outcome (see Box 7.7 for an example of this) in a study and this occurs *to a different extent in the two study groups* (cases and controls or exposed and unexposed) then the study results can be biased either up or down, i.e. towards or away from the null value, and it is often impossible to know which way the bias would have gone or how large the effect might be. This type of misclassification can be very difficult to deal with because, unless you have some idea of how much misclassification is occurring and where it is occurring, you cannot work out what the true results should have been.

Table 7.7 The effects of differential systematic misclassification: 20% of unexposed cases, but *not* controls, are misclassified as exposed.

	Cases	Controls	Total
Exposed	300 + 20 = 320	250	570
Unexposed	100 − 20 = 80	150	230
Total	400	400	800

$$OR = \frac{320 \times 150}{80 \times 250}$$
$$= 2.40$$

Box 7.7 Misclassification of the outcome

This can be a particular issue in cohort studies, especially if they rely on self-reporting of events. If those who are exposed are more (or less) likely to report the outcome, perhaps because of preconceived beliefs about what causes the outcome, then the association may be over- (or under-) estimated. For example, when followed-up by telephone, American veterans who had served in Vietnam (the exposure of interest) reported higher rates of a variety of medical conditions than did non-Vietnam veterans. However, when a subset of the veterans was examined more thoroughly, there was little real difference between those who had and had not served in Vietnam (CDC, 1988). Note that the analysis presented in Box 7.3 was based on routine statistics and not on self-report by the veterans themselves, so it is not subject to the same types of error.

Misclassification of the outcome is also possible in case–control studies if the disease is quite common and can only be reliably diagnosed (or ruled out) by an invasive test, for example some pre-cancerous conditions like endometriosis and Barrett's oesophagus. In this situation it is usually impossible to check all of the controls to ensure that they are truly free of disease and if the control group does include a proportion of people with undiagnosed disease, then any association between exposure and disease will appear weaker than it really is.

Sources of measurement error

As you will have gathered, almost every study will be subject to some degree of measurement error. One common but easily avoidable source of bias is the use of different instruments or measuring systems for different study groups or parts of groups. Examples of this include the use of different laboratories to analyse biological specimens, different locations for interviews of cases and controls (e.g. hospital versus home) and different interview methods (face-to-face versus telephone interview or postal questionnaire). Other particularly troublesome sources of error are the possibilities of recall bias and interviewer or observer bias.

Recall bias

Some degree of recall error is inevitable in any epidemiological study that requires participants to remember their past exposures. If this error is random and if it occurs equally in all study groups (i.e. it is non-differential) then the effects will usually be to bias the effect estimates towards the null. What can be more problematic is *recall bias* which, as we noted above, can occur in case–control studies and cross-sectional studies if cases (or those with disease in a cross-sectional study) are systematically more likely to over- or underestimate their exposure than controls. For example, if an exposure is thought to cause disease, then cases might be more likely to recall or to exaggerate their past exposure than controls, leading to overestimation of the effect of that exposure on disease (as in the passive smoking example above). The opposite effect would occur if cases tended to underestimate their exposure because they feel guilty about it. This could occur, for example, in a study of the effects of sunburn in childhood on the occurrence of childhood skin cancer. If mothers are asked whether their children have ever been sunburnt, the mothers of children with cancer might tend to underestimate (or under-report) the occurrence of sunburn in their children if they felt guilty for allowing their children to get burned when they were young. This could lead to falsely low estimates of the frequency of sunburn in cases and consequently a weakened association between sunburn and skin cancer.

It is difficult to know, even qualitatively, the extent to which recall bias may operate in any given study, so a great deal of effort is put into designing information collection systems to limit the likelihood of it occurring. Examples include the use of highly structured questionnaires, standard prompts and so forth. Recall bias has been a major concern in the field of melanoma epidemiology because of the growing public awareness of the risks of sun exposure. However, an analysis of data from a case–control study nested within an existing cohort, where exposure information was collected both *before* and *after* the cases were diagnosed, did not give any consistent evidence of substantive recall bias being present for a range of sun-related exposures (Gefeller, 2009). Nonetheless, this does not mean that we can ignore the need to capture data as objectively as possible to minimise this potentially important measurement flaw.

Interviewer or observer bias

Differential error may also occur if data collectors ask questions or record information in a different way for cases and controls (or for exposed and unexposed groups in a cohort study or randomised trial). For instance, an interviewer who knows the case/control status of a subject may probe more deeply with the cases than with the controls, resulting in differences in the quality of exposure data obtained for the two groups. Similarly, if in a cohort study or trial the observers know whether or not a person is exposed or unexposed (or treated/untreated), they may be more or less likely to diagnose the outcome of interest. A logical way to avoid these possibilities is to blind the interviewers/observers to the subject's status, although this is often not possible. Again, the use of objective criteria for outcome assessment, structured questionnaires and interview schedules, training and tape-recording interviews for quality control all help minimise interviewer bias.

Control of measurement error

It is difficult to get rid of measurement error once it has occurred and so it is important to minimise the potential for error at the design stage of the study. Whether you are conducting your own research or reading the reports of others, some important things to consider include the following.

Definitions

Everything that is measured in a study needs to be carefully defined. If the exposure is smoking, what makes someone a smoker? Anyone who has ever smoked a cigarette? 10 cigarettes? 100 cigarettes? A cigarette a day for six months? Are we only interested in current smokers? Those who have smoked within the last few years? Or anyone who has smoked at any time? Or does it matter how many cigarettes someone smoked each day? In practice most people probably try a cigarette at one time or another, so to classify them all as smokers would not be sensible. Common definitions that have been used are that someone should have smoked at least 100 cigarettes in their lifetime or that they should have smoked at least one cigarette a day for a defined period, usually a few months. If we want to estimate the effect of increasing dose (amount) of smoking we might want to measure lifetime exposure in 'pack-years' where one pack-year is equivalent to smoking a pack of 20 cigarettes daily for a year.

In addition to the important distinctions of exposed/unexposed (and of case/non-case in a cohort study or trial), it is also essential to have clear definitions and good measurements of the cofactors being measured. These are other factors that may influence (or 'confound' – see Chapter 8) the results of a study, e.g. age, SES, smoking, etc.

Choice of instrument

Instruments in epidemiological studies can include sophisticated laboratory tests, detailed questionnaires, or even simple observations. Inevitably the method of measurement used will influence the degree of error in the data. A set of scales that weigh to the nearest 100 g would be more accurate than scales that weigh to the nearest kilogram. It is relatively easy to collect dietary data from large numbers of people using a food frequency questionnaire (FFQ) which asks people to report how often they ate various food items over the previous months. However, people find it hard to accurately report their average consumption of a long list of foods. Diet diaries avoid this problem by asking people to record exactly what they ate over a few days, but they are more costly to administer, harder to analyse and, while they may give an accurate picture of what someone has eaten recently, this may not represent their usual diet.

Ideally the instrument used should be that which minimises both *random* and *systematic* error. Consideration should also be given to the circumstances of time and place of use of the instrument, as these may also affect the results obtained. For example, a face-to-face interview with a trained interviewer might elicit more reliable information than a questionnaire completed by the study participants themselves, but it would also be more expensive. And there are always exceptions – use of self-completed computer-based questionnaires may well capture more reliable data on use of illicit or socially stigmatised behaviours than in-person interviews.

Quality control

Whatever measuring devices are used, they need to be standardised. Instruments need regular calibration against a standard value and interviewers need training in a standard approach to obtaining data. Structured questionnaires help here, too. If the study continues for some time, consistency should also be monitored and maintained.

Assessment of measurement error

The two main issues in measurement are (i) is the instrument accurate (i.e. no systematic error), and (ii) is it precise (minimal random error)?

Assessing accuracy

In some situations accurate measuring devices or tests are available but too complex or costly to use on everyone in the study, so the investigators have to use a simpler or cheaper and less-accurate tool. In this situation it is good practice to conduct a *validation study* in which both the accurate expensive ('gold standard') test and the simpler, potentially less accurate test are used on a subset of people in the study and the results are compared (see e.g. Willet *et al.*, 1985 and 'Measuring & validating dietary data' online). It may then be possible to 'correct' the results of the study for any inaccuracies in the cheaper test (we will not consider the mechanics of this here).

Assessing precision

Another desirable way to test how well a measuring device performs is to measure its 'repeatability' or precision. If the same thing is measured on two different occasions or by two different people, how well do the two measurements compare? This might simply be a case of repeating laboratory tests on

Measuring & validating
dietary data

some samples, or it might involve asking some study participants to complete a study questionnaire twice on two different occasions to see how well their answers agree. In a cohort study that has repeated measures over time (such as the Nurses' Health Study), the values can be averaged over time to give better precision.

Assessing the likely effects of measurement error on the results of a study

By now it will be clear that there will always be some random measurement error in any data and thus if subjects have been classified into different exposure groups, there will always be some misclassification, the extent of which will depend on the variable being studied and the tool used to measure it. Things like age and height do not change (or change predictably) and can be measured fairly easily. In contrast, we have alluded to the fact that complex factors like diet and physical activity are very hard to measure and so will be associated with a lot more misclassification. On top of this there may also be systematic error such as recall bias, particularly when we use case–control and cross-sectional designs.

The important thing is to assess the likely impact of any such error on the results of the study. Is it possible that an observed association is entirely due to error, or would the association still exist (and perhaps be even stronger) if the error could be eliminated? As shown in Figure 7.3, *the key question in a survey is whether the error is random or systematic.* Random errors should not lead to biased estimates of descriptive statistics such as means, but systematic errors will. In contrast, when looking for associations between exposure and outcome *the central issue is whether any error and resulting misclassification is likely to be non-differential or differential*; i.e. is it likely to have occurred to the same extent in all study groups or to a differing extent in different groups? As

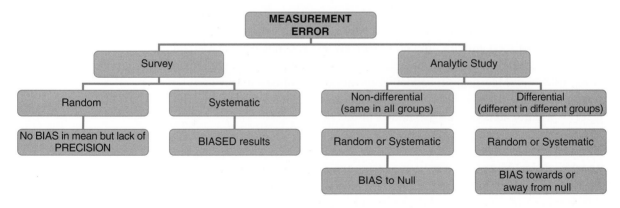

Figure 7.3 An overview of the types and consequences of measurement error.

Table 7.8 The likely effects of misclassification on the results of a case–control study.

Type of error/ misclassification	True odds ratio (OR)	Study results	Type of bias
Non-differential	2.0	≥ 1.0 but < 2.0	Result biased towards null but not below
	1.0	1.0	No effect if there is no association
	0.5	> 0.5 but ≤ 1.0	Result biased towards null but not above
Differential – cases overestimate (or controls underestimate) exposure	2.0	> 2.0	Result biased upwards with no upper limit. An inverse association (OR < 1.0) could appear to be a positive association (OR > 1.0)
	1.0	> 1.0	
	0.5	> 0.5	
Differential – cases underestimate (or controls overestimate) exposure	2.0	< 2.0	Result biased downwards. A positive association (OR > 1.0) could appear to be a inverse association (OR < 1.0)
	1.0	< 1.0	
	0.5	< 0.5	

you have seen, the likely effects of non-differential misclassification (either random or systematic) are to bias the estimates of effect (RR or OR) towards the null, making associations look weaker than they really are or, in some situations, masking them altogether. However, differential misclassification can bias estimates upwards or downwards, towards or away from the null. If information from a validation study is available, it may be possible to 'correct' the results of a study to allow for the fact that the measurements were not perfect, although any such correction will also be imperfect. *Sensitivity analysis* involves repeating the data analysis using different assumptions in the same way as we did to assess the effects of loss to follow-up above (look back to Box 7.5): if a proportion of subjects were misclassified, what effect would this have had on the results? As noted above for selection bias, *quantitative bias analysis* can also be used to assess the likely presence and effects of measurement bias (Lash *et al.*, 2009, 2014).

At the very least, it is essential to assess the likely degree of measurement error and/or misclassification and then make some judgements as to how this might have affected the results. Table 7.8 summarises the likely effects of misclassification on the estimates of an odds ratio under different scenarios. We will come back to this challenge in Chapter 9.

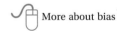 More about bias

Summary

No epidemiological study will be perfect. The important thing, therefore, is to minimise errors and then evaluate the likely effect of any remaining error, and we will come back to this again when we look at how to read (or write) and interpret epidemiological papers in Chapter 9. For now, we can summarise the problem of error as follows: errors can be *random* or *systematic* and can relate to *subject selection* or to *measurement* of exposure and/or outcome. The effects of *random sampling error* can be assessed from a confidence interval, but *systematic selection bias* is not so easily assessed, and is therefore a major concern in surveys. It can also be a problem in case–control studies, particularly with regard to selection of the control group. In cohort studies or clinical trials selection bias is more likely to occur if people are lost to follow-up and loss is related to both exposure and outcome. In a survey, *systematic measurement error* is a bigger problem than random error. In analytic studies, the important distinction is between *non-differential error* (it occurs equally in all study groups), which will usually bias the study results towards the null, and *differential error* (it occurs to a different extent in the different study groups), which can bias the study results either towards or away from the null.

We have now considered two of the three possible 'alternative explanations' for an observed association, namely chance and bias. In the next chapter we will discuss the third major threat to the internal validity of epidemiological and other health research: confounding.

Questions

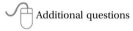
Additional questions

1. Imagine that a research team wanted to estimate the prevalence of vegetarianism in the community by means of a short questionnaire distributed with a women's health magazine. Would this give an accurate picture of the percentage of people who were vegetarians?

2. In a case–control study of liver disease and alcohol consumption, all patients in a community who had been newly diagnosed with liver disease were recruited as cases and people without liver disease were selected at random from the community to act as controls. All of the cases and controls were then asked about their alcohol intake. Only 25% of the controls selected from the community agreed to take part in the study.
   (a) Do you think that people with a high alcohol intake would be more or less likely to agree to take part in the study than average?
   (b) Is alcohol consumption in the controls likely to be higher, the same as, or lower than in the whole community?
   (c) What effect would this have on the estimate of the association between alcohol and liver disease?

3. Look back at the hypothetical study shown in Table 7.4 and imagine that the measurement instrument *systematically* overestimated people's exposure and, as a result, 15% of all unexposed people, both cases and controls, were misclassified as exposed.
   (a) Is this misclassification differential or non-differential? Why?
   (b) In the presence of this misclassification is the observed odds ratio likely to be an overestimate or an underestimate of the true odds ratio?

   (c) How many of (i) the 100 unexposed cases and (ii) the 150 unexposed controls would have been wrongly misclassified as exposed?

   (d) So, in total, how many (i) cases and (ii) controls would have been classified as exposed and how many as unexposed using the flawed measuring tool?

   (e) What would the odds ratio have been?

4. Now imagine that cases underestimated their exposure and, as a result, 20% of exposed cases were falsely classified as unexposed, but that the classification of controls was not affected.

   (a) Is this type of misclassification random or systematic? Is it differential or non-differential? Why?

   (b) What effect would it have had on the results of the study?

   (c) Compare your answer to (b) with that in Table 7.7, where cases systematically *overestimated* their exposure.

5. Imagine that in a cohort study 10% of *all exposed people* were misclassified as unexposed.

   (a) Is this misclassification random or systematic? Non-differential or differential? And why?

   (b) What effects would the misclassification have on the incidence of disease in (i) the exposed cohort and (ii) the unexposed cohort?

   (c) What effect would this have on the observed relative risk?

6. Imagine that all of the cases in a case–control study had their blood pressure measured by a single doctor at the local hospital but, for practical reasons, the controls had their blood pressure measured by their local doctor. In this situation it is likely that there would be less random error in the blood pressure readings for cases that came from a single doctor than in those for controls that came from a number of different doctors.

   (a) Recalculate the results of the hypothetical case–control study shown in Table 7.4 assuming that the measurement of exposure among cases was perfect but 20% of exposed controls were randomly misclassified as unexposed, and vice versa.

   (b) Is this misclassification differential or non-differential and why?

   (c) What effect has it had on the odds ratio and why?

   (d) What would the effect have been if we had misclassified cases instead of controls?

REFERENCES

Carter, K. N., Imlach-Gunasekara, F., McKenzie, S. K. and Blakely, T. (2012). Differential loss of participants does not necessarily cause selection bias. *Australian and New Zealand Journal of Public Health*, 36: 218–222.

CDC (Centers for Disease Control). (1988). Health status of Vietnam veterans. II. Physical health. *Journal of the American Medical Association*, 259: 2708–2714.

Dobson, A. J., Alexander, H. M., Heller, R. F. and Lloyd, D. M. (1991). Passive smoking and the risk of heart attack or coronary death. *Medical Journal of Australia*, 154: 793–797.

Gefeller, O. (2009). Invited commentary: Recall bias in melanoma – much ado about almost nothing? *American Journal of Epidemiology*, 169: 267–270.

Kinsey, A. C. (1948). *Sexual Behavior in the Adult Male*. Philadephia, PA: W. B. Saunders.

Krumholz, H. M., Ross, J. S., Presler, A. H. and Egilman, D. S. (2007). What have we learnt from Vioxx? *British Medical Journal*, 334: 120–123.

Lash, T. L., Fox, M. P. and Fink, A. K. (2009). *Applying Quantitative Bias Analysis to Epidemiologic Data*. New York, NY: Springer. Spreadsheets for conducting bias analysis can be downloaded from https://sites.google.com/site/biasanalysis/, accessed 25 February 2015.

Lash, T. L., Fox, M. P., MacLehose, R. F., Maldonado, G., *et al.* (2014). Good practices for quantitative bias analysis. *International Journal of Epidemiology*, 43: 1969–1985.

Maslow, A. H. and Sakoda, J. M. (1952). Volunteer error in the Kinsey study. *Journal of Abnormal Psychology*, 47: 259–262.

Pandeya, N., Williams, G. M., Green, A. C., *et al.* (2009). Do low control response rates always affect the findings? Assessments of smoking and obesity in two Australian case–control studies of cancer. *Australian and New Zealand Journal of Public Health*, 33: 312–319.

Willett, W. C., Sampson, L., Stampfer, M. J., *et al.* (1985). Reproducibility and validity of a semiquantitative food frequency questionnaire. *American Journal of Epidemiology*, 122: 51–65.

Wilson, E. J., Horsley, K. W. and van der Hoek, R. (2005). *Australian Vietnam Veterans Mortality Study 2005*. Canberra: Department of Veterans' Affairs.

RECOMMENDED FOR FURTHER READING

- More about quantitative bias analysis and tools for doing it:

    Lash, T. L., Fox, M. P. and Fink, A. K. (2009). *Applying Quantitative Bias Analysis to Epidemiologic Data*. New York, NY: Springer. Spreadsheets for conducting bias analysis can be downloaded from https://sites.google.com/site/biasanalysis/, accessed 25 February 2015.

    Lash, T. L., Fox, M. P., MacLehose, R. F., Maldonado, G., *et al.* (2014). Good practices for quantitative bias analysis. *International Journal of Epidemiology*, 43: 1969–1985.

Muddied waters: the challenge of confounding

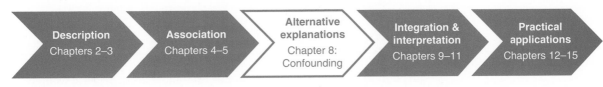

Description	Association	Alternative explanations	Integration & interpretation	Practical applications
Chapters 2–3	Chapters 4–5	Chapter 8: Confounding	Chapters 9–11	Chapters 12–15

Box 8.1 Are university admissions biased towards men?

Table 8.1 shows that in one year a prestigious university admitted 52% of male applicants compared with only 45% of female applicants, suggesting that there was a bias in favour of men. When quizzed about this, the two main faculty heads said that it couldn't be true, they had both admitted a higher proportion of women than men: the success rate in arts was 38% for women and only 32% for men and that in science was 66% for women compared with only 62% for men. How can this be?

    This is an example of *Simpson's paradox*, an extreme form of confounding where an apparent association observed in a study is in the

(*continued*)

Box 8.1 (*continued*)

Table 8.1 University admissions.

Faculty	Men Applicants	Admitted	Percentage	Women Applicants	Admitted	Percentage
Arts	4,100	1,300	32	8,250	3,150	38
Science	8,200	5,100	62	2,900	1,900	66
Total	12,300	6,400	52	11,150	5,050	45

direction to the true association. In this example it arose because women were much more likely to apply to arts courses, for which applicants had a lower overall success rate.

(Based on an analysis of graduate admissions data conducted at the University of California, Berkeley (Bickel *et al.*, 1975).)

In Chapters 6 and 7 we considered two reasons why the results of a study might not be the truth, namely chance and error or bias. In this chapter we will consider a third possible 'alternative explanation' – confounding.

Confounding refers to a mixing or muddling of effects that can occur when the relationship we are interested in is confused by the effect of something else. It arises when the groups we are comparing are not completely *exchangeable* and so differ by factors other than their exposure status (whether they are 'exposed' or 'not exposed'). If one (or more) of these other factors is a cause of both the exposure and the outcome, then some or all of an observed association between the exposure and outcome may be due to that factor. For example, if in a cohort study we observe that people with yellow fingers have a higher incidence of lung cancer compared to those who do not have yellow fingers, does this mean that having yellow fingers causes you to get lung cancer? Of course, the reason we see this association is because the exposure 'yellow fingers' and the outcome 'lung cancer' share a common cause – tobacco smoking (Figure 8.1). The exposure groups we are comparing (those with and without yellow fingers) are therefore not exchangeable because people with yellow fingers are more likely to be smokers than people who do not have yellow fingers. As a result, they are also more likely to get lung cancer. *Even if an exposure does not cause a disease, it will appear to be associated with the disease if both it and the disease are caused by a third factor*, in this case smoking. The relation between yellow fingers and lung cancer is therefore *confounded* by smoking.

Confounding can be a major problem and has to be addressed in all non-randomised research and in some randomised trials as well, especially if they

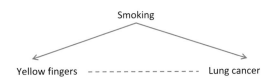

Figure 8.1 The relation between smoking, yellow fingers and lung cancer.

Figure 8.2 A hypothetical case–control study of alcohol and lung cancer (blue = drinkers, black = non-drinkers).

are small. As in previous chapters, we will mainly discuss confounding in the context of studies of the causes of a disease but, as with all epidemiological methods, everything that we say will apply equally to any study looking at associations.

The following hypothetical case–control study of alcohol and lung cancer illustrates how easily confounding can arise and how it can be diagnosed. It also suggests how confounding can be dealt with and we will discuss this in more detail later in the chapter.

An example of confounding: is alcohol a risk factor for lung cancer?

Imagine a (very small) case–control study with 20 cases (people with lung cancer ☹) and 20 controls who do not have lung cancer (☺). Is drinking alcohol associated with the risk of lung cancer? If all the cases and controls were asked about their alcohol consumption we could classify people as 'drinkers' (☹,☺) or 'non-drinkers' (☹,☺) (Figure 8.2) and calculate an odds ratio to estimate the strength of the association between alcohol and lung cancer.

What is the odds ratio for the association between alcohol and lung cancer?

Can we conclude that alcohol consumption is associated with lung cancer?

As Table 8.2 shows, the odds ratio for the association between alcohol and lung cancer is 3.0, suggesting that the risk of developing lung cancer in people who drink alcohol is three times that in non-drinkers.

However, we know that smokers are much more likely to develop lung cancer than non-smokers, and it is possible that they are also more likely to drink alcohol than non-smokers. Could smoking have affected the association

Table 8.2 Calculation of the odds ratio for the association between alcohol and lung cancer.

	Cases	Controls
Alcohol drinkers	10	5
Non-drinkers	10	15

$$Odds\ Ratio = \frac{a \times d}{b \times c} = \frac{10 \times 15}{5 \times 10} = 3.0$$

Smokers

Cases	Controls
☹ ☹ ☹ ☹ ☹	☺ ☺ ☺
☹ ☹ ☹ ☹	☺
☹ ☹ ☹	

Non-smokers

Cases	Control
☹	☺ ☺
☹ ☹ ☹ ☹ ☹	☺ ☺ ☺ ☺ ☺
☹ ☹	☺ ☺ ☺ ☺ ☺
	☺ ☺ ☺ ☺

Figure 8.3 Separating smokers and non-smokers (blue = drinkers, black = non-drinkers).

we saw between alcohol and lung cancer? To investigate this we need to separate the smokers from the non-smokers and look at the association between alcohol and lung cancer – the 'alcohol effect' – in each group. Figure 8.3 shows that 12 of the 16 smokers were also alcohol drinkers compared with only 3 of the 24 non-smokers.

Calculate the odds ratio for alcohol and lung cancer separately for (i) smokers and (ii) non-smokers. (Hint: first draw up the appropriate 2 x 2 tables.)

Is alcohol associated with lung cancer among smokers? Among non-smokers?

How do you explain the change in the pattern of the alcohol–lung cancer relationship?

The odds ratio for the association between alcohol and lung cancer among smokers is 1.0. Fewer of the non-smokers drink alcohol, but again the odds ratio is 1.0 (see Table 8.3). This process in which we divide or *stratify* the study participants into two or more separate groups (*strata*) is known as **stratification**.

So, although there appears to be an association between alcohol and lung cancer in the whole study population, it disappears when we consider smokers and non-smokers separately. We could then go on to combine the odds ratios in smokers and non-smokers to calculate a *pooled* odds ratio that

Table 8.3 Calculation of the odds ratio for the association between alcohol and lung cancer, stratified by smoking status.

		Cases	Controls	
Smokers	Alcohol drinkers	9	3	$Odds\ Ratio = \dfrac{9 \times 1}{3 \times 3} = 1.0$
	Non-drinkers	3	1	
Non-smokers	Alcohol drinkers	1	2	$Odds\ Ratio = \dfrac{1 \times 14}{2 \times 7} = 1.0$
	Non-drinkers	7	14	

is *adjusted* for the effects of smoking. In this example, the adjusted odds ratio is also 1.0. (We will not discuss the methods for calculating an adjusted odds ratio here, but a common method, developed by Mantel and Haenszel (1959), is shown in Appendix 8.)

The apparent (*crude*) overall relationship we saw between alcohol and lung cancer arose because while those with lung cancer were indeed more likely to drink alcohol than those without lung cancer, alcohol and smoking go together so they were also more likely to be smokers than those without lung cancer. The increased risk of lung cancer among alcohol drinkers was in fact due entirely to their smoking.

This situation, in which an apparent relationship between an exposure and an outcome is really due, in whole or in part, to a third factor that is associated both with the exposure and with the outcome of interest is known as confounding. In the example, smoking is said to be a **confounder** of the alcohol–lung cancer link. Confounding is a *mixing of effects* because the effect of the exposure we are interested in (e.g. alcohol) is mixed up with the effect of some other factor (e.g. smoking). To look at the real effect of the exposure we have to first deal with the effect of the confounder.

Characteristics of a confounder

As you saw above, a confounder is a factor that is associated with both the exposure and the outcome. Strictly speaking, these associations should be causal as in the yellow fingers example at the start of the chapter – smoking causes both yellow fingers and lung cancer. However, in practice the confounder may just be a *proxy* for the true cause and this is the situation in the smoking and alcohol example. Smoking does not cause someone to drink alcohol in the usual sense of the word, but instead both behaviours probably result from a complex interplay of genes, socioeconomic status (SES) and environment. Importantly, the confounder must not be a consequence of either the exposure or the outcome. So, to summarise, for something to be a confounder it must:

- be a risk factor for disease (among those who are not exposed to the factor of interest),
- be associated with the exposure of interest (in the source population or among the controls in a case–control study) and
- not be an intermediary between exposure and the outcome (i.e. it must not lie on the causal pathway).

Look back to Figure 8.3 and check that smoking has these attributes in the alcohol and lung cancer example.
- *Among non-drinkers* what proportion of (i) cases and (ii) controls smoked?
- *Among the controls* what proportion of (i) smokers and (ii) non-smokers drank alcohol?
- Is alcohol likely to *cause* smoking? (That is, could smoking lie on a causal pathway between alcohol and lung cancer?)

In the alcohol example, smoking was a confounder for the following reasons.

(1) *It was associated with lung cancer*: among people who did not drink alcohol, 3 out of 10 cases were smokers (30%) compared with only 1 of 15 controls (7%). That is, among non-drinkers, the cases were more likely to smoke than were the controls.

(2) *It was associated with alcohol among the controls*: 3 out of 4 controls who smoked also drank alcohol (75%), compared with only 2 out of 16 controls who did not smoke (12.5%). That is, among the controls, smokers were more likely to drink alcohol than were non-smokers.

(3) *It is not on a causal pathway between alcohol and lung cancer*: although alcohol and smoking often go together, drinking alcohol does not 'cause' someone to be a smoker.

An example of an intermediary is seen in the association between obesity and heart disease. High blood pressure is related both to obesity (the exposure) and to heart disease (outcome) and could, therefore, be a potential confounder of this association. However, because raising blood pressure is part of the causal path through which obesity acts to increase the risk of heart disease (obesity → increased blood pressure → heart disease), it would be misleading to adjust for this, as it would remove part of a real causal effect of being heavy.

Figure 8.1 illustrates these criteria, showing how when a confounder is causally related both to the exposure and to the outcome of interest, the exposure may appear to be related to the disease even when it is not. Because having yellow fingers is associated with (caused by) smoking and smoking causes lung cancer, yellow fingers and lung cancer appear to be associated.

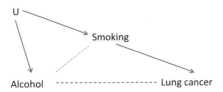

Figure 8.4 A DAG showing how smoking confounds the relation between alcohol and lung cancer.

Figure 8.1 is an example of a **directed acyclic graph** or DAG. DAGs are a very helpful way to visualise the relationships among the different factors that might affect an outcome and also to identify potential confounding variables (see Box 8.2 for more information about DAGs). We could also draw a DAG for the alcohol and lung cancer example but, as we noted above, while tobacco smoking clearly causes lung cancer, it is not so obviously a 'cause' of alcohol consumption. In practice, it is likely that tobacco smoking is a proxy for some unmeasured factor or factors (designated 'U') that are a common cause of both smoking and alcohol consumption and this is illustrated in Figure 8.4. In this example, smoking fulfils the criteria for a confounder because alcohol is associated with smoking (because they share the common cause U) and smoking is associated with lung cancer.

The effects of confounding

In the example above, the apparent effect of alcohol on lung cancer was entirely due to the effect of smoking, but confounding does not necessarily create an apparent effect where really there is none. Confounding can lead to either overestimation or underestimation of the size of a real effect, it can completely hide a real association that exists and in very extreme situations it can even reverse the direction of an effect, making it appear that a cause of a disease actually protects against it. (This is known as *Simpson's paradox* and it explains the apparent contradiction in the university admissions data at the start of the chapter).

Age, sex and SES are common confounders. As an example, many diseases occur more frequently in older people. If the exposure of interest also occurs more commonly in the elderly, e.g. a poor diet, then the confounding effects of age would have to be considered.

Authors of early studies that looked at the relation between diet and heart disease found that the more a person ate, the lower their risk of heart disease. This apparent association was all the more surprising because we know that obesity is a risk factor for heart disease. However, one factor that the studies did not take into account was physical activity and, on average, people who are physically active eat more than those who are inactive, i.e. physical activity is potentially a cause of high energy intake and physical activity also reduces risk of heart of disease. Could this have affected the results of the studies?

Table 8.4 Results of a hypothetical case–control study of high energy intake and heart disease, stratified by level of physical activity.

Energy intake	Total		High physical activity		Low physical activity	
	Heart disease	Controls	Heart disease	Controls	Heart disease	Controls
High	730	600	520	510	210	90
Low	700	540	100	150	600	390

Table 8.4 presents the results of a hypothetical case–control study evaluating the association between energy intake and heart disease.

Is physical activity associated with energy intake in this study?

Draw a DAG showing the likely relationships between energy intake, physical activity and heart disease.

Is physical activity likely to confound the relationship between high energy intake and heart disease? Why?

Table 8.4 clearly shows that people who are more active consume more energy than those who are less active (510 ÷ 660 = 77% of active controls have high energy intake compared to only 90 ÷ 480 = 19% of inactive controls). Figure 8.5 shows a DAG for this example, suggesting that physical activity is a common cause of both energy intake and heart disease and so is likely to confound the association between them.

What is the odds ratio for the *crude* association between high energy intake and heart disease?

What is the odds ratio for the association between high energy intake and heart disease in people with (i) high and (ii) low levels of physical activity?

Is the association between high energy intake and heart disease confounded by the level of physical activity?

Figure 8.5 A DAG showing how physical activity will confound the relation between energy intake and heart disease.

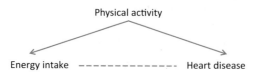

The crude odds ratio for the association between high energy intake and heart disease in this study is (730 × 540) ÷ (700 × 600) = 0.9, i.e. those with high energy intake appear to have a 10% *lower* risk of coronary heart disease (CHD). When we stratify by physical activity the odds ratio is $(520 \times 150) \div (100 \times 510) = 1.5$ among the physically active and $(210 \times 390) \div (600 \times 90) = 1.5$ among the inactive. Thus, when we remove the confounding effects of physical activity by stratification, high energy intake is associated with a 50% *higher* risk of CHD (OR = 1.5). In this example the confounding meant that the observed odds ratio (OR = 0.9) was an underestimate of the true association between obesity and CHD (OR = 1.5).

Although this example was a case–control study, confounding can occur in exactly the same way in a cohort study (see the questions at the end of the chapter for an example of this).

How can we tell if an association is confounded?

If a factor has the characteristics of a confounder (see above) and when you stratify or adjust for it the effect estimate changes, then confounding is present. In the lung cancer example at the start of the chapter the odds ratio dropped from 3.0 to 1.0 when we adjusted for smoking, indicating that smoking was a strong confounder. In the heart disease example the estimate increased from 0.9 to 1.5 when we adjusted for physical activity, so again this was confounding the association. A commonly used rule is that if, when you adjust for a potential confounder, the crude and adjusted effect estimates differ by 10% or more, then the crude estimate is confounded to some degree and it is more appropriate to present the adjusted value.

When will a possible confounder actually be a confounder in practice?

There are many things that could confound an association between an exposure and outcome, but in practice they might not actually do so.

Table 8.5 shows the characteristics of a group of women at the time of recruitment into a cohort study of oral contraceptives (OCs) and CHD.

Assume that all the factors are known risk factors for CHD. Which of them might be confounders of the OC–CHD relationship? Why?

For something to be a confounder it has to be associated both with the exposure of interest (OC use) and with the outcome of interest (CHD). All of the factors listed are known risk factors for CHD, so they are all associated with CHD. Some are also associated with OC use – we can see from Table 8.5 that, compared with non-users, OC users are:

• twice as likely to be under the age of 30 as non-users (60% versus 30%),
• slightly more likely to be of low SES (50% versus 40%),
• slightly more likely to be current smokers (17% versus 12%),

Table 8.5 Characteristics of women at time of recruitment into a study of oral contraceptive use and coronary heart disease.

	Oral contraceptive use	
	Yes	No
Percentage aged less than 30 years	60	30
Percentage of low SES	50	40
Percentage smoking >15 cigarettes/day	17	12
Mean body mass index (weight (kg)/height (m)^2)	26.5	27.0
Percentage with a history of:		
Hypertension	1	1
Stroke	0.03	0.3
Venous thromboembolism	1	8

(Figures adapted from Vessey and Lawless, 1984.)

- 10 times less likely to have had a stroke (0.03% versus 0.3%) and
- 8 times less likely to have had a venous thromboembolism (1% versus 8%).

So will these factors confound the association between OC use and CHD?

In practice, it turns out that only age, history of thromboembolism and, to a lesser extent, smoking are likely to affect the results appreciably. Because CHD rates increase with age, the rate in the OC users will be lower than in the non-users simply because they are younger. If OC use truly increased the risk of CHD, say the true RR = 3.0, then the effect of confounding by age might reduce the observed RR (unadjusted for age) to about 2.5 (Table 8.6), thus reducing the (real) difference between the groups. Similarly, the eightfold difference between the OC users and non-users in terms of their history of thromboembolism, a strong risk factor for CHD, will also bias the observed RR downwards to about 2.4. Conversely, CHD rates are higher in smokers and OC users are slightly more likely to be smokers than non-users, thus the effect of confounding by smoking would be to increase the apparent RR, making the effect look stronger than it really is.

This contrasts strikingly with the confounding influence of a history of stroke. Theoretically this looks sure to be an important confounder, given the 10-fold difference between OC users and non-users in terms of their past stroke experience, i.e. a very strong association between OC use and stroke (note that this occurs because women who have had a stroke would not normally be prescribed the OC pill), and the very strong known link between stroke and heart disease (due to their common set of risk factors). However, because stroke is so rare in young women, this imbalance affects only a tiny proportion of the total study group, and so has a trivial effect on the crude RR, biasing it downwards by <5%, from 3.0 to 2.9. Even if a history of stroke had been five times more

Table 8.6 Likely effects of potential confounders in a study of oral contraceptive use and coronary heart disease when the true RR = 3.0.

	Oral contraceptive use		Likely
	Yes	No	Observed RR[a]
Percentage aged less than 30 years	60	30	2.5
Percentage of low SES	50	40	3.2
Percentage smoking >15 cig/day	17	12	3.3
Mean body mass index (weight (kg)/height (m)^2)	26.5	27.0	2.9
Percentage with a history of:			
Hypertension	1	1	3.0
Stroke	0.03	0.3	2.9
Venous thromboembolism	1	8	2.4

[a] Estimated RR for OC use and CHD, assuming that the RRs for the associations between the potential confounders and CHD are: 2.0 for age, 2.0 for SES, 4.0 for smoking, 4.0 for BMI, 10.0 for stroke and 5.0 for venous thromboembolism.

common in the study groups (0.015% and 1.5%), the RR would have been biased downwards by only about 10%, from 3.0 to 2.7. More predictably, strong independent risk factors for CHD such as low SES and BMI also fail to confound when their distributions in the groups being compared are reasonably similar, i.e. the groups are still exchangeable with respect to these factors. So for something to be a confounder in practice it must not only be associated quite strongly with the exposure and the outcome, it must also be reasonably prevalent in the population.

As another example, consider the case–control study of energy intake and heart disease shown in Table 8.4. In this study the prevalence of the confounder (physical activity) in the population was very high – 660 of the 1140 controls or 58% were physically active. What would have happened to our analysis if the population had been much less active? Table 8.7 shows results from a similar study for a population in which only 6% of controls were physically active. (To obtain these numbers we have just divided the numbers in the physically active group by 10 and multiplied the numbers in the inactive group by 2.) The stratum-specific odds ratios, and thus the *adjusted* odds ratio, are unaffected but the crude odds ratio is now 1.3 instead of 0.9; i.e. it is much closer to the unconfounded value of 1.5 and there is much less confounding by physical activity because this is now much less common.

We can summarise this by saying the following.

- If the association between a potential confounder and *either* the exposure *or* the outcome is weak, then the confounder is unlikely to have much effect on the results of a study.

Table 8.7 Results of a hypothetical case–control study of high energy intake and heart disease, stratified by level of physical activity (present in only 6% of the population).

Energy intake	Total		High physical activity		Low physical activity	
	Heart disease	Controls	Heart disease	Controls	Heart disease	Controls
High	472	231	52	51	420	180
Low	1210	795	10	15	1200	780
OR	**1.3**		**1.5**		**1.5**	

- If a potential confounder is either *rare* or almost *ubiquitous* then it is unlikely to have much effect on the results of a study because these will be driven by the large number of people who are not exposed to the rare confounder or by the many who are exposed to the very common confounder.

The most important confounders are therefore those that are both *relatively common* and strongly related to the exposures and health outcomes of interest. The typical confounders that we mentioned above – sex, age and SES – fulfil all of these criteria. Another common confounder is smoking: it is still quite common despite large declines in smoking rates in many countries; it is strongly associated with many lifestyle factors, including high alcohol and coffee consumption, a less healthy diet (less fresh fruit and vegetables) and low levels of physical activity; and is also a major risk factor for many diseases. There are also many other disease-specific confounders: sun exposure is a major confounder in studies of other risk factors for skin cancer, obesity may be a confounder in studies looking for causes of type-2 diabetes, and so on. Although note that, in this latter example, it is also possible that obesity may lie on the casual pathway for diabetes, for example in studies of physical activity where it is likely that lower physical activity → obesity → diabetes. In this situation we have to think carefully about whether obesity is simply a confounder or if it might explain some of the effects of physical activity on diabetes risk.

Control of confounding

Once we have identified the potential confounders of an exposure–outcome relationship (see Box 8.2 for further discussion of the use of DAGs for this), what approaches can we take to remove or reduce the effects of any confounding? There are two strategies for dealing with confounding. The first is to try to prevent it from occurring in the first place and this can be done at the

Box 8.2 Defining pathways to disease outcomes: directed acyclic graphs

The examples we discussed above mainly relate to a single factor that might confound an association between an exposure and an outcome but in reality there is likely to be a multitude of potential confounders that could be common causes of both the exposure and the outcome. There may also be intermediate steps between an exposure and an outcome, or between a confounder and the exposure or outcome. Diseases are rarely (if ever) the result of a single causal factor (we will discuss this further in Chapter 10), but usually arise as the result of a complex interaction of an array of variables, some of which we can never measure. How then can we make sense of this complexity? And how can we use this information to determine those factors that are more or less important in understanding whether an observed association is 'confounded'? One approach is to use causal diagrams or *Directed Acyclic Graphs* (DAGs) to show the relationship between an exposure, confounders, intermediaries and an outcome. This is an a priori approach that allows epidemiologists to both clearly articulate the assumptions they have made about how variables are inter-related, and decide how best to account for the effects of confounding in an analysis. Figure 8.6 expands on the DAG shown in Figure 8.5 to include some other factors that are likely to be important if we want to assess the relation between energy intake and heart disease.

In this example, energy intake is associated with heart disease through what are called 'unblocked paths' via physical activity, age and smoking, so these are all potential confounders of the energy–heart disease relationship. In practice, it turns out that we only need to worry about age and physical activity because controlling for these two factors will block all the indirect (non-causal) pathways from energy intake to heart disease. If there are no other important confounders (and in practice it is likely there are), then any association remaining after we control for age and

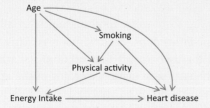

Figure 8.6 A more complete DAG looking at potential confounders of the relation between energy intake and heart disease.

(*continued*)

physical activity could be attributed to a direct effect of energy intake on heart disease.

So, how do you decide what variables should be included in a DAG? This is a very important question and it relies on the content knowledge and hypotheses of the epidemiologist, the type of study design and, most importantly, evidence from the literature. One strength of DAGs is that they display causal assumptions that are not captured by conventional statistical models, but this is also a limitation, as the variables included in a DAG are chosen by the epidemiologist who has their own biases and prejudices about what is (and is not) important. We will not discuss DAGs further here, but more detailed information, examples and suggestions for further reading are available (see Greenland *et al.*, 1999 and online).

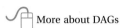 More about DAGs

study design stage by *randomisation*, *restriction* or *matching*. The alternative is to deal with it when it occurs by using analytic techniques such as stratification and statistical modelling. The effectiveness of all of these strategies except randomisation depends on the ability to identify and measure any confounders accurately.

Control of confounding through study design

Confounding occurs when a confounding variable is distributed unevenly across our study groups (e.g. in the lung cancer example at the start of the chapter, cases were more likely to be smokers than controls). One way to avoid confounding is therefore to design a study so that all groups are similar with respect to any potential confounders.

Randomisation

The most effective way to prevent confounding is to allocate people to the different study groups *at random*. Clearly, this is possible only in an intervention study and it is for this reason that randomised trials are usually considered to provide the strongest evidence of any of the epidemiological study designs (note that non-randomised trials are particularly prone to a type of confounding called **confounding by indication** – see Box 8.3). When a trial is large enough, random allocation will generally ensure a balanced distribution of all characteristics between the intervention (exposed) and control (unexposed) groups, i.e. it will ensure they are highly exchangeable. *However, even*

Box 8.3 Confounding by indication

If in a trial the participants are *not* randomly allocated to the various treatment groups then confounding is still a major problem, particularly what is often called **confounding by indication** (Miettinen, 1983). This arises because, even among a group of people who all have the same medical condition, those who choose to take or who are prescribed a particular medication may well differ from those who do not take it or who are not prescribed it. Those who take the drug might tend to have more (or less) severe disease than those who do not take it and, conversely, anyone who has a medical condition or exposure that is contraindicated for the drug should certainly not be taking it. As a result, the outcomes of those who take the drug may well differ from the outcomes of those who do not in a way that has nothing to do with the treatment itself, i.e. they might differ simply because those taking the group are less sick or do not have other major health conditions (comorbidities). The obvious solution to this problem is a randomised trial in which people are allocated to the various treatment groups at random. If a randomised study is not possible then *propensity scores* can sometimes be used to control for potential confounding by indication in observational studies (see Box 8.6).

randomisation cannot guarantee the absence of confounding, especially in smaller studies, so it must always be looked for. The analysis of a randomised study must then include all participants in the groups to which they were originally randomised (regardless of whether they actually received the intervention). This is known as **intention to treat** analysis and we will discuss the importance of this further in Chapter 15 when we consider randomised evaluations of screening programmes.

A major advantage of randomisation over other forms of control of confounding is that it deals not only with confounders that we know and can measure, but also with other unrecognised and unmeasured (or unmeasurable) confounders. These too will, on balance, be evenly distributed by the randomisation process. Such *unknown confounders* (e.g. aspects of personality that affect complex lifestyle patterns) cannot be dealt with by any other method.

Restriction

Because randomisation is not possible in the majority of epidemiological studies, are there any alternatives? One option is to *restrict* the study sample to people with or without the confounding characteristic. This can be done by restricting a study to a particular age or socioeconomic group, thereby removing confounding by age or SES, or by restricting a study to non-smokers if smoking is a potential confounder. For example, we know that infection with human papillomavirus (HPV) is a major factor (potentially a **necessary cause**, see Chapter 10) in the development of cervical cancer and we also know that HPV infection is strongly associated with a number of other lifestyle factors such as smoking and the use of oral contraceptives. This makes it very difficult to evaluate the association between smoking and cervical cancer because it is hard to be sure that any association observed is not simply due to confounding by HPV infection. (Smokers are more likely to be HPV-positive than are non-smokers, so this could explain why they are more likely to develop cervical cancer.) By restricting a study to include only HPV-positive women, any confounding by HPV status would be removed making it possible to evaluate the effects of other cofactors, such as smoking. Restriction is, however, of limited practical value when it is necessary to control for more than one or two likely confounders.

Matching

The third possibility is to select study subjects so that major known confounders are evenly distributed across the study groups. This is achieved by matching subjects on the presence or absence of the confounding variable(s). This is most often done in case–control studies in which controls are selected to match the cases in some predetermined way, e.g. by age and sex. Matching can be done on an individual basis, with one or more controls matched to each case so that, for instance, each control is matched by sex and year of birth to a specific case. Alternatively, *frequency matching* aims to select controls to match the general distribution of the confounding variable in cases. For example, adenocarcinoma of the oesophagus is about seven times more common in men than in women so in a study of this cancer, controls might be selected to give a similar ratio of males to females (i.e. 7:1). If, in this situation, controls were simply selected as a random sample of the population, it is likely that about half would be female and half male. There would therefore be many more female controls than female cases but many fewer male controls than male cases. Sex would be a potential confounder in the analysis (because it is associated with the disease and many of the potential risk factors), but any adjustment for sex would be statistically inefficient because of the large sex imbalance between cases and controls.

Matching can also be used in the same way in cohort studies. This has historically been much less common but, with the increasing use of record linkage to conduct historical cohort studies, it is likely to become more common in the future. For example, a group used records from blood donation centres in the USA to identify a cohort of 10,259 adults whose blood samples tested positive for hepatitis C virus (HCV) antibodies between 1991 and 2002 and another 10,259 blood donors who tested negative. The HCV-negative group were frequency-matched to the HCV-positive group by age, sex, year of blood donation and postcode (as a surrogate marker for ethnicity and SES). They then used record linkage to the National Death Index to identify the dates and causes of death of people in the two groups. They found that after an average of 7.7 years follow-up, the risk of dying was three times higher in the HCV-positive group than in the HCV-negative group (hazard ratio = 3.1, 95% CI 2.6–3.8) (Guiltinan *et al.*, 2008).

> The **hazard ratio** is a measure of relative risk. It is essentially the same as an incidence rate ratio and is often calculated in cohort studies.

While it may seem tempting to match cases and controls (or the exposed and unexposed groups in a cohort study) on as many factors as possible in the hope of removing all possible confounders, this can lead to *over-matching*, which greatly decreases the efficiency and increases the cost of a study. It is much harder to find a suitable control who matches a long list of criteria than it is to find someone who is only the same age and sex as the case (and even that is not always as easy as it sounds).

Finally, in a case–control study *it is essential that any matching factors are accounted for in the analysis*. The process of matching does not itself remove confounding – it can actually introduce different confounding, which must then be allowed for. If the matching factor is associated with the exposure of interest then, even if it is *not* associated with disease and so is not a true confounder (see characteristics of a confounder above), the fact that cases and controls have been matched for that factor *will make it a confounder in the study*. In general, if a matching factor is positively associated with the exposure, the matching process will make cases and controls look more similar than they should. This means that, if the matching is not taken into account in the analysis, the calculated odds ratios will underestimate the true association between exposure and disease (they will be closer to 1.0) as shown in the example in Box 8.4. If frequency matching has been used it is sufficient to treat the matching factors as normal confounders (see 'Control of confounding' below), but there are special techniques for analysing individually matched data (see Box 8.4). The only exception to this rule is if, in practice, it turns out that a matching factor is *not* associated with exposure in a case–control study. In this situation, matching cases to controls on that factor will not have introduced any additional confounding and the factor need not be allowed for in the analysis.

Matching was a primary technique for control of confounding in the early decades of the modern case–control study (from the mid twentieth century

Box 8.4 Analysis of individually matched data

To analyse the data from a simple matched case–control study you have to compare each case with their matched control (or controls if more than one control is selected for each case). In Table 8.8 the numbers no longer represent individual people but 155 matched pairs of cases and controls, so there are 40 pairs for which both the case and the control are exposed, 25 pairs for which only the case was exposed, and so on.

Table 8.8 Analysing data from an individually matched case–control study.

		Controls		
		Exposed	Unexposed	
Cases	Exposed	40	25	Matched odds ratio
	Unexposed	10	80	= 25 ÷ 10 = 2.5

If a case and their matched control are both exposed (or both unexposed) that pair (or set) cannot tell us anything about the association between exposure and disease. The interesting case–control pairs are those for which one member is exposed and the other is unexposed. The matched odds ratio is calculated by simply dividing the number of pairs for which the case was exposed and the control unexposed by the number of pairs for which the control was exposed and the case unexposed:

$$\text{Matched OR} = \frac{\text{\# of pairs where the case was exposed and the control unexposed}}{\text{\# of pairs where the control was exposed and the case unexposed}} \quad (8.1)$$

Note that, if we had not taken the matching into account in the analysis, we would have said that 65 (40 + 25) out of the 155 cases were exposed and 90 (10 + 80) were unexposed compared with 50 (40 + 10) exposed and 105 (25 + 80) unexposed controls, giving an unmatched odds ratio of (65 × 105) ÷ (90 × 50) = 1.5, which is considerably less than the matched value of 2.5.

until the 1980s). The ready availability now of flexible and reasonably straight-forward computing packages that allow effective control for confounding at the stage of data analysis (either by stratified or multivariable analysis) has somewhat lessened its importance, although it continues to be used to increase efficiency in a variety of situations.

Does increasing the size of a study help?

Increasing the size of an observational epidemiological study will not make any difference to the amount of confounding. (To convince yourself of this, go back to one of the earlier examples and try doubling the numbers of people in each group. This will not alter the odds ratios or rate ratios, nor will it get rid of the confounding.) The only time study size does matter is in the context of a randomised controlled trial. The bigger a randomised trial is, the more likely it is that any confounders (known and unknown) will be balanced across the study groups (i.e. that we get closer to complete exchangeability between the different arms of the trial) and the less likely it is that there will be any confounding.

Control of confounding in data analysis

If you have designed a study using restriction or matching to reduce the effects of confounding, it is no longer possible to study the effects of those confounding variables. For example, if you have restricted your study to people aged between 60 and 70 years, or have matched cases and controls individually for age, it would no longer be possible to look at the direct effects of age on disease. This means that it is often preferable to collect information on potential confounders and then to control for these in the analysis. The aim of the analysis is exactly the same as the design options mentioned above, namely to ensure that the confounders are balanced across the groups, and in practice this is achieved by comparing exposure–disease patterns within narrow ranges of one or more confounders. These approaches apply equally to case–control and cohort studies and also to intervention studies if they are not randomised or if, in a randomised study, the randomisation did not lead to an equal balance of important confounders across the study groups.

Stratification

This is the method that we used in the alcohol and lung cancer example where we stratified by smoking status, and the steps are shown in Figure 8.7 (where RR stands for relative risk and may be a rate, risk or odds ratio). Study subjects are split into groups, or strata, based on levels of the confounding variable. The association between the exposure and outcome of interest is then measured separately in each stratum because if the people in each stratum are homogeneous (the same or similar) with respect to the confounding variable, there can no longer be any confounding by that factor. An analysis could be done separately for men and women to remove confounding by sex, for different age groups, for smokers and non-smokers (as in the example of alcohol and lung cancer) and so on.

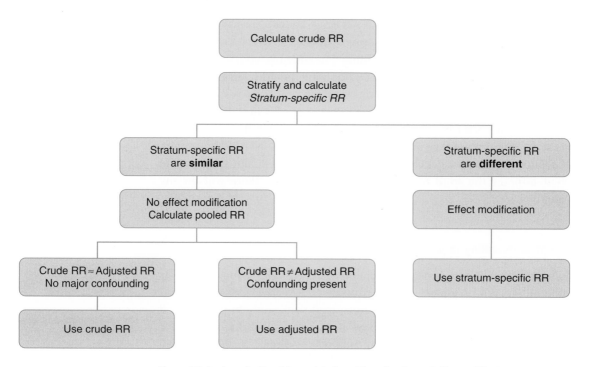

Figure 8.7 A scheme for identifying and dealing with confounding and effect modification.

In the examples we have looked at so far, the stratum-specific odds ratios were exactly or almost exactly the same, but this is rarely the case in practice. If the stratum-specific estimates are similar then it is reasonable to assume that the small differences between them are simply due to chance. In this situation it is possible to combine the estimates from each separate stratum to summarise the overall effect in the whole group. There are several ways to do this and the effect is then said to be 'adjusted' for the confounder (see Appendix 8). This process is analogous to the standardisation that you met in Chapter 2. If the adjusted measure of association is *different* from the original crude measure, then we know that the crude association was confounded. In the alcohol and lung cancer example the crude OR was 3.0 and the adjusted OR was 1.0, showing that the crude OR was heavily confounded by smoking.

If, however, the stratum-specific estimates are quite different, then there may be ***effect modification***, or in other words the 'effect' (the association between exposure and outcome) may be truly different in the different strata. For example, regular physical activity might reduce the risk of a particular disease among people who are overweight, but it might confer no benefit for those of normal weight. In this situation obesity *modifies* the effect of physical activity on disease and it would be inappropriate to treat obesity as a confounder (see Figure 8.7). In practice, however, there is always some variation in the odds ratios across the different strata and it can be very difficult to know whether this indicates a meaningful difference or just random variation. There are statistical tests (tests for heterogeneity) that can be used to help decide whether the variation could just be due to chance. However, these are not very powerful and are unlikely to detect variation unless the difference is very great (in which case it would be apparent without a statistical test) or the study is very large. In this situation it is still possible to use statistical packages to 'adjust' for the effect modifier, but it is important to consider whether this is appropriate. If the effects in different groups really are different then combining them will just average out the differences and give a measure that may not reflect the true association in any of the groups. See Box 8.5 for more about effect modification.

Box 8.5 More about effect modification (EM)

The presence of effect modification depends on the effect measure used. If the relative risk (RR) does not differ between groups then the risk difference or absolute risk (AR) will differ and vice versa. To see this use the data in Table 8.9 to calculate the AR and RR for the relationship between smoking and (i) disease A and (ii) disease B, separately for normal and overweight/obese individuals. Is the association between smoking and (i) disease A and (ii) disease B modified by body size?

Table 8.9 Risks of two hypothetical diseases by smoking status and body size.

	Risk of disease A (per year)		Risk of disease B (per year)	
	Non-smokers	Smokers	Non-smokers	Smokers
Normal weight	0.2%	0.5%	0.2%	0.5%
Overweight/obese	0.5%	0.8%	0.5%	1.25%

Among people of normal weight the AR and RR for smoking and disease A are 0.3% (0.5% – 0.2%) and 2.5 (0.5% ÷ 0.2%), respectively, compared to 0.3% (0.8% – 0.5%) and 1.6 (0.8% ÷ 0.5%) among those who are overweight/obese. This suggests there is effect modification of the RR (i.e. on a multiplicative scale) but not of the AR (additive scale). In contrast, the AR and RR for disease B are 0.3% and 2.5 among normal weight people and 0.75% and 2.5 among the overweight/obese. In this example, the ARs differ but the RRs do not. The fact that the presence of EM depends on the measure being used has led to suggestions that a more appropriate term would be **effect measure modification**. For a more detailed discussion of the issues of EM and biological interaction see Rothman (2012).

Finally, it is important to note that although stratification can also be used for studies in which cases and controls have been frequency-matched, it is generally not appropriate for individually matched studies. These should be analysed using a special 'matched' analysis (see Box 8.4) or modelling techniques (see below).

Multivariable modelling

Stratification may be impractical when a study is small or you need to control for several confounders simultaneously, because you are likely to end up with small numbers in any one stratum. If, for example, you wanted to control for sex, age with five 10-year age groups (20–29, 30–39, 40–49, 50–59 and 60–69) and smoking (non-smoker versus smoker), you would end up with 20 different strata (five age groups for smokers and five for non-smokers for each sex). On average, each stratum will contain only 5% of your study population and, with small numbers, it can be difficult to obtain precise estimates of the stratum-specific associations. An alternative is to use statistical modelling techniques to estimate the strength of the relationship of interest while controlling for all of the potential confounders. The most commonly used multivariable approach for unmatched (or frequency-matched) case–control studies is *multiple logistic regression*. Individually matched case–control data can be analysed by a variation of this called *conditional logistic regression*, which takes the individual matching between cases and controls into account. A common technique used to analyse person-time data from a cohort study is *Cox proportional hazards regression*. (Note that this generates *hazard ratios* which are essentially the same as incidence rate ratios.) We will not discuss the details of these procedures here – they can be found in any standard medical statistics text. See also Boxes 8.6 and 8.7 for examples of some more complex approaches to controlling for confounding.

It is very likely that you will come across the output from regression models in the form of tables and figures in epidemiological reports and papers. Table 8.10 shows a typical example of results from a conditional logistic regression model used to analyse data from a population-based case–control study of suicide in young adults in New South Wales (Australia). Exposure information on suicide cases was obtained from interviews with key informants for the suicide case, and this information was compared to key informant interviews for live age-matched controls. The main question was whether a history of substance use disorder in the previous 12 months was associated with an increased risk of suicide. The investigators also indicated a priori that there were two main potential confounders of this relationship, namely SES and sex.

When it is not possible to interview people directly (e.g. because the cases have died), information may be collected from **key informants** who are familiar with the case. To ensure comparability and minimise bias, key informants were also used for controls although they were still alive and could have been interviewed.

Table 8.10 Relative risk of suicide associated with a history of substance use disorders in young adults (18–34 years, New South Wales, Australia)

	Cases		Controls		Crude		Adjusted	
	N^a	%	N^a	%	OR (95% CI)	p^b	OR (95% CI)	p
Substance use disorder[c] in the last 12 months								
No	48	57.1	219	87.3	1.0		1.0	
Yes	36	42.9	32	12.7	4.9 (2.7–8.9)	<0.001	3.3 (1.7–6.4)	<0.001
Sex								
Female	13	15.5	148	59.2	1.0		1.0	
Male	71	84.5	102	40.8	7.5 (3.9–14.3)	<0.001	6.9 (3.5–13.7)	<0.001
Socioeconomic status								
High	14	16.7	66	26.8	1.0		1.0	
Middle	23	27.4	77	31.3	1.8 (0.9–4.0)	0.1	1.6 (0.7–3.8)	0.2
Low	47	56.0	103	41.9	3.8 (1.8–7.7)	<0.001	3.8 (1.7–8.5)	0.001

(Modified from Page *et al.*, 2014)
[a] Note, numbers may not sum to the total because of missing data.
[b] *P*-value from a statistical test of whether the OR is significantly different from 1.0.
[c] As defined by the 10th edition of the International Classification of Diseases (ICD-10).

How strong was the *crude* (unadjusted) association between substance use disorder and suicide?

How likely is it that this crude association might be confounded by (a) sex and (b) SES and why?

How strong was the *adjusted* association between substance use disorder and suicide?

What was the effect of adjusting for confounders on the association between substance use disorder and suicide?

What have we learnt overall about risk factors for youth suicide?

The unadjusted or *crude* association between substance use and suicide is quite strong. Those with a history of a substance use disorder were 4.9 times more likely to die by suicide than those without a substance use disorder (the 'reference' group in the comparison, indicated by OR = 1.0). The 95% confidence interval indicates how precise this estimate is (see Chapter 6), although in this case the range from 2.7 to 8.9 suggests quite a bit of uncertainty. The *p* value (<0.001) suggests there was a less than 1 in 1000 chance that an association this strong would have occurred by chance.

As is often done, the authors have also shown us the associations between the potential confounders and suicide so we can see from the crude ORs that being male and being in a low SES group are also both much more common among cases than controls and so are strongly associated with suicide. This makes them likely confounders of the association between substance use disorder and suicide. **Adjusted** estimates have been obtained by simultaneously including the confounding variables and the exposure variable into a single regression model. The OR for history of a substance use disorder drops from 4.9 (crude) to 3.3 (adjusted). That is, the strength of the association was reduced by approximately 30% after adjusting for sex and SES. In contrast, the associations between the confounders and suicide do not change substantially after adjustment. From this output we can conclude that some of the association between substance use and suicide is attributable to the higher risk of suicide among males and among those from a lower SES group. If the analyses had not been adjusted for these confounders, the investigators would have overestimated the strength of the association between substance use disorder and suicide. Nonetheless, even after controlling for this confounding, substance abuse and suicide remain strongly associated, and sex and SES also have strong independent effects.

A word of caution, however; multivariable modelling can be performed very easily with modern statistics software but it is important to know what you are doing. The models can be complex and they are based on a number of underlying assumptions. If you are not familiar with the techniques it is wise to seek advice from a statistician before diving in. Furthermore, it is important to have a very clear research question in mind and to be familiar with your data before starting any modelling, and nothing can replace simple stratified analyses, as outlined above, for this.

Residual confounding

In practice it is rarely possible to remove all confounding so we will be left with some **residual confounding**. For example, in a study of US health professionals the crude RR (0.56; 95% CI 0.38–0.84) suggested that men who consumed high levels of fruit and vegetables had almost half the risk of lung cancer of those who ate little fruit and vegetables (Feskanich *et al.*, 2000). When the authors adjusted their analysis for a simple measure of smoking status (never, past, current smoker) the RR increased to 0.86 (95% CI 0.58–1.29), suggesting that the crude RR was confounded by smoking. When they also adjusted for more detailed measures of smoking, including time since stopping and current amount smoked, the RR increased still further to 1.07 (95% CI 0.71–1.61). This shows convincingly that the simple adjustment for smoking status was not sufficient to remove all of the confounding by smoking and there was considerable residual confounding. If they had not adjusted for the additional smoking variables the results would have left some room for optimism that improving diet might confer some benefit, whereas the fully adjusted result

Box 8.6 More complex ways to identify and control confounding

Propensity scores are mainly used in non-randomised trials when the probability that an individual receives a particular treatment may depend on multiple characteristics of the individual, such as other comorbidities, that might themselves affect the outcome. The first step is to calculate how individual characteristics (potential confounders of the relation between treatment and outcome) affect the probability that someone receives the treatment of interest. It is then possible to calculate, for each individual, their probability of receiving treatment based on their particular characteristics. If we then match or stratify study participants on the basis of this '*propensity score*', the net effect is to balance the *measured* confounders between the study groups, thereby increasing their exchangeability and reducing the effects of confounding (Joffe and Rosenbaum, 1999).

  Instrumental variables are also used for non-randomised treatment studies and for other observational studies. In this case the aim is to find a variable that is associated with treatment selection but not with outcome. This instrumental variable must be associated with the exposure (treatment) and must affect the outcome only via this exposure, i.e. it must not have any independent effect on outcome. It must also not share any common cause with the outcome, and must not be associated with confounders of the exposure (Figure 8.8). This variable can then be used in the analysis instead of the treatment variable. The strength of this approach over propensity scores is that it controls for both *measured* and *unmeasured* confounders. The major challenge is to find an appropriate variable that meets all of the criteria for an instrumental variable. For example, observational treatment data from the US Surveillance Epidemiology and End Results (SEER) programme were used to assess whether chemotherapy improved survival from advanced lung cancer in the elderly. The authors did not look at whether the individuals themselves received chemotherapy or not, but instead used the probability that the health care centre the patient attended would offer chemotherapy. This fitted the criteria of an instrumental variable because, by definition,

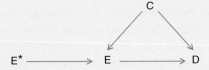

Figure 8.8 DAG showing the relationships between an instrumental variable (E*), the exposure (E), confounders (C) and the outcome (D).

(*continued*)

Box 8.6 (*continued*)

it would affect whether someone received chemotherapy but should not otherwise be related to outcome. The results suggested that chemotherapy did increase one-year survival by approximately 9% (Earle *et al.*, 2001).

Genetic markers are increasingly being used as instrumental variables, taking advantage of what is known as ***Mendelian randomisation*** (see Box 8.7).

Box 8.7 Mendelian randomisation

More about Mendelian randomisation

Gregor Mendel, an Austrian monk, conducted pioneering work with pea plants that laid the foundation of modern genetics. Based on the patterns of inheritance of plant traits, he developed his Laws of Inheritance: the laws of 'segregation', 'random assortment' and 'dominance'. The first two of these laws are what epidemiologists take advantage of when applying Mendelian randomisation to observational studies. Mendel's original paper *Experiments in Plant Hybridization* (1865) has been archived at http://www.mendelweb.org/archive/Mendel.Experiments.txt

The principle of Mendelian randomisation is that genetic markers are passed on between generations independently of other genetic characteristics, and of other environmental factors (Davey Smith and Ebrahim, 2003; Davey Smith, 2011; Davey Smith and Hemani, 2014). For example, whether you inherit a genetic variant of the *FTO* gene that predisposes you to obesity occurs independently of any other genetic predisposition you may have; and is also unrelated to your propensity to, say, smoke or drink alcohol (given our usual ignorance of which genetic variants we carry). This principle of Mendelian randomisation allows an observational study examining, for example, whether the *FTO* variant is associated with renal cancer to approximate a randomised controlled trial. While a standard study looking at the relation between obesity (E in Figure 8.8) and renal cancer (D) could be confounded by a multitude of lifestyle factors (C) such as diet that could affect both obesity and cancer risk, the genetic variants (E*) that affect observed weight are unlikely to be related to the potential confounders. This genetic variant provides an instrumental variable that can be used to estimate the unconfounded relation between obesity and renal cancer showing, in this case, that obesity was associated with increased risk of renal cancer (Brennan *et al.*, 2009).

Studies using Mendelian randomisation (MR) have highlighted how confounding in observational studies can lead to misleading conclusions, with some apparently clear associations shown to be null, or even reversed, by MR analyses. For example, cohort and case–control studies had reported that plasma fibrinogen was associated with an increased risk of coronary heart disease (CHD; RR = 1.8, 95% CI 1.6–2.0), but residual confounding could not be excluded with certainty as higher fibrinogen levels are also associated with other CHD risk factors. Subsequently, MR analyses have shown that there is no association between variants of the

(*continued*)

Box 8.7 (continued)

β-fibrinogen gene that predict higher fibrinogen levels and CHD (RR = 1.0, 95% CI 0.92–1.04), suggesting the apparent association seen in observational studies was largely attributable to confounding (Davey Smith et al., 2005).

The challenges with studies of this type are first the need to find genetic variants that fulfil the requirements of an instrumental variable (an association with the exposure of interest and no independent association with the outcome that is not mediated by the exposure) and, second, that the genetic effects on lifestyle traits such as obesity are often quite weak and so we need very large sample sizes (typically thousands or tens of thousands) to see an association. (There are also additional issues specific to genetic research, e.g. linkage disequilibrium and population stratification, which can be problematic; see Davey Smith and Ebrahim, 2003; Davey Smith 2011.)

suggests that unfortunately this is not the case. It also indicates the importance of measuring confounding variables well, i.e. to minimise misclassification of confounders as well as the exposure of interest, if we are to achieve effective control of confounding. In general, if adjustment changes an observed odds ratio quite markedly, e.g. it reduces it from 5.4 to 2.6, then it is likely that, if we could have controlled for the confounding perfectly, the true odds ratio would have been even less than 2.6. We then have to decide whether we think that there is a *true* association between the exposure and disease or whether all the *observed* association could be due to confounding. However, if the control for confounding only changed the odds ratio from 5.4 to 5.1 then it is likely that, even if we could have controlled completely for confounding, the true odds ratio would still have been close to 5.0, suggesting that this is more likely to be a real association.

Confounding: the bottom line

Confounding is almost ubiquitous in practice and almost any paper that reports associations between two factors will say that the authors have 'adjusted' for this, that and the other to control for confounding. If a paper does *not* mention adjustment for confounding then it is important to consider whether this is a possibility; we will discuss this further in the next chapter.

As we discussed in the previous chapter, it can be hard to know what effects bias might have on the results of a study; in contrast, *known* confounders can be identified and addressed *if information about the confounders has been collected.*

Even if an analysis has 'adjusted for confounders' there is likely to be *residual confounding* either by measured confounders or by unmeasured/ unknown confounders. For *known confounders*, a big difference between the unadjusted and adjusted measures suggests that there may be considerable residual confounding; a small difference implies that residual confounding is not a big problem. Unless we are talking about a randomised trial we will not know anything about the likely effects of any *unknown or unmeasured confounders*, but if we see a strong association between exposure and outcome then the confounding would have to be enormous (very strong associations between the confounder and both the exposure and the outcome) to explain the whole association. In practice we might hope that we would know about such strong confounders.

We have now covered the three main issues that we have to consider before we conclude that the results of a study are real: namely chance, bias and confounding. In the next chapter we will bring these altogether to look at how we can make sense of the epidemiological literature.

Questions

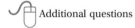 Additional questions

Table 8.11 shows some data from a study of injuries involving moped riders in Spain. The authors obtained information from the Spanish Registry of Traffic Crashes regarding 187,353 moped riders injured in traffic accidents between 1990 and 1999. They then compared the group with head injuries (cases) with those with other types of injury (controls).

1. What is the crude odds ratio for the association between not wearing a helmet (exposed) and head injury?

Table 8.11 Results of a study of head injury and helmet use.

	Driver		Passenger		Total	
	Head injury	Other injury	Head injury	Other injury	Head injury	Other injury
No helmet	17,869	51,900	3052	12,522	20,921	64,422
Helmet	7,342	86,212	485	7,971	7,827	94,183
Total	25,211	138,112	3,537	20,493	28,748	158,605

(Lardelli-Claret *et al.*, 2003)

2. What is the odds ratio for the association between not wearing a helmet and head injury among (i) moped drivers and (ii) moped passengers?
3. Was the crude association between not wearing a helmet and head injury confounded by position on the moped?
4. Does the position of the rider (driver or passenger) on the moped affect their chances of sustaining a head injury? (Hint – first calculate the crude odds ratio for the association between moped position and head injury and then consider whether this could be confounded by helmet use.)
5. If we are interested in the association between drinking coffee and incidence of heart disease, which of the following factors are likely to be confounders and why:
   (a) age and sex
   (b) smoking
   (c) physical activity
   (d) fruit and vegetable intake?
6. Imagine that, when we were interested in the association between energy intake and heart disease we had conducted a cohort study instead of a case–control study. The results of this study are shown in Table 8.12.
   (a) What is the crude rate ratio for the association between high energy intake and heart disease?
   (b) What is the rate ratio for the association between high energy intake and heart disease in people with (i) high and (ii) low levels of physical activity?
   (c) Is the association between high energy intake and heart disease confounded by the level of physical activity?
7. Go back to Table 8.7 and recalculate the crude (overall) and stratum-specific odds ratios assuming that the study had (i) half as many people (i.e. divide all the numbers of cases and controls by 2) and (ii) twice as many people. What effect does changing the size of a study have on the confounding effect of physical activity?

Table 8.12 Results of a hypothetical cohort study of high energy intake and heart disease, stratified by level of physical activity.

Energy intake	Total		High physical activity		Low physical activity	
	Person-years	Developed heart disease	Person-years	Developed heart disease	Person-years	Developed heart disease
High	60,000	720	50,000	500	10,000	220
Low	55,000	700	15,000	100	40,000	600

REFERENCES

References

Bickel, P. J., Hammel, E. A. and O'Connell, J. W. (1975). Sex bias in graduate admissions: data from Berkeley. *Science*, 187: 398–404.

Brennan, P., McKay, J., Moore, L., *et al.* (2009). Obesity and cancer: Mendelian randomization approach utilizing the *FTO* genotype. *International Journal of Epidemiology*, 38: 971–975.

Davey Smith, G. (2011). Use of genetic markers and gene-diet interactions for interrogating population-level causal influences of diet on health. *Genes and Nutrition*, 6: 27–43.

Davey Smith, G. and Ebrahim, S. (2003). 'Mendelian randomization': can genetic epidemiology contribute to understanding environmental determinants of disease? *International Journal of Epidemiology*, 32: 1–22.

Davey Smith, G. and Hemani, G. (2014). Mendelian randomization: genetic anchors for causal inference in epidemiological studies. *Human Molecular Genetics*, 23: R89–R98.

Davey Smith, G., Harbord, R., Milton, J., Ebrahim, S. and Sterne, J. A. (2005). Does elevated plasma fibrinogen increase the risk of coronary heart disease? Evidence from a meta-analysis of genetic association studies. *Arteriosclerosis, Thrombosis and Vascular Biology*, 25: 2228–2233.

Earle, C.C., Tsai, J. S., Gelber, R. D., *et al.* (2001). Effectiveness of chemotherapy for advanced lung cancer in the elderly: instrumental variable and propensity analysis. *Journal of Clinical Oncology*, 19: 1064–1070.

Feskanich, D., Ziegler, R. G., Michaud, D. S., *et al.* (2000). Prospective study of fruit and vegetable consumption and risk of lung cancer among men and women. *Journal of the National Cancer Institute*, 92: 1812–1823.

Greenland, S., Pearl, J. and Robins, J. M. (1999). Causal diagrams for epidemiologic research. *Epidemiology*, 10: 37–48.

Guiltinan, A. M., Kaidarova, Z., Custer, B., *et al.* (2008). Increased all-cause, liver, and cardiac mortality among hepatitis C virus-seropositive blood donors. *American Journal of Epidemiology*, 167: 743–750.

Joffe, M. M. and Rosenbaum, P. R. (1999). Invited commentary: propensity scores. *American Journal of Epidemiology*, 150: 327–333.

Lardelli-Claret, P., Luna-del-Castillo, J. D. D. and Jimenez-Moleon, J. J. (2003). Position on the moped, risk of head injury and helmet use: an example of confounding effect. *International Journal of Epidemiology*, 32: 162–164.

Mantel, N. and Haenszel, W. (1959). Statistical aspects of the analysis of data from retrospective studies of disease. *Journal of the National Cancer Institute*, 22: 719–748.

Miettinen, O. S. (1983). The need for randomization in the study of intended effects. *Statistics in Medicine*, 2: 267–271.

Page, A., Morrell, S., Hobbs, C., *et al.* (2014). Suicide in young adults: psychiatric and socio-economic factors from a case–control study. *BMC Psychiatry*, 14: 1–9.

Rothman, K. J. (2012). *Epidemiology: An Introduction*. New York, NY: Oxford University Press.

Vessey, M. P. and Lawless, M. (1984). The Oxford Family Planning Association contraceptive study. *Clinical Obstetrics and Gynaecology*, 11: 743–757.

RECOMMENDED FURTHER READING

- For more about DAGs:

  Greenland, S., Pearl, J. and Robins, J. M. (1999). Causal diagrams for epidemiologic research. *Epidemiology*, 10: 37–48.

- For more about Mendelian randomisation:

  Davey Smith, G. (2011). Use of genetic markers and gene-diet interactions for interrogating population-level causal influences of diet on health. *Genes and Nutrition*, 6: 27–43.

  Davey Smith, G. and Ebrahim, S. (2003). 'Mendelian randomization': can genetic epidemiology contribute to understanding environmental determinants of disease? *International Journal of Epidemiology*, 32: 1–22.

  Davey Smith, G. and Hemani, G. (2014). Mendelian randomization: genetic anchors for causal inference in epidemiological studies. *Human Molecular Genetics*, 23: R89–R98.

9

Reading between the lines:
reading and writing epidemiological papers

Description
Chapters 2–3

Association
Chapters 4–5

Alternative explanations
Chapters 6–8

Integration & interpretation
Chapter 9:
Reading papers

Practical applications
Chapters 12–15

The over-arching goal of public health is to maximise the health of the population and for this we need evidence about what works and what doesn't work. In Chapters 4, 6, 7 and 8 we looked at the different epidemiological study designs and examined the various misfortunes that can befall them. Good studies are difficult to design and implement, and interpretation of their results and conclusions is not always as straightforward as we might hope. How, then, can we make the best use of this information? In the next three chapters we will look at ways to identify, appraise, integrate and interpret the literature to generate the evidence we need to inform policy and practice. In this chapter we will focus on interpreting the results from a single study, while Chapter 10 will consider some of the issues involved when we try to decide if an observed association might be causal. Finally, Chapter 11 will look at how we conduct and interpret reviews and how we can bring all of this information together to make evidence-based recommendations.

The central question we have to answer when we read a study report is '*Are the results of the study valid?*' If the authors report an association between exposure and outcome, is it real? If they find nothing, do we accept this? Or could there be an alternative explanation for the results, namely chance, bias and/or confounding? Then, if we think the results are valid, we should ask 'so what?' – are the results clinically or socially important? And 'to whom do these results apply' – can we assume that they will apply more generally than in that particular study population?

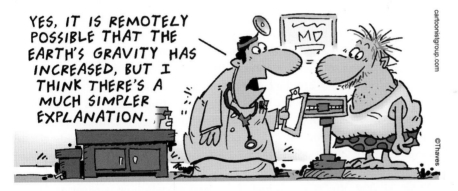

Much of the following discussion will pick up and integrate the core epidemiological issues covered in the previous chapters. We will concentrate mainly on analytic studies looking for associations between 'cause' and 'effect', the study designs that you met in Chapter 4, but the same general principles apply equally to descriptive epidemiology. To extract the maximum information from a paper we need a systematic approach to identifying its strengths and weaknesses. Some quite detailed sets of guidelines for 'critical appraisal' of the health literature exist already (e.g. see Box 9.2 on page 259) and we do not intend to add to this list (although we do offer a flowchart for more general guidance). Instead, we will focus on the essence of the challenge: what are the practical effects of the ways in which subjects

It is obviously easier to assess the results of a study if they are presented in a clear and systematic way. A number of **checklists** have been developed to assist authors with this; we will discuss these under 'Writing papers'.

were selected and information collected, and the likely influence of confounding and chance on the results we see? While the elements of the general strategy we propose are universal, the approach can (and should) be tailored to suit your own personal style. In practice you will almost certainly have to read individual papers and reports and, if you are involved in research, you may write some of your own. Both activities demand a very practical approach and this is what we will focus on here. We will emphasise the perspective of the reader, but the writer should be thinking about exactly the same things, because good writing demands that the readers' needs and perspectives are kept firmly in mind.

The research question and study design

When reading a paper, the first step is to identify the *research question* that the authors set out to answer and then the strategy they used to attempt to answer that question. Was the *study design* appropriate to answer the question posed? This involves consideration of what the *ideal* type of study would be and also what would be *practical* in that particular situation.

As you have seen, the *ideal* study to answer a question of cause and effect would usually be some sort of randomised trial, as this is the best way to ensure that the groups we are comparing are exchangeable, but in many situations this will be impossible for numerous ethical and/or practical reasons. Next best would generally be a cohort study in which exposure is measured prior to the development of disease, but again the resources, time and money required to conduct a large enough study often make it unfeasible. So from a practical viewpoint, the key question should be '*Was the research design the best that could have been done in the circumstances to answer that particular question?*' If it was not the best, can it still provide useful information? Are there other studies addressing the same issue that were of better design?

Many studies are not conducted to give a definitive answer to direct questions about causation, but because they can answer other more indirect questions of interest. For example, the results from the ecological study of *Helicobacter pylori* infection and stomach cancer rates in China shown in Figure 3.8 cannot directly answer the question 'Does *H. pylori* infection cause stomach cancer?', but they can answer the question 'Are stomach cancer rates higher in areas where *H. pylori* infection is more common?' If *H. pylori* infection does cause stomach cancer then we would expect this to be the case and evidence to this effect supports the hypothesis that the relation is causal. Although non-randomised studies provide more circumstantial evidence than RCTs, if the results are valid each can increase our understanding of the relation between an exposure and outcome. As an example, ecological and migrant studies conducted across countries with widely differing levels of solar ultraviolet (UV) radiation have consistently revealed an association between sun exposure in childhood and melanoma rates. In contrast, case–control studies, which have generally been conducted within a single country or region with a narrow range of UV exposures, have not given consistent results (Whiteman *et al.*, 2001). In this particular situation ecological studies with their wide variety of exposure levels provide a valuable addition to the case–control studies.

Internal validity

Internal validity is the extent to which the results of a study reflect the true situation *in the study sample.* So how do we decide whether the results of a study are internally valid? We have to consider the three main alternative explanations that we discussed in the preceding chapters: chance, bias (both the *selection of participants* for the study and the *information* that was *measured* or collected from or about them) and confounding.

The study sample: selection bias

Who was included in the study, how were they selected and are there possible sources of selection bias? Specific questions to ask when reading a paper include those below.

- *Is the comparison group appropriate?*
  In a case–control study are the controls really representative of the population from which the cases arose? In a cohort study where the comparison cohort was recruited separately from the exposed cohort, are the two groups really comparable (i.e. are they *exchangeable*)?
- *What proportion of eligible participants actually took part in the study and, if appropriate, what proportion was lost to follow-up?*
  Low participation or follow-up rates may be cause for some concern. If the rates are lower than 80% or 90%, could participation (or loss to follow-up) be related to either the exposure or the outcome of interest? That is, could those who refused to take part (or who were lost to follow-up) have differed in some way from those who did take part? If so, might this have led to an overestimation or underestimation of the level of exposure and/or outcome? Most importantly, could this have differed between study groups?
- *Finally, what is the likely effect of any selection bias on the results of the study?*
  Ideally, the authors of the paper will have considered all of these issues in their discussion, but if they have not then it is up to the reader to decide whether bias might be present and, if so, what effect it may have had on the

As you saw in Chapter 7, high **participation rates** are very important for cross-sectional and case–control studies, but high **follow-up rates** are more important in cohort studies and trials.

results. In practice there will almost certainly be some potential for selection bias. Participation rates are never 100% and in many developed countries it is becoming increasingly hard to persuade people to take part in research, especially when they see no benefit to themselves. This is a major issue in case–control studies when the motivation for a 'case' to take part may be much greater than that of an unaffected 'control'. Also, people are becoming increasingly mobile, so follow-up in a cohort study that runs for more than a few years is never likely to be 100%. However, remember that selection bias will only affect the validity of the results if, in a case–control or cross-sectional study, the likelihood that someone agrees to take part differs by both case–control *and* exposure status or, in a cohort study, the likelihood of someone being lost to follow is related to both their exposure *and* their probability of developing the disease of interest.

If we were to reject all studies with less than 100% participation or follow-up rates, we would be left with nothing to review. In practice, participation or follow-up rates greater than 80% or 90% are generally considered to be good, but rates lower than this do not necessarily invalidate the findings (see Example 2 below). This is especially true for cohort studies and trials where low participation rates are less of a problem *as long as the follow-up rate is high*. The challenge for both investigator and reader is to think practically and to decide whether any potential biases related to selection might have compromised the study results (the **internal validity**) and, if so, how and to what degree the results might be biased. It is often impossible to quantify this, but **sensitivity analyses** making various assumptions about the size and direction of possible bias can be informative (see Chapter 7).

Example 1: case–control studies of blood transfusion and Creutzfeldt–Jakob disease

In five case–control studies of Creutzfeldt-Jakob disease (CJD) the controls were more likely to report having had a blood transfusion than cases (Riggs *et al.*, 2001). Does this tell us that blood transfusions might protect against CJD (a finding contrary to the causal hypothesis)? If we consider the control groups, we find that in three of the five studies they were selected from among hospitalised patients and in another study more than 12,000 telephone calls were made in order to recruit just 784 controls.

The use of hospital controls and the very low participation rate among controls should ring alarm bells. Why?

People who are in hospital are more likely to have had a blood transfusion than those who are not; in addition, given the publicity surrounding 'mad cow disease', people who have had a blood transfusion may well have been more likely to agree to take part in a study of CJD. Indeed, in these four studies approximately 20% of controls reported having had a blood transfusion – an improbably high proportion, probably due at least in part to these selection pressures. So what can we conclude about the association between transfusion and CJD from these studies? Not much. The high transfusion rate in controls almost certainly overestimates the base rate in the population from which the cases came. Unless we have some knowledge of how common transfusion really is in the population, we have no idea whether the true background rate is similar to that in cases (i.e. there is no association) or lower than in cases (i.e. there is a positive association). Our next example shows how external information was used to help resolve such a dilemma.

Example 2: a case–control study of oesophageal cancer and smoking in Australia

In an Australian case–control study of oesophageal cancer, the authors considered the relation with smoking. In this study approximately 70% of eligible cases but only 49% of the controls who were contacted agreed to participate – this is a fairly typical response rate in many countries these days, but far from ideal. The authors found that current smoking rates were higher among cases with oesophageal adenocarcinoma than controls (OR compared to never smokers = 2.7; 95% CI 1.9–3.9), but could this be due to selection bias?

In general, smokers are less likely to agree to take part in a study than non-smokers. What effect might this have had on the odds ratio?

If smokers were less likely to take part the prevalence of smoking in the control group would be *lower* than that in the general population. This would exaggerate the difference between cases and controls and so increase the odds ratio, making it look as if smoking is associated with oesophageal adenocarcinoma when in reality it might not be. To address this issue the authors used data from a National Health Survey conducted at about the same time. If they assumed that the whole control population had a smoking rate equal to that seen in the national survey, they found that the odds ratio for the association between smoking and oesophageal adenocarcinoma was slightly weaker but still significantly greater than 1.0 (imputed OR = 2.4; 95% CI 1.7–3.4). This suggested that even though only about half of the controls invited to take part in the study actually agreed to participate, the overall results for the association with smoking were not seriously biased (Pandeya *et al.*, 2009).

Measuring disease and exposure: measurement bias

We also have to consider the information collected from or about the people in the study – particularly the measurement of 'outcome' and 'exposure' but

More about low participation rates: Investigators compared prevalence estimates and ORs for the association between selected exposures and health conditions calculated using baseline data from a cohort study with a participation rate of only 18%, with those from a population survey with a 60% response rate. The results suggested that any bias due to the low response rate in the study was minimal (Mealing *et al.*, 2010).

also measurement of other factors that might be important confounders. Attention to unbiased measurement of outcome is crucial for cross-sectional, cohort and intervention studies. It is of relatively less importance in a case–control study, in which cases are selected because they have already experienced the outcome of interest (although a clear definition of what constitutes a case is still essential). Accurate measurement of exposure is important in every study, and in a case–control study it is critical to ensure that there are no systematic differences in measurement between cases and controls. Good measurement of confounders is often overlooked, but this is essential to enable optimal control of confounding in the analysis (see comments on residual confounding in Chapter 8).

Some questions to ask when reading a paper are the following.

- Have all relevant outcomes and/or exposures and/or confounders been included and, if not, how important are those omitted?
- Were the outcome/exposures/confounders clearly defined, and how were they measured?
- Were the same definitions and methods of measurement used in all of the study groups?
- Is measurement error likely to be a problem and, if so, could there be **non-differential misclassification**?

Non-differential misclassification is particularly problematic in dietary studies because measurement of diet is very challenging and, as a result, misclassification is likely to be high. Furthermore the real effects are likely to be small.

No measurement is perfect and some measurements are very poor. The effect of the ubiquitous random error and consequent non-differential misclassification must always be considered. The practical implication of this is that effects (OR, RR) estimated in the face of equal measurement error in the compared groups will usually appear *weaker* than they truly are, e.g. if the observed OR is 1.8 then, in all probability, the real association is even stronger, i.e. >1.8. Thus a finding of a positive association, despite poor measurement, should not be dismissed because of this – the true association is likely to be more impressive. On the other hand, a null finding or a very weak effect in the presence of non-differential misclassification is uninformative because it may reflect the imprecise measurement (thereby masking a true association) or there may truly be no effect. (Note that non-differential misclassification is unlikely to make it appear that an association exists when in reality there is none.)

- Is the extent of any measurement error likely to differ between groups (e.g. could there be *recall* or *interviewer bias* in exposure measurement in a case–control study) and so could there be **differential misclassification**?

If so, is it possible to predict what the differences might have been? For example, are cases more or less likely to have over-reported exposure? If cases overestimate their exposure then the OR is likely to be biased upwards, conversely if they underestimate their exposure (or controls overestimate theirs) then the bias is likely to be downwards. Could the observed association be due to misclassification? Or might the real association be stronger than that observed? Differential misclassification can bias results in either direction, it can make an association appear where there is none, it can make it seem that there is no association when in reality there is one and it can even make a positive association look like an inverse association, and vice versa. It is particularly important to consider this possibility in cross-sectional and case–control studies when exposure is measured after the outcome has occurred. In analytic research it is generally easier to distinguish clearly between outcome states (diseased versus non-diseased) than it is to measure exposures precisely, but the avoidance of differential outcome assessment is central to the integrity of cohort studies and trials, and again for cross-sectional studies.

- Finally, what *practical effects* might any measurement bias (outcome or exposure) have had on the results of the study?

Example 3: a case–control study of body mass index (BMI) and asthma in Mexico

A significant association between asthma and obesity[1] based on self-reported weight and height was observed among women (adjusted OR = 1.7; 95% CI 1.1–2.7), with a weaker non-significant association (adjusted OR = 1.3; 95% CI 0.6–2.9) among men (Santillan and Camargo, 2003); but how reliable are self-reported data on body size, and could measurement error have affected the results? The authors specifically addressed this question by weighing and measuring all of the participants. They found that, on average, people tended to report that they were taller and lighter than they really were, particularly the men. As a result, the *true* prevalence of obesity based on measured BMI was higher than that based on self-reported BMI and the difference was somewhat greater for cases (40% versus 24% for men and 44% versus 38% for women) than for controls (28% versus 22% for men; 24% versus 23% for women).

Is the error in the self-reported information on body-size differential or non-differential?

Assuming that the measured BMI values are correct, is the *true* association between obesity and asthma likely to be stronger or weaker than that seen for self-reported obesity?

---

[1] In this study, as in most, obesity was defined as a body mass index (BMI, calculated as weight in kg divided by the square of height in m) ≥ 30 kg/m^2.

In this example there is *differential* error because cases, particularly men, were more likely to underestimate their weight and overestimate their height than controls. The effect of these errors would be to reduce the association seen and this is what happened. When the authors calculated the association between asthma and *measured* obesity, the OR was 2.3 (95% CI 1.5–3.8) for women and 2.5 (95% CI 1.1–5.9) for men, i.e. the associations were much stronger than those based on self-reported BMI above. By measuring height and weight they have removed the possibility of recall bias and any subsequent *differential* misclassification, and they have also reduced the potential for *non-differential* misclassification. The OR based on measured BMI is therefore likely to be a more accurate estimate than that based on self-reporting. (Note that even this may still slightly underestimate the 'true' effect because there may be some remaining non-differential random misclassification.) Validation studies such as this can provide valuable insights into the accuracy of study results as can sensitivity analyses such as that described in Box 9.1.

Box 9.1 Sensitivity analysis: pet flea treatment and autism spectrum disorders

Laboratory studies suggest prenatal exposure to the insecticide imidacloprid may induce neurobehavioural deficits in animals. To assess whether it might have a similar effect in humans, researchers conducted a case–control study to assess the relationship between use of pet flea and tick treatments containing imidacloprid and autism spectrum disorders (ASD) in young children. Mothers of children with and without ASD were asked how often they used flea or tick products before, during and after their pregnancy. The results did not show a significant association between imidacloprid use and ASD (OR = 1.3; 95% CI = 0.79–2.2). However, because of the high potential for recall bias, the researchers performed a range of sensitivity analyses where they assumed different proportions of children were misclassified as exposed or unexposed. Depending on the level of misclassification and whether it occurred in cases and/or controls, the OR varied from about 0.6 (suggesting no increase in risk) up to about 4.0 – suggesting a very strong association. The authors concluded that their results suggested an association could result from misclassification alone, but they also noted that their estimates were higher among consistent users and for use during pregnancy and suggested further studies were warranted.

(Keil *et al.*, 2014)

Confounding

The next major issue to consider is that of confounding.

- Have the authors considered all important confounders and controlled for them in their analysis?
- Could there be residual confounding by variables that have not been considered or because of incomplete adjustment for factors that have?
- If so, what effect might this have had on the study results?

As we discussed in Chapter 8, it can be helpful to draw a directed acyclic graph or DAG to show the relationships between all of the factors that need to be considered as potential confounders. There are then formal methods to help identify which factors are likely to be confounders and which can be ignored. Again, the important thing is to think practically: in which direction is any residual confounding likely to operate? If adjustment brings a RR towards 1.0 then in the presence of residual confounding the true RR is likely to be even closer to 1.0. Conversely, if the adjusted RR is further from 1.0 than the crude RR, then the true RR is likely to be even more extreme. In the former situation our confidence in a positive effect estimate would decrease, unless it was very large. A large effect is less likely to be wholly due to confounding because, to explain away a very strong RR (e.g. 10.0), the confounder itself would have to be an even stronger risk factor for the disease. If this is the case then it is likely to be known already, and hence should have been measured and controlled for.

Example 4: a cross-sectional study of risk factors for depression in the UK

Among 14,217 adults aged over 75 years, the risk of depression appeared to be somewhat higher among women than among men (crude OR = 1.3, 95% CI 1.1–1.5) (Osborn *et al.*, 2003). After adjustment for potential confounding factors including age, marital status, living alone, smoking and alcohol consumption, the adjusted OR was 1.1 (95% CI 1.0–1.3).

What do these results suggest about the association between sex and risk of depression?

The adjustment has reduced the OR, bringing it closer to 1.0. It is also likely that there is further residual confounding, which might bring the true OR even closer to 1.0, suggesting that sex is not associated with depression (at least in this study). This example also highlights the need to consider the clinical or practical significance of the results of a study. A very large study can show what appears to be a very small effect with great precision (a narrow confidence interval); even though the result might be statistically significant ($p < 0.05$), the key question is whether such a small difference is meaningful.

Example 5: a cohort study of statin use and atrial fibrillation in the USA

A cohort of patients with coronary artery disease was followed for a minimum of 12 months to document the incidence of atrial fibrillation (AF, an abnormal heart rhythm); 263 of the patients were using statins (cholesterol-lowering drugs) and 186 had never used them (Young-Xu *et al.*, 2003). (Note that this was an observational study – a prognostic cohort – not a randomised trial.) Overall, the rate of AF was lower among the group taking statins, giving a crude relative risk of 0.5 (95% CI 0.3–0.8). When the authors adjusted for potential confounding factors including age, systolic blood pressure, alcohol consumption, history of heart failure and total serum cholesterol level, the RR was 0.4 (95% CI 0.2–0.8).

Assuming that there are no important selection or measurement errors, what conclusions can we draw about the association between statin use and AF?

It appears that there was some confounding by the other factors such as age because the RR dropped from 0.5 to 0.4 after adjustment, indicating that the real effect of statin use was even stronger than the crude RR suggested. However, doctors prescribe treatment partly on the basis of prognostic judgements, which are difficult to measure. There may thus be other unknown and unmeasured confounders that have not been controlled for, so we would still need to be cautious about this particular result. Large, well-conducted RCTs remove this potential problem which, as you saw in Chapter 8, is called **confounding by indication**.

Interpreting results from RCTs

Although RCTs are less susceptible to confounding than other study designs, it is important to remember that they are not immune to bias and problems can occur even in the best trials. It is for this reason that the Cochrane Collaboration developed their 'risk of bias' tool to assess the quality of RCTs (see Box 9.2).

Example 6: the Women's Health Initiative (WHI) trial of menopausal hormone therapy

The WHI comprised a number of studies including a double-blind RCT where about 16,600 menopausal women aged 50–79 years were randomly allocated to receive oestrogen plus progesterone (combined hormone therapy, HT) or placebo. After five years of follow-up the results suggested that rather than improving women's health, those randomised to combined HT experienced higher rates of some outcomes, including breast cancer. The conclusion was that combined HT increased a woman's risk of developing breast cancer (Rossouw *et al.*, 2002) and the trial was stopped. However, although the trial was conducted according to rigorous standards, women randomised to combined HT often experienced bleeding requiring investigation to rule out uterine cancer and this meant that a high proportion (> 40%) became 'unblinded' and so knew which tablet they were taking, compared to only 7% of women in the placebo

Box 9.2 The Cochrane collaboration (www.cochrane.org)

This was established to promote evidence-based decision making in health. It does this by conducting systematic reviews to bring together all of the relevant evidence in a given health area (we will discuss systematic reviews in Chapter 11). To facilitate the review process, the Cochrane Collaboration has developed standardised methods for reviewing the literature including a 'risk of bias' tool to help a reviewer assess the quality of evidence from RCTs (Higgins *et al.*, 2011). (As the focus is on evaluating health interventions, the best information usually comes from RCTs.) The tool covers six domains including issues relating to: randomisation (what they term *selection bias**), blinding of participants and personnel (*performance bias*) and of outcome assessment (*detection bias*), loss to follow-up and exclusions (*attrition bias*), completeness of reporting (*reporting bias*) and any *other bias*. The probability that each type of bias has occurred is rated as high, low or unclear. A parallel tool, ROBINS-I (previously ACROBAT-NRSI) (www.riskofbias.info) has been developed for assessing risk of bias in non-randomised studies of interventions by comparing them to an idealised RCT of the same intervention (Sterne *et al.*, 2014).

*This is another example where those working in a more clinically oriented environment use somewhat different terms from epidemiologists working in public health.

group. If women who knew they were taking HT were more likely to examine their own breasts or to seek breast screening, it is possible they were more likely to be diagnosed with breast cancer than control women. As a result, some have suggested that although combined HT might increase breast cancer, the results of the WHI trial did not conclusively establish this (Shapiro *et al.*, 2011).

Chance

Finally, it is important to consider the role of chance. Have the authors included confidence intervals for their estimates? How narrow (good precision) or wide (poor precision) are they? Have they conducted any statistical tests and presented the resulting p-values? If an association is seen, how likely is it that there is really no effect (i.e. the association arose by chance)? As you saw in Chapter 6, if the probability of getting a result as strong as or stronger than that observed is $< 5\%$ ($p < 0.05$, i.e. one time in 20) then, by convention, we would consider it unlikely to be due to chance. However, in many modern studies the investigators study multiple associations so the probability that one will arise by chance is greatly increased. Although some authors recommend correcting results for this problem of 'multiple testing' (see Box 6.3 in Chapter 6), we and many others prefer to rely more on a common-sense approach that places less emphasis on the question of statistical significance and more on the overall strength, coherence and plausibility of an observed association. (We will discuss some of these issues further in Chapter 10.) If there is no clear association (e.g. if the confidence limits are very wide and include 1.0 or $p > 0.05$), is it possible that there is a real effect but the study was simply too small to detect it? Is the study useful or are the results inconclusive?

Overall internal validity

Once we have considered all of these aspects (summarised in Figure 9.1) we can make an overall judgement of the internal validity of the study results. Have the authors discussed the limitations of their study? What conclusions do they draw with respect to the research question? Are these conclusions justified? Does the study appear to be internally valid or could the results be due to chance, bias or confounding? These 'alternative explanations' have been the focus of this and the preceding chapters.

The prime objective of study design, implementation, analysis and interpretation is to generate an answer to the research question that is as close to the truth as possible. However, in public health we are dealing with real people and complex exposures that are often difficult to measure and/or impossible to control adequately and we are, quite rightly, constrained as to what we can do by codes of ethics. Any study is thus likely to fall short of perfection and it is important to realise this. Research should be appraised in the light of what it has been able to achieve – there will be deficiencies but, given the particular circumstances, could things realistically have been improved? The evidence reported in a research paper might not always be strong but, if it is the best that is likely to be available, we should not discount it because of the flaws. Rather we should draw from it what information we can.

So what? Are the results important?

We discussed the need to consider whether the results could have arisen by chance above, but as well as *statistical significance* it is also important to consider whether the results are *socially* or *clinically* significant (see *Statistical versus clinical significance* in Chapter 6). A large study may give an association that is statistically significant, for example the odds ratio of 1.1 (95% CI 1.0–1.3) seen for the association between sex and depression in Example 4 above, but we then have to ask whether a 10% higher risk of depression in women than men is a meaningful difference. As you saw in Chapter 5, the relative risk is not the only measure we can look at to assess the importance of a relationship, and relative and absolute risks can often give a very different picture. A modest RR can equate to a high population attributable fraction if

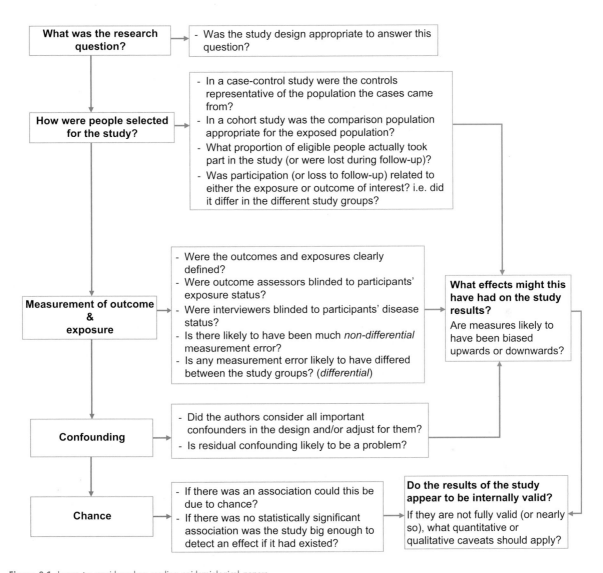

Figure 9.1 Issues to consider when reading epidemiological papers.

the exposure is common but, conversely, if the exposure is rare the PAF may be low, despite a high RR. Similarly, if the background rate of disease is low, a small absolute increase will appear to be a large relative increase. The question of clinical significance becomes particularly problematic when the cost of achieving a statistically significant, but sometimes very small, clinical benefit is high. This is a particularly thorny issue for governments who have to grapple with decisions whether to subsidise expensive new drugs (see Box 9.3).

Box 9.3 How much is life worth?

More than 90% of new anti-cancer agents approved by the US Food and Drug Administration between 2005 and 2009 cost more than US$20,000 for a 12-week course of treatment. However, many show only marginal gains in survival: new therapies approved for non-small cell lung cancer, for example, cost an average of US$91,000 per patient and increase median survival by only 1.2 months; others for pancreatic cancer cost $16,000 and increase median survival by only 10 days. This equates to costs of up to US$800,000 per year of life gained compared to $129,090 for something like renal dialysis and raises the question of what represents a clinically significant improvement and how much we should we pay for this (Fojo and Grady, 2009).

Generalisability (external validity)

It is important to remember that the aim of the 'causal arm' of epidemiology is to discover general scientific truths about cause and effect. If the results of a study of, for example, American men aged 50–65 appear to be internally valid, can they be generalised to all American men in that age group? What about older or younger men? Women? Non-Americans? (Note that internal validity must always be the primary goal, *if a study is not internally valid, then the results should not be applied to anyone.*)

There are no firm rules to help with generalising from a study to the wider population but the first step is to consider whether the results obtained from the study population can be generalised to the source population that they came from (see Figure 3.4) and this will depend both on how potential participants were identified for the study, and on the response rate. In case–control comparisons, population-based studies are the ideal in order to reduce the possibilities of selection bias and, as a result, it might not require such a leap of faith to extrapolate the study results to the source population. The second step is to consider whether the results might also apply to other populations and this process is not simply a matter of statistical representativeness, but is more fundamentally one of biological insight. The question then is 'How relevant (biologically) is a result for a given population?' Can a study in a very select population (e.g. urban-living Japanese, Czech women, Brazilian men) inform us about disease causation more generally? Well, we certainly hope so. As an example, careful follow-up of the survivors of the atomic bomb blasts in Hiroshima and Nagasaki, Japan, has yielded volumes of information regarding the relation between exposure to ionising radiation and subsequent risks of mortality, cancers and other diseases. While this information comes only from the Japanese, no one would argue that radiation would not have similar effects in other nationalities, and we certainly do not want to see this 'unnatural experiment' repeated. While this generalisation is perhaps easier than many because of the magnitude and timing of the effects and the well-understood physical and biological properties of ionising radiation, the principle is identical for other abstract causal speculation.

Generalising from clinical and other trials raises additional issues. For practical reasons, many clinical trials are conducted on highly selected groups of people. This can make the results of the specific trials easier to interpret (good internal validity), but means it can be hard to know exactly how well the intervention will work in the general population. Post-marketing surveillance systems such as those you met in Chapter 4 (see Record linkage and Box 4.6) are increasingly being established to monitor new interventions for unexpected adverse events.

> **Generalising from RCTs:** trials of new drugs are often restricted to younger more healthy patients. It is then hard to know whether the drugs will also work for older people who often have significant comorbidities and who may comprise the majority of the patient group.

Descriptive studies

The discussion above has focussed on papers evaluating associations between exposure and outcome and that, therefore, address the 'Why?' of epidemiology. It is equally important to evaluate the results of descriptive studies that provide the 'Who?', 'Where?' and 'When?' information that is essential to make a community diagnosis and, as you will see in Chapter 14, is also important for evaluating the effects of public health interventions. In practice this requires us to consider exactly the same issues: selection and measurement error, confounding and chance.

- How was the survey sample selected? Is it representative of the wider population?
  It is important to note that, although representativeness is not the primary issue in studies of aetiology, it is critical for most descriptive research as you saw in Chapter 7 (Box 7.1). If the sample of people surveyed to identify the health needs of an area does not represent the whole population, the results could be very misleading. For example, if they were unusually healthy then the needs of the population might be greatly underestimated, and vice versa. For this reason, national censuses and, in some countries like Australia, the government-run national health surveys are supported by legislation that legally obliges people to take part.
- How was the factor of interest measured? Is it likely to be over- or under-reported?
- If we are making comparisons, are we comparing like with like (are the groups we are comparing *exchangeable*?) or is there a need for standardisation (to remove confounding by, for example, differences in the age structure of populations)?

- Could any observed excesses (or deficits) of disease in different populations, in different places or at different times be due to chance? For example, it is unlikely that several cases of a rare disease would occur in the same small community (what is known as a 'cluster' – see Chapter 13), but it is not impossible for this to occur by chance. Similarly, rates of disease (particularly rare diseases) will naturally vary from year to year, so could an apparent increase or decline just be due to chance?

Writing papers

We have concentrated on the information that you need to look for when reading a paper and, as we suggested at the start of this chapter, it goes without saying that this is also the information that you need to provide when writing a paper. In general, a research paper should be structured with a brief *abstract* followed by an *introduction* to show why the research question is of interest; a *methods* section to explain how the work was done; a summary of the *results*; and, finally, the *conclusions* or a *discussion* where the results are interpreted, any threats to validity considered and causal conclusions drawn. To improve the reporting of health research, specific standards have been developed for a wide range of study types and many journals now require authors to complete the relevant checklist prior to submitting their paper for publication. Many of these guidelines are available via the EQUATOR (Enhancing the QUAlity and Transparency Of health Research) Network (www.equator-network.org/) and Table 9.1 summarises some of the most useful.

Table 9.1 Guidelines for reporting the results of health research.

Guideline	Area
CONSORT: Consolidated Standards of Reporting Trials (Shulz *et al.*, 2010)	Randomised controlled trials
TREND: Transparent Reporting of Non-randomised Designs (Des Jarlais *et al.*, 2004)	Behavioural and public health interventions with non-randomised designs
STROBE: Strengthening the Reporting of Observational Studies in Epidemiology (von Elm *et al.*, 2007)	Cohort, case–control and cross-sectional studies
STREGA: Strengthening the Reporting of Genetic Association Studies (Little *et al.*, 2009)	A modification of STROBE for genetic studies
STARD: Standards for the Reporting of Diagnostic Accuracy Studies (Bossuyt *et al.*, 2003)	Diagnostic tests
CARE: Case Reporting (Gagnier *et al.*, 2013)	Consensus-based guideline for clinical case reports and reports of patient encounters
SAMPL: Statistical Analyses and Methods in the Published Literature (Lang and Altman, 2013)	Basic statistical reporting for articles published in biomedical journals

Box 9.4 The Francis field trial of inactivated poliomyelitis vaccine or 'Salk vaccine trial' – a practice changer

Regular poliomyelitis epidemics in the USA, with over 58,000 affected in 1952 alone, led to widespread fear of the disease and its consequences (paralysis, death). In response, the National Foundation for Infantile Paralysis, a voluntary foundation, proposed, initiated and largely funded a massive project in the early 1950s to evaluate the preventive benefits of a vaccine developed by Dr Jonas Salk. This single trial, which you first met in Chapter 4, initiated the modern era of vaccine evaluation, and was a national event, with intense public scrutiny.

Thomas Frances (epidemiologist) saw the need for a randomised placebo-controlled trial with independent evaluation to ensure that the result would be accepted by scientists and the community. However, he also understood that many saw randomisation as unethical although they supported the need to assess the vaccine. Thus, a randomised trial was conducted in parallel with an observational study. In the randomised component, all children in grades 1–3 in 84 counties in 11 states were randomised to either vaccine (200,745) or placebo (201,229) injections. In the observational arm, participating grade 2 children in 127 areas in 33 states were vaccinated and compared to children in grades 1 and 3.

The speed with which the project was designed, implemented, analysed and reported was phenomenal by current standards. Vaccine and placebo were given to participants between April and June 1954, after which intensive surveillance of all 1.8 million children continued throughout that summer. Clinical and laboratory diagnoses were confirmed and data analyses undertaken over the next 6 months and the results were reported at a national press conference in April 1955.

Attack rates of paralytic polio (per 100,000) were 54.7 for the placebo arm and 16.4 for the vaccine arm of the trial, RR = 0.3. This success led to the immediate licensing of the vaccine for national use. By 1961 polio rates in the US were $< 1/100,000$, and international vaccination campaigns are now close to eliminating polio globally.

(From: Francis *et al.*, 1955 and Meldrum, 1998; see also https://sph.umich.edu/polio/)

Summary: one swallow doesn't make a summer

As we have discussed, the ultimate aim of much public health research is to change practice or policy to improve health outcomes, but even if a well-written paper that is (largely) free from major sources of bias and confounding

One swallow doesn't make a summer is an old proverb meaning that one instance of something is just one instance, it does not indicate a trend. Swallows fly south for the European winter and return when the weather warms up, but the sight of one swallow in the sky does not necessarily mean that summer has arrived.

finds what appears to be a statistically and practically significant association between an exposure and health outcome, we cannot rush out to act on this. Despite our best efforts and those of the investigators, it is still possible that statistically significant results can arise by chance. With the possible exception of a large randomised trial (see Box 9.4 for one that did change practice), no practical or policy decision should be made on the basis of the results of a single study, however good. As you have seen, individual studies can never be perfect, so it is important to consider all of the evidence on a given subject before attempting to make policy or practical decisions. We will come back to the ways in which you can do this in Chapter 11.

Questions

 Additional questions

Questions and answers (covering a range of study designs) for this chapter can be found on the accompanying website (www.cambridge.org/9781107529151).

In addition, the Epidemic Intelligence Service of the US Centers for Disease Control and Prevention has developed an excellent exercise 'Cigarette smoking and lung cancer' that draws on many of the issues covered in this and the previous chapters. This and other similar exercises are freely available from http://www.cdc.gov/eis/casestudies.html.

REFERENCES

References

Bossuyt, P. M., Reitsma, J. B., Bruns, D. E., *et al.* (2003). Towards complete and accurate reporting of studies of diagnostic accuracy: the STARD initiative. *British Medical Journal*, 326: 41–44.

Des Jarlais, D. C., Lyles, C., Crepaz, N. and the TREND Group. (2004). Improving the reporting quality of non-randomized evaluations of behavioral and public health interventions: the TREND statement. *American Journal of Public Health*, 94: 361–366.

Fojo, T. and Grady, C. (2009). How much is life worth: Cetuximab, non-small cell lung cancer, and the $440 billion question. *Journal of the National Cancer Institute*, 101: 1044–1048.

Francis, T. Jr, Korns, R. F., Voight, R. B., *et al.* (1955). An evaluation of the 1954 poliomyelitis vaccine trials: summary report. *American Journal of Public Health*, 45: 1–50.

Gagnier, J. J., Kienle, G., Altman, D. G., *et al.* (2013). The CARE Guidelines: consensus-based clinical case reporting guideline development. *Journal of Medical Case Reports*, 7: 223.

Higgins, J. P., Altman, D. G., Gøtzsche, P. C., *et al.* (2011). The Cochrane Collaboration's tool for assessing risk bias in randomised trials. *British Medical Journal*, 343: 1–9.

Keil, A. P., Daniels, J. L. and Hertz-Picciotto, I. (2014). Autism spectrum disorder, flea and tick medication, and adjustments for exposure misclassification: the CHARGE (CHildhood Autism Risks from Genetics and Environment) case–control study. *Environmental Health*, 13: 1–10.

Lang, T. A. and Altman, D. G. (2013). Basic statistical reporting for articles published in biomedical journals: the "Statistical analyses and methods in the published literature" or the SAMPL guidelines. In: Smart, P., Maisonneuve, H. and Polderman, A. (eds). *Science Editors' Handbook*. European Association of Science Editors.

Little, J., Higgins, J. P. Y., Ioannidis, J. P. A., *et al.* (2009). STrengthening the REporting of Genetic Association Studies (STREGA) – an extension of the STROBE statement. *PLoS Medicine*, 6(2): e1000022.

Mealing, N. M., Banks, E., Jorm, L. R., *et al.* (2010). Investigation of relative risk estimates from studies of the same population with contrasting response rates and designs. *BMC Medical Research Methodology*, 10: 1–12.

Meldrum, M. (1998). 'A calculated risk': the Salk polio vaccine field trials of 1954. *British Medical Journal*, 317: 1233–1236.

Osborn, D. P. J., Fletcher, A. E., Smeeth, L., *et al.* (2003). Factors associated with depression in a representative sample of 14,217 people aged 75 and over in the United Kingdom: results from the MRC trial of assessment and management of older people in the community. *International Journal of Geriatric Psychiatry*, 18: 623–630.

Pandeya, N., Williams, G. M., Green, A. C., *et al.* (2009). Do low control response rates always affect the findings? Assessments of smoking and obesity in two Australian case–control studies of cancer. *Australian and New Zealand Journal of Public Health*, 33: 312–319.

Riggs, J. E., Moudgil, S. S. and Hobbs, G. R. (2001). Creutzfeld–Jakob disease and blood transfusions: a meta-analysis of case–control studies. *Military Medicine*, 166: 1057–1058.

Rossouw, J. E., Anderson, G. L., Prentice, R. L., *et al.* (2002). Risks and benefits of estrogen plus progestin in healthy postmenopausal women: principal results from the Women's Health Initiative randomized controlled trial. *Journal of the American Medical Association*, 288: 321–333.

Santillan, A. A. and Camargo Jr, C. A. (2003). Body mass index and asthma among Mexican adults: the effect of using self-reported versus measured weight and height. *International Journal of Obesity*, 27: 1430–1433.

Schulz, K. F., Altman, D. G., Moher, D. for the CONSORT Group. (2010). CONSORT 2010 Statement: updated guidelines for reporting parallel group randomised trials. *PLoS Medicine*, 7(3): e1000251.

Shapiro, S., Farmer, R. D., Mueck, A. O., Seaman, H. and Stevenson, J. C. (2011). Does hormone replacement therapy cause breast cancer? An application of causal principles to three studies Part 2. The Women's Health Initiative: estrogen plus progestogen. *Journal of Family Planning and Reproductive Health Care*, 37: 165–172.

Sterne, J. A. C., Higgins, J. P. T. and Reeves, B. C. on behalf of the development group for ACROBAT-NRSI. (2014). A Cochrane Risk Of Bias Assessment Tool: for Non-Randomized Studies of Interventions (ACROBAT-NRSI), Version 1.0: 1–56. www.riskofbias.infom, accessed 23 January 2015.

von Elm, E., Altman, D. G., Egger, M., *et al.* (2007). The Strengthening the Reporting of Observational Studies in Epidemiology (STROBE) Statement: guidelines for reporting observational studies. *PLoS Medicine*, 4(10): e296.

Whiteman, D. C., Whiteman, C. A. and Green, A. C. (2001). Childhood sun exposure as a risk factor for melanoma: a systematic review of epidemiologic studies. *Cancer Causes and Control*, 12: 69–82.

Young-Xu, Y., Jabbour, S., Goldberg, R., *et al.* (2003). Usefulness of statin drugs in protecting against atrial fibrillation in patients with coronary artery disease. *American Journal of Cardiology*, 92: 1379–1383.

RECOMMENDED FOR FURTHER READING

- Studies assessing the practical effects of bias:

  Mealing, N. M., Banks, E., Jorm, L. R., *et al.* (2010). Investigation of relative risk estimates from studies of the same population with contrasting response rates and designs. *BMC Medical Research Methodology*, 10: 1–12.

  Pandeya, N., Williams, G. M., Green, A. C., *et al.* (2009). Do low control response rates always affect the findings? Assessments of smoking and obesity in two Australian case–control studies of cancer. *Australian and New Zealand Journal of Public Health*, 33: 312–319.

- For historical interest – More about the Salk polio vaccine trial:

  Meldrum, M. (1998). 'A calculated risk': the Salk polio vaccine field trials of 1954. *British Medical Journal*, 317: 1233–1236.

- Guidelines for reporting observational studies:

  von Elm, E., Altman, D. G., Egger, M., *et al.* (2007). The Strengthening the Reporting of Observational Studies in Epidemiology (STROBE) Statement: guidelines for reporting observational studies. *PLoS Medicine*, 4(10): e296.

Who sank the boat? Association and causation

| Description
Chapters 2–3 | Association
Chapters 4–5 | Alternative
explanations
Chapters 6–8 | Integration &
interpretation
Chapter 10:
Causality | Practical
applications
Chapters 12–15 |

Box 10.1 Who sank the boat?

As the story goes, there were five animals living by the sea, a cow, a donkey, a sheep, a pig and a mouse. One fine day they decided to go rowing on the bay.

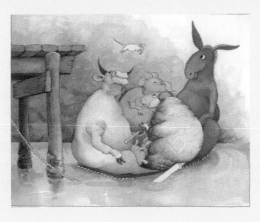

(continued)

269

Box 10.1 *(continued)*

First the cow got into the boat, it rocked a bit but she settled herself down comfortably at the back. Then the donkey got in carefully and sat down at the front to balance the boat. Next the pig climbed in, clutching her umbrella – the boat is low in the water by now. Then the sheep climbed in carrying her knitting and she sat down opposite the pig.

The boat is still afloat, but only just. Finally the little mouse jumped aboard and – disaster! The boat capsized and the animals had to swim to the shore.

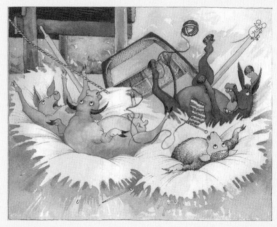

So who sank the boat?

(Storyline (adapted) and pictures from *Who Sank the Boat?* by Pamela Allen, Copyright 1982. Published by Penguin Books Australia. Reproduced courtesy of Tim Curnow Literary Agent and Consultant, Sydney.)

The search for the causes of disease is an obvious central step in the pursuit of better health through disease prevention and Box 10.1, abstracted from a wonderful children's picture book, illustrates perfectly the complexity of assigning causation. In the previous chapters we have looked at how we measure health (or disease) and how we look for associations between exposure and disease. Being able to identify a *relation* between a potential cause of disease and the disease itself is not enough, though. If our goal is to change practice or policy in order to improve health then we need to go one step further and decide whether the relation is causal because, if it is not, intervening will have no effect. As in previous chapters we will discuss causation mainly in the context of an exposure causing disease but, as you will see, when we come to assessing causation in practice, the concepts apply equally to a consideration of whether a potential preventive measure really does improve health.

What do we mean by a cause?

It is tempting to think that a cause is a single condition or event that inevitably leads to a particular effect or outcome; i.e. that there is a one-to-one relationship such that wherever or whenever the cause occurs the effect will follow. If we consider this more closely, it quickly becomes apparent that things are not so simple and that everyday causal phenomena are rather more complicated than they might seem at first. For example, while it might appear that all we need to do to turn on a computer is press the 'on' button, we know better: what if the wiring is faulty, there is no power supply or the hard drive has died an untimely death? To 'cause' the computer to come on we need power, good wiring, a functioning hard drive and relevant software in addition to the pressure of our finger on the button. We could describe each of these separate requirements as **component causes**, because they are all part of the one **sufficient cause** that will inevitably lead to the effect – in this case the computer turning on. In this situation they are also **necessary causes** because in the absence of just one of these things the computer will not work.

In the same way, disease rarely occurs as the result of a single event or exposure. Even though it might seem that an infectious agent would be a sufficient cause in its own right, not everyone develops disease following exposure to a particular bug. The real-life food-poisoning example in Chapter 1 made this clear – although people who ate the cold chicken were 3.8 times more likely to suffer from food poisoning than those who did not, almost one-quarter (23%) of those who ate the cold chicken suffered no ill effects. Whether someone does become ill depends both on their susceptibility to the agent and on the dose they receive. For tuberculosis (TB), for example, a person's susceptibility is determined by whether they have been infected before and are now immune, and also their overall level of health at the time. The infectious agent, the tubercle bacillus, is only a component of the total or sufficient cause that will lead to TB. It is, however, a *necessary* cause in that, by definition, TB cannot occur without it. We will look at infectious diseases in more detail in Chapter 13.

Some definitions

There are many definitions of a cause, but the following, from Rothman (1986, p. 11), is appealing because of the brevity with which it captures the concept:

a cause is 'an event, condition or characteristic [or a combination of these factors] that plays an essential role in producing an occurrence of the disease'

A more modern definition (Parascandola and Weed, 2001) that picks up on the concept of the 'counterfactual' that we discussed in Chapter 4 is that a cause is

something that makes a difference in the outcome (or the probability of the outcome) when it is present compared with when it is absent, while all else is held constant

The key to this second definition is that 'all else is held constant', something that is almost always impossible to achieve in real life. It also allows that a 'cause' may not always produce disease but may just increase (or reduce) the chance that disease will develop.

There are also many ways in which such entities (causes) can be classified, but the following subdivision serves well.

- A **sufficient** cause is a factor (or more usually a combination of several factors) that will inevitably produce disease.
- A **component** cause is a factor that contributes towards disease causation but is not sufficient to cause disease on its own.
- A **necessary** cause is any agent (or component cause) that is required for the development of a given disease (for example, the specific infectious agent).

In terms of working out 'who sank the boat' we can say that each one of the animals was a *component* cause and that together they created the *sufficient* cause that caused the disaster. Probably none was actually *necessary* to sink the boat – any group of similarly sized animals would have had a similar effect. The ordering of the events, i.e. whether the mouse got in first or last, also did not matter; it was the sum of the weights that caused the boat to sink. This may also be true in much disease causation, but sometimes the component causes will have to occur in a specific order or they will have to be present at the same time. For example, TB infection will occur only if the individual is susceptible at the time they are exposed to the infection; and thrombosis (blood clotting) in an artery leading to a heart attack or stroke rarely occurs unless the blood vessel is already damaged or partly blocked.

A useful model for considering causal mechanisms is the 'pie' diagrams used by Rothman (1976) and shown in Figure 10.1. In this scheme:

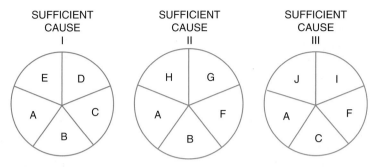

Figure 10.1 A conceptual scheme for the causes of a hypothetical disease. (*From:* Rothman, Causes, *Am. J. Epidemiol.*, 1976; 104: 589, by permission of the Society for Epidemiological Research.)

- I, II and III are three different *sufficient causes* for a disease;
- A is a *necessary cause* for the disease because it is present in all three sufficient causes (assuming there are no other sufficient causes that do not include A); and
- A, B, C, D, E, F, G, H, I and J are all *component causes* of one or other of the sufficient causes.

So, for example, if 'A' were the cow, 'B' the donkey, 'C' the pig, 'D' the sheep and 'E' the mouse, we would have sufficient cause I, while the other 'pies' show that different combinations of animals or other objects would also have led to the boat overturning.

In practice, when considering causes of disease we mostly find ourselves dealing with component causes. Aside from something like a major disaster such as an earthquake or nuclear explosion, it is hard to imagine identifying a single factor that is truly necessary and sufficient to cause disease. We also have to accept that, other than for something like an injury, we are unlikely to know either the precise nature of any sufficient cause or many of the possible component causes of disease. This need not matter – we do not have to eliminate all components of a particular cause in order to prevent disease due to that cause. If any one of them is identified and removed (e.g. B in the example above), then we will prevent cases of disease due to sufficient causes that contain component B (i.e. I and II). Some disease will still occur, however, as a result of sufficient cause III.

The causes of many diseases, and especially those like cancer that develop over many years, are going to be complex and we may never identify all their components. It is thus encouraging to know that by just identifying one or two we may still prevent a large proportion of the disease. If we could have stopped any one of the animals, even the mouse, from getting into the boat then it would not have turned over at that point in time. However, if the wind blew up or a wave came along once they had pushed off then they may have sunk later: a different sufficient cause leading to a similar outcome. Searching for

> To be strictly accurate, we will only prevent the disease occurring *at that point in time*. In practice we may not prevent it completely, but might simply delay the onset. This is most obvious if we consider premature mortality; while we may be able to help someone live longer, e.g. by stopping them from smoking, we cannot prevent death completely.

Table 10.1 The percentage of DALYs due to cardiovascular and circulatory diseases which can be attributed to various risk factors, shown separately for developing and developed countries, 2010.

	Percentage of DALYs attributable to various risk factors		
	Developing	Developed	Global
Dietary risks	65	66	65
High blood pressure	56	58	57
Tobacco smoking	27	25	26
Ambient particulate matter pollution	21	11	18
High body mass index	13	29	17
Physical inactivity	15	20	16
Household air pollution from solid fuels	21	2	16

(Data from Institute for Health Metrics and Evaluation (IHME), 2013, accessed 7 May 2015.)

modifiable causes that are associated with a large population attributable risk, i.e. those which cause a large number of cases of disease, will give the greatest benefit in terms of public health. (We will take this up again in Chapter 14.)

Look at Table 10.1. The proportions of DALYs for cardiovascular and circulatory diseases attributable to the various risk factors sum to more than 100%. Why is this so? Is it a problem?

If we assume that each of the causes of cardiovascular and circulatory disease shown can be represented by one of the letters in Figure 10.1 (for example, if dietary risks were cause 'A', high blood pressure were cause 'B' and smoking were cause 'C'), we can immediately see that the total amount of disease attributable to each component cause will be much greater than 100%. Ensuring that everyone had an adequate diet (i.e. removing cause 'A') would prevent all disease due to sufficient causes I, II and III. However, if we have already removed the problem of high blood pressure (cause 'B') and so prevented disease due to sufficient causes I and II, then the extra benefit of improving diet could only prevent the extra disease due to sufficient cause III. Similarly, although stopping everyone smoking would prevent some disease on its own, once we have removed the problems of diet and high blood pressure it would have little extra benefit.

In thinking about how component causes might act together, we need to keep in mind that in no sense need they be similar: one component might be the absence of a protective factor, and another the presence of a quite different harmful factor. For instance, if we consider the underlying causes of lung cancer we would probably find that cigarette smoke is a component in most sufficient causes. However, because not all smokers develop lung cancer we can surmise that smoking is not a sufficient cause on its own but also requires other factors (for example, weakened DNA-repair capacity) to complete a sufficient cause. Similarly, because lung cancer can develop in the absence of smoking, we can presume that there is at least one sufficient cause that does not have personal smoking as a component cause.

Association versus causation

In preceding chapters we have considered how we can determine whether a particular exposure is *associated* with the outcome of interest. The next stage is to determine whether such an association may be causal. Just because a particular exposure is associated with the development of a disease does not automatically imply cause and effect. We must attempt to draw appropriate causal inferences explicitly from our data, in the light of other evidence.

In London during the cholera epidemics of the nineteenth century one common belief, the 'miasma' theory, was that cholera was caused by noxious vapours in the air. While John Snow was conducting his pioneering work implicating contaminated water, William Farr, director of the Office of the Registrar General, was also interested in the transmission of cholera. He had noticed that cholera mortality seemed to be higher in lower-lying areas and so collected mortality data for a number of districts in London at different elevations. This revealed a dramatic inverse relation between elevation and mortality, and Farr was able to calculate a formula that could accurately predict the mortality rate for any given elevation. Figure 10.2 shows a graph of actual cholera death rates for various levels of elevation above the River Thames as well as the death rates predicted by Farr's theory. These data were taken as strong evidence in favour of the miasma theory, under which it was felt that the vapours would be most concentrated and, therefore, most dangerous at lower elevations.

However, as you saw in Chapter 3, like most ecological research (the graph compares rates of cholera in areas at various elevations, not individual data), these observations provide weak evidence for a true causal association, and we must consider whether other differences between people living at different elevations could explain them. As it happened, people living closest to the river were also more likely to be exposed to contaminated water than their neighbours in the higher areas. This confounding factor could explain the apparent association between elevation and cholera mortality entirely, and today it is John Snow, not William Farr, whom we recognise as having solved

Figure 10.2 Actual (——) and predicted (- - - -) cholera death rates at various levels of elevation above the River Thames in London, England, 1849. (*Data source:* Farr, 1852.)

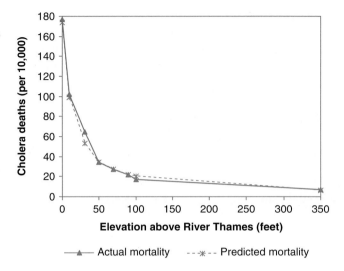

Figure 10.2 Actual (——) and predicted (- - - -) cholera death rates at various levels of elevation above the River Thames in London, England, 1849. (*Data source:* Farr, 1852.)

the mystery of cholera. Ironically, in trying to prove his own 'airborne' theory, Farr also provided much of the crucial evidence that ultimately supported Snow's theory of contaminated water.

This example highlights the necessity of not accepting the results of any study, however exciting, at face value. There are two substantial steps to be taken before we can reasonably promote an exposure–disease relation as warranting serious attention with respect to disease control. We must first thoroughly consider alternative non-causal explanations for an association: could it be an artefact due to chance, bias or confounding? We need to apply the approach outlined in Chapter 9 to decide whether the results we are looking at (our own or those reported by someone else) are believable. In the cholera example we have postulated that confounding by water supply is the most likely explanation for the close association seen in Figure 10.2, and that the relation with elevation is an artefact. If, however, the answer to the question 'Is it real?' is at least a qualified 'yes', then we can move on to the next step – a formal evaluation of whether the observed relation could be causal.

Evaluating causation

How should we do this? The nature of causation has been a central theme of philosophy for centuries (see Box 10.2) and in recent times has been given a fair bit of attention by epidemiologists as well (see Box 10.3). This has given a useful perspective, but epidemiologists are fundamentally pragmatic and seek

Box 10.2 Some potted philosophy

Do we learn about the world from observation and experience or by
reason? This was the major tension in Western causal thinking for many
centuries. Broadly speaking, observation or learning from our own
experience (*induction*) gradually replaced more abstract reasoning about
how the world worked (*deduction*). The practical inductive approach fits
pretty well with public health and epidemiology – we collect facts, decide
what they mean and then act accordingly – but, of course, it is not perfect.
Starting with David Hume in eighteenth-century Scotland, many
philosophers have demonstrated that induction can never *prove* a cause-
and-effect relationship (this became known as Hume's problem). Just
because we observe that the computer turns on the first 99 times we press
the button does not mean that it will turn on again the 100th time (we are
all familiar with this phenomenon). Final proof is thus unobtainable by
this process. In Europe in the middle decades of the twentieth century,
Karl Popper in a sense turned Hume's problem around and said that,
although induction based on supportive observations could never finally
confirm a hypothesis, contrary data could be used to *refute* one. Consider
the statement 'all swans are white'. We may see only white swans but can
never prove that this statement is true – it just takes one black swan to
disprove it. The hypothesis stood for millennia in Europe until Dutch
explorers saw their first black swan in Western Australia in 1697.

We will never know anything with absolute certainty and this is
something we have to learn to live with comfortably. You will note that the
subsequent guidelines to causal reasoning incorporate both judgement

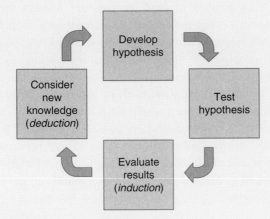

Figure 10.3 An integrated cycle of causal reasoning.

(*continued*)

Box 10.2 *(continued)*

and probabilistic elements, reflecting that we cannot demand certainty. If we did we would never act, the antithesis of the remit of public health. In pursuit of making good judgements on how and when to act, epidemiologists have long sought to bring good evidence to bear on a question. In the past decade or so this has come into sharper focus with research increasingly aiming to test critical elements of causal belief or hypothesis along the lines proposed by Popper and his followers last century. This has led to an integrated cycle of causal reasoning that essentially combines both induction and deduction (Figure 10.3).

practical tools. Unfortunately, in the causal realm our tools are not as precise as we might like and views on how to apply them differ somewhat.

As we discussed in Chapter 4, the best way to assess whether an exposure is truly associated with a given outcome is in the context of a randomised controlled trial (RCT). Assuming that the trial is of high quality, it would be reasonable to assume in this situation that the exposed and unexposed groups were *exchangeable* and thus that the exposure caused the outcome – at least among the type of people included in the study.[1] However, in the absence of good trial data, and these are rare in the field of public health, we often have to make decisions about causation using observational data. As we noted at the end of the previous chapter, no practical decisions should be made on the basis of a single study – it is important to consider all of the available evidence. We will come back to look at how we conduct reviews to integrate this evidence in Chapter 11, but first we will look more closely at how we might decide whether an observed association really is causal. Various sets of guidelines have been proposed to assist our causal evaluations in this situation. There are many similarities among them, and arguably the best known – certainly the best written – were set forth by a British statistician, Sir Austin Bradford Hill, in an after-dinner speech. He put forward a list of nine aspects of an association to be considered when assessing whether it was likely to be causal (Hill, 1965). He was adamant that these should serve only as '*aids to thought*' and were not absolute requirements to be met before an exposure could be considered to cause a disease. Various modifications of this list have

---

[1] As we noted previously, RCTs often have very strict inclusion and exclusion criteria so their results may only apply to the (sometimes small) subset of the population that meet the same criteria.

Box 10.3 The counterfactual (potential) outcomes model of causation

This more recent way of thinking about causation (see e.g. Hernán, 2004) comes from the counterfactual definition of a cause that we presented earlier. If, at the simplest level, we consider a perfectly measured exposure that is either present or absent and its relation to a single disease, there are two potential outcomes for each individual: they will either get the disease or they won't. In the counterfactual world that we described in Chapter 4 we could look to see who developed disease when they were exposed and, in a hypothetical parallel universe, who would develop it when they were not exposed. If someone would develop disease when they were exposed but not if they were unexposed, then we could confidently say that the exposure caused their disease.

The left panel in Table 10.2 shows some hypothetical data relating an exposure to disease. It appears that five men were exposed and three of them (60%) developed disease compared to one of the three men who were unexposed (33%). This suggests the exposure may have increased the risk of disease in the exposed group, but we don't know what would have happened to them if they had not been exposed or what would have happened to the unexposed men if they had been exposed. By invoking the idea of a parallel universe we could look to see what would have happened to the same people if they had all been exposed and then if none had been exposed. The right panel in Table 10.2 shows that their outcomes would have been identical regardless of whether or not they were exposed: half or 50% of the men would have developed disease in

Table 10.2 Potential outcomes (0 = no disease, 1 = disease) from an exposure.

	Real world			A world with parallel universes	
	Exposed	Unexposed		Exposed	Unexposed
Alfred	1		Alfred	1	1
Bob		0	Bob	0	0
Charles	0		Charles	0	0
David		1	David	1	1
Edward		0	Edward	0	0
Fred	1		Fred	1	1
George	0		George	0	0
Harry	1		Harry	1	1

(*continued*)

> **Box 10.3** (*continued*)
>
> each case. Therefore, although in the 'real world' shown in the left panel the exposure appeared to be *associated* with the disease, in this example it did not actually *cause* the disease.
>
> The problem in real life is that we do not know what would have happened to someone if their exposure level had been different so we only know one of their two potential outcomes: what would happen if they were exposed *or* what would happen if they were unexposed. The other *counterfactual* outcome (it is counter to fact because it does not actually occur) is unknown. This means we cannot say for sure whether the exposure actually caused the disease in that individual. However, we can estimate whether the exposure appears to be causing disease at the population level and this is what we set out to achieve in epidemiological studies by trying to ensure that our exposed and unexposed groups are *exchangeable* (i.e. they are as similar as possible in every way except the exposure) even if they are not exactly the same people.

been suggested, and many of the elements remain cornerstones of judgement on whether an exposure really does cause a disease, or whether an intervention is effective in preventing or treating disease. These elements are discussed below.

Temporality

For an exposure to cause a disease it must precede the development of the disease. This might seem obvious, but in some instances, say for a condition like cancer that is often present for many years before diagnosis, it can be difficult to decide whether an exposure really did occur before the true origin of disease. If we find that people with stomach cancer have lower levels of vitamin C in their blood than those without stomach cancer, can we be sure that the low levels of vitamin C really preceded the growth of the cancer? Or might the lower vitamin C levels be a result of the disease process? As you will recall from Chapter 4, these questions can frequently be answered only by performing cohort studies and, even then, it may be difficult to establish the order of exposure and effect with certainty. *Of all Bradford Hill's factors this is the only one that is an absolute requirement.*

Strength of association

The stronger an association is (usually as described by the relative effect, OR or RR), the less likely it is to be due solely to either bias or confounding.

A strong association is thus more suggestive that the effect is real. However, just because a relation is weak does not mean that it cannot be causal, only that it is harder to eliminate study error as a possible explanation for the apparent effect.

What constitutes a 'weak' or a 'strong' effect? There is no universal agreement on this, but we might generally consider an effect (OR, RR) greater than 2.0 to be moderately strong and an effect greater than 5.0 to be strong. Note, however, that a small effect observed consistently in many studies, especially if these are of different designs and performed in different settings, may well give stronger evidence of causation than an effect that is strong in one or two studies but not found in others (see 'Consistency', below, and Chapter 11). It is important not to be too dismissive of 'weak' effects, as these can be of great public health importance when the exposure is common and the consequences severe. For example, smoking is well accepted as an important cause of coronary heart disease but, as you saw in Table 5.4, the RR for CHD among smokers compared to non-smokers in the British Doctors' Study was only 1.6.

Consistency

An effect found consistently across a range of studies of different types and/ or in different populations gives some reassurance that it is not an artefact. Figure 10.4 summarises the results of 10 studies that looked at the relation between frequency of aspirin use and risk of colorectal cancer. If we look first at the square boxes that represent the relative risks, we see that, while there is some variability, all are less than 1.0 and in six the association is statistically significant (i.e. their 95% confidence intervals do not cross 1.0). When the data from all 10 studies were combined the overall 'pooled' RR was 0.80 (95% confidence interval 0.75–0.85), suggesting that there was a 20% reduction in risk among those who took aspirin most frequently. The results are, therefore, quite consistent and so increase belief that the association between aspirin use and colorectal cancer might be 'causal' (note in this case the relationship is reversed and aspirin prevents colo-rectal cancer).

However, lack of consistency need not in itself rule out causation. Differing results could reflect variation in study design or quality, or an exposure could have a different effect in people with a different genetic make-up or with different exposures to other factors that might modify (interact with) the possible cause of interest. As you will see in the next chapter, it is important to give thoughtful consideration to why studies might give different results (heterogeneity) when reviewing the evidence for an association; indeed, this is essential for a good review.

Figure 10.4 The relation between frequency of aspirin use (high vs. low) and risk of colorectal cancer. The squares represent the relative risk, with the size of the square being proportional to the size of the study, and the horizontal lines represent the 95% confidence intervals. The open diamond represents the relative risk and 95% confidence interval from all 10 studies combined.

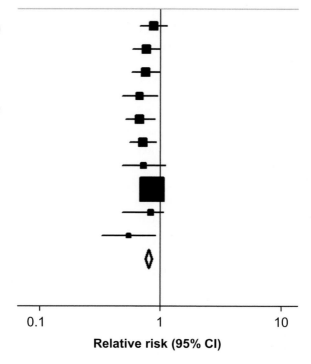

Dose–response relationships

If a factor does cause a disease, then the risk of developing the disease is likely to be related to the amount or 'dose' of exposure. This is often a function of both *level* and *duration of exposure*. Figure 10.5 shows some data from the first eight years of follow-up of the US Nurses' Health Study. The investigators calculated the age-adjusted relative risk that a woman would develop type-2 diabetes on the basis of her body mass index (BMI; weight/height^2) and found that the risk of diabetes increased dramatically with increasing body size, particularly for women with a BMI greater than 25 kg/m^2 (the upper limit of what is usually considered to be 'normal'). Among the heaviest women, those with a BMI of 35 kg/m^2 or greater, the risk of diabetes was almost 60 times that of women with a BMI less than 22 kg/m^2. Similarly, we saw that the risk of lung cancer increases sharply with increasing numbers of cigarettes smoked (Figure 1.1). Patterns like these add credence to the idea that an association is causal. Note, however, that measurement of dose is not always straightforward. In the British Doctor's Study discussed in previous chapters, Doll and Hill used a simple measure of dose of smoking, namely 'average number of cigarettes smoked per day'. This clearly worked very well, but does not capture

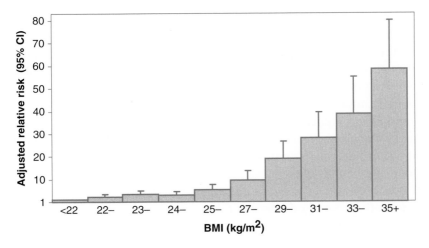

Figure 10.5 Age-adjusted relative risks and 95% confidence intervals for type-2 diabetes in relation to body mass index. (*From*: Colditz *et al.*, Weight as a risk factor for clinical diabetes in women. *Am. J. Epidemiol.*, 5, 1990; 132: 505, reprinted by permission of the Society for Epidemiological Research.)

other important information such as the number of years that someone has smoked. These days this additional information would almost always be included in any assessment of effects of smoking, often in a combined variable called 'pack-years', where one pack-year is equivalent to smoking 20 cigarettes a day for 1 year (or 10 cigarettes a day for 2 years, etc.).

Of course, some genuine cause-and-effect relationships will not give such a regular pattern. For instance, there may be a 'threshold' effect, whereby any exposure above a certain level will lead to disease. For example, infectious diseases often show a threshold effect as exposure to a number of organisms below the 'infectious dose' is unlikely to cause disease but exposure to a higher number of organisms will. The actual dose required for infection will, however, differ depending on a person's age, immune and nutritional status, etc. (see Chapter 13). A dose–response relationship can therefore add weight to an evaluation of causation, but its absence need not count against a causal link.

Biological plausibility

A causal hypothesis should obviously be viewed in the light of its plausibility. If there is a likely biological mechanism through which an exposure might cause the disease, this can add substantial weight to a causal argument. Lack of plausibility does not necessarily rule out causation, because increasing know-ledge of disease mechanisms may make an association appear more credible in time. The characteristic of plausibility is also tempered by the realisation that scientists are ingenious by nature and can probably come up with a plausible-sounding hypothesis in most situations if they believe an association to be causal!

Specificity

Bradford Hill presented this concept somewhat less clearly than the others on his list – he suggested that, if an association were limited to a specific outcome, then this would argue in favour of causation. He went on to say that this characteristic should not be overemphasised because factors could cause more than one disease and diseases might have more than one cause. This concept was crudely interpreted as 'one cause – one disease' in attempts to argue that cigarette smoking did not cause lung cancer: cigarettes were linked to many different diseases, therefore their effects were not specific, therefore they caused none of them.[2]

When we recall that many diseases are based on similar underlying pathologies (e.g. vascular diseases of the brain, heart and other organs frequently stem from atherosclerosis) it is hardly surprising that a single exposure (e.g. a high-fat diet) can be linked to a variety of different conditions. Nonetheless, we would still not expect an exposure to be linked to *all* outcomes; thus there must be some degree of specificity that we can use to inform an evaluation of causation (Weiss, 2002). For example, bicycle helmets would be expected to reduce the risk of head injury but not of other types of injury (specificity of outcome). If results of studies suggested that helmet use did indeed reduce the risk of injuries to the head only, then this would strengthen belief that it was a causal (or in this case protective) association. An association seen only for one particular type of analgesic (as in the Phenacetin study described in Box 4.4) could again strengthen belief in causation (specificity of exposure). Similarly, individuals might be susceptible to an exposure only if they have a particular genetic make-up, so, if the relation is seen only for those with the specific genotype (specificity of susceptibility), then belief in causation is again strengthened.

Pulling it all together

Bradford Hill also suggested that consideration should be given to any *experimental data* – these could come from studies in animals or other organisms or from intervention studies in humans. Such evidence in humans is of course crucial to assessing the benefits of interventions. The final two characteristics that he put forward are sensible but of less direct help than the others: *coherence* – a cause-and-effect interpretation should not conflict with the known facts; and *analogy* to existing known causal associations. An additional aspect to consider is that, if a relation is causal, then removal of the exposure

---

[2] In fact, cigarette smoke has been shown to have multiple components, some of which do show specificity of action at various sites.

should lead to a reduction in the effect – as was seen in the time trends of cigarette sales and lung cancer mortality in Figure 3.7.

Consideration of these issues can help us decide whether an association is likely to be causal. Sometimes the decision may be clear-cut, but it is equally likely to be controversial, and in this situation there can be no 'right' answer. It is important to remember that these elements do not provide an infallible checklist that will lead to the correct decision. Rather, they provide a framework for an evaluation of causation.

Bradford Hill (1965) summarised the questions that should guide a consideration of causation as follows:

Is there any other way of explaining the set of facts before us, is there any other answer equally, or more likely than cause and effect?

An example: does *H. pylori* cause stomach cancer?

In the next chapter we will look at how we can review evidence to make causal judgements in practice, but before we do this we will end this chapter with an example of how we might consider the issues raised by Bradford Hill to decide whether an observed association really is causal. You have seen in earlier chapters that there appears to be a link between infection with *H. pylori* (a bacterium that infects the stomach) and stomach cancer rates. Many case–control studies have been conducted to evaluate this, but these are fraught with problems, in particular because people with stomach cancer may test negative for *H. pylori* even if they have been infected in the past. As a result, there is the potential for differential misclassification of cases as *H. pylori*-negative, thereby biasing the odds ratio towards the null. Cohort studies are impractical because of the logistics of testing thousands of cohort members for *H. pylori*. The best evidence therefore comes from well-designed *nested case–control studies* (see Chapter 4) in which blood samples were collected prior to the diagnosis of cancer. In 2001, a group pooled the data from 12 such studies to evaluate this association (*Helicobacter* and Cancer Collaborative Group, 2001). (We will discuss *pooled* studies further in Chapter 11.) In all of the studies the cases and controls were matched for age and sex and there were no other major confounders; there were also no obvious sources of selection or measurement bias. Authors of all 12 studies reported an increased risk of stomach cancer associated with infection, which was statistically significant (i.e. unlikely to be due to chance) in nine. The odds ratio from all 12 studies combined was 2.4 (95% CI 2.0–2.8).

So could the relation be causal? The association is quite *strong* and also *consistent* across these better studies. In all of them the blood samples used for testing for *H. pylori* were collected before diagnosis of cancer, suggesting that infection does indeed *precede* cancer. Because, by and large, someone is either infected or not infected, it is not possible to look for a *dose–response* relationship, but the association appears to be fairly *specific* for some types of stomach cancer, and laboratory studies have shown that some types of *H. pylori* may be more carcinogenic than others. Further *experimental evidence* comes from studies that have shown that *H. pylori* infection induces cancer in some animal models. A relation is also biologically *plausible* because the bacterial infection directly affects the stomach, which is where the cancer occurs. Taken together, there is thus good evidence for the conclusion, now widely accepted, that *H. pylori* infection is indeed a cause of stomach cancer.

Conclusion

Although wholly reliable criteria for truly establishing causation do not exist, modern society often requires a black-and-white answer. Clinicians need to know what treatment to offer their patients and public health physicians need to know what advice they should give the population to prevent disease. Also, increasingly, rapid 'proof' is required for legal reasons when an individual sues the government or a corporation claiming they have been exposed to something that made them sick. Unfortunately, as you will have gathered, this yearning for certainty can rarely be fulfilled. As we have discussed, it is impossible to prove something definitively so, ultimately, absolute proof is almost impossible but the clearer our thinking and our insight into the evidence, the better our judgements will be.

So, to conclude this chapter, if we had stopped the mouse from jumping into the boat (i.e. removed one component cause) it would not have overturned at that precise point in time (we would have prevented that particular outcome). But who is to say what would have happened if the other animals had ventured out into the rougher water in the middle of the lake ...

Questions

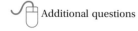 Additional questions

1. Your case–control study has shown a halving of risk of stroke among people who eat cauliflower three or more times weekly. Before you can claim this association is causal, which of the following alternative explanations must you consider?
   (a) chance,
   (b) random misclassification of exposure,
   (c) random misclassification of the stroke diagnosis,
   (d) increased forgetfulness of stroke patients.
2. What other alternatives to a causal explanation for the association must always be considered?

3. If your finding is robust and none of the above alternatives seem likely, what other factors would you consider when determining whether the association between cauliflower and stroke is likely to be causal and why?

REFERENCES

Allen, P. (1982). *Who Sank the Boat?* Thomas Nelson Australia. Republished by Penguin Books Australia Ltd, 1998.

Farr, W. (1852). Influence of elevation on the fatality of cholera. *Journal of the Statistical Society London*, 15: 155–183.

Helicobacter and Cancer Collaborative Group. (2001). Gastric cancer and *Helicobacter pylori*: a combined analysis of 12 case-control studies nested within prospective cohorts. *Gut*, 49: 347–353.

Hernán, M. A. (2004). A definition of causal effect for epidemiological research. *Journal of Epidemiology and Community Health*, 58: 265–271.

Hill, A. B. (1965). The environment and disease: association or causation? *Proceedings of the Royal Society for Medicine*, 58: 295–300.

Institute for Health Metrics and Evaluation (IHME). (2013). *GBD Compare.* Seattle, WA: IHME, University of Washington, 2013. Available from http://vizhub.healthdata.org/gbd-compare (accessed 7 May 2015).

Parascandola, M. and Weed, D. L. (2001). Causation in epidemiology. *Journal of Epidemiology and Community Health*, 55: 905–912.

Rothman, K. J. (1976). Causes. *American Journal of Epidemiology*, 104: 587–592.

Rothman, K. J. (1986). *Modern Epidemiology.* Boston, MA: Little Brown & Co.

Weiss, N. S. (2002). Can the "specificity" of an association be rehabilitated as a basis for supporting a causal hypothesis? *Epidemiology*, 13: 6–8.

 References

RECOMMENDED FOR FURTHER READING

- Hill's classic and very readable exposition on things to consider when thinking about causation:
  Hill, A. B. (1965). The environment and disease: association or causation? *Proceedings of the Royal Society for Medicine*, 58: 295–300.
- A classic paper that presents the 'causal pies' model of causation:
  Rothman, K. J. (1976). Causes. *American Journal of Epidemiology*, 104: 587–592.
- A good introduction to the concept of the counterfactual in assessing causation:
  Hernán, M. A. (2004). A definition of causal effect for epidemiological research. *Journal of Epidemiology and Community Health*, 58: 265–271.

Assembling the building blocks: reviews and their uses

While it is important to be able to read and interpret individual papers, as we have noted previously the results of a single study are never going to provide the complete answer to a question. To move towards this we need to review the literature more widely. There can be a number of reasons for doing this, some of which require a more comprehensive approach than others. If the aim is simply to increase our personal understanding of a new area then a few papers might provide adequate background material.

Traditional *narrative reviews*, which give less emphasis to complete coverage of the literature and tend to be more qualitative, have value for exploring areas of uncertainty or novelty, but it is harder to scrutinise them for flaws. In contrast, a major decision regarding policy or practice should be based on a *systematic review* and perhaps a *meta-analysis* of all the relevant literature and it is this systematic approach that we will focus on here.

What is a systematic review?

A systematic review should be a helpful synthesis of all of the relevant data – highlighting patterns but not hiding differences. Although its primary data units are whole studies rather than individuals, it should still have a clearly formulated research question and be conducted with the same rigour as its component studies. So how should we go about conducting a systematic review? This is a major undertaking and excellent guidelines are widely available for would-be reviewers (see e.g. the Cochrane Collaboration website www.cochrane.org) so we will not attempt to cover all of the issues here. But, in brief, it involves:

- identifying *all* potentially relevant primary research studies that address the question of interest and including or excluding them according to predetermined criteria;
- abstracting the data in a standard format and critically appraising the included studies;
- summarising the findings of the studies, this might include a formal meta-analysis to combine the results of all of the studies into a single summary estimate; and
- an overall evaluation of the evidence with appropriate conclusions.

It follows from this that such a review should be structured in the same way as a primary paper: an *introduction* to show why the research question is of interest; a *methods* section to explain how studies were identified, included/excluded and appraised, and how the data were abstracted; the *results* where patterns are highlighted and differences assessed; and, finally, a *discussion* where the results are interpreted, threats to validity considered and causal conclusions drawn. Box 11.1 shows a condensed excerpt from the methods section of a Cochrane systematic review of the use of antibiotics for treating acute laryngitis, giving a sense of the detailed approach required. In the next few pages we will discuss the various stages of the review process as a guide to both reading and writing a systematic review.

Box 11.1 Are antibiotics effective for treating acute laryngitis?

Objectives

To assess the effectiveness and safety of different antibiotic therapies in adults with acute laryngitis.

Search strategy

We searched the Cochrane Central Register of Controlled Trials (CENTRAL 2014, Issue 11), MEDLINE (January 1966 to November week 3, 2014), EMBASE (1974 to December 2014), LILACS (1982 to December 2014) and BIOSIS (1980 to December 2014). The CENTRAL and MEDLINE search strategies are provided. We imposed no language or publication restrictions.

We employed other strategies including the searching of references of review articles and books related to infections of the respiratory tract, and handsearches of journals, etc. We searched grey literature such as conference abstracts/proceedings, published lists of theses and dissertations, etc., and other literature outside of the main journal literature, where possible.

Trial selection

Randomised controlled trials (RCTs) comparing any antibiotic therapy with placebo or another antibiotic in the treatment of acute laryngitis. The primary outcome was an improvement in recorded voice score assessed by an expert panel.

Data extraction

Two review authors (names provided) independently:

- retrieved the articles and assessed their eligibility from the title and abstracts,
- assessed the full text of all studies identified as possibly relevant,
- assessed the risk of bias (see Box 9.2) for each study and resolved disagreements by discussion.

Data synthesis

We used Review Manager 5.3 to create 'Summary of findings' tables. We produced a summary of the intervention effect and a measure of quality for each of the above outcomes using the GRADE approach (see 'Drawing conclusions', below).

(Excerpted from Reveiz and Cardona, 2015.)

Identifying the literature

The first challenge when conducting a systematic review is to identify all of the relevant literature. The potential sources of data are numerous. MEDLINE is probably the most commonly used source for epidemiological papers. At June 2016 it contained more than 23 million references to articles published since 1946 in 5,600 life sciences journals worldwide. It is freely accessible through the US National Library of Medicine search engine PubMed® at www.ncbi.nlm.nih.gov/pubmed/. EMBASE® is not so widely available but has some advantages over MEDLINE in that it includes many additional journals as well as conference abstracts. Another valuable database, particularly for systematic reviews of trials of the effects of healthcare interventions, is that of the Cochrane Collaboration (CENTRAL, www.cochrane.org). There are also many other electronic databases that may be valuable sources of literature depending on the question you are researching (e.g. PsycINFO® has an obvious specialised focus).

No electronic literature search is ever likely to be complete, so it is important to use multiple strategies. Once several relevant articles have been identified, it can help to check the papers that they cite, and also to look in the other direction, i.e. for papers that have cited them (e.g. via PubMed which lists other articles in PubMed that have cited the selected paper). Other sources include personal communication with experts in the field who may know of additional published articles (and unpublished material); theses, seminars, internal reports and non-peer-reviewed journals (sometimes described as the 'grey literature'); and other electronic information including topic-specific Internet databases.

Publication and related biases

When searching the literature it is important to bear in mind that studies with positive and/or statistically significant findings may be more likely to be published than those without significant results. This **publication bias** is related not only to selective acceptance by journals, but also to selective submission to journals by researchers who may decide not to submit reports from research that either finds no association at all (i.e. a null finding) or in which the results are not statistically significant.

> It is possible to check the existence of **publication bias** by drawing what is called a *funnel plot*. In the absence of bias, this should be a roughly symmetrical inverted funnel shape.

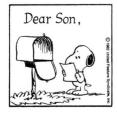 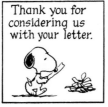 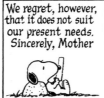 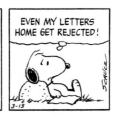

Another problem is the preferential detection of articles in English. For an English speaker there are several barriers to the inclusion of non-English studies in a review, including the difficulties associated with translation and the fact that non-English articles may be published in local journals that are not indexed by major bibliographic databases. This is more likely to be the case for less exciting findings. It is also important to be aware that there may be multiple publications from one study and, if these are included as separate studies in the review, this could bias the conclusions.

Study inclusion and exclusion

Studies should be selected for inclusion in the review on the basis of pre-defined criteria. Depending on the research question, it might be appropriate to restrict the review to specific research designs, for example only random-ised trials, or to those with specific methodological features. Such features might include:

- the study size (e.g. only those studies with more than a certain number of cases),
- the participants (e.g. a particular age range or sex),
- a specific outcome or the way in which the outcome was measured (e.g. histological or serological confirmation),
- the way in which the exposure was measured or classified (e.g. a particular type of blood test to measure an infection, more than two levels of alcohol intake) and
- the duration of follow-up (e.g. more than 12 months).

Appraising the literature

The amount and types of literature generated by a search will vary enormously depending on the subject area. For a review of a specific treatment the studies may all be clinical trials, whereas an aetiological review is likely to include observational studies of all types from case reports to cohort studies, with few or no trials. As you have seen, different types of study answer different types of questions, or may be subject to different biases when answering the same question, so it is sensible to group them separately, at least to start with. This grouping may then provide a logical framework to help organise the data within the review.

Key information including aspects of the study design and conduct, the potential for error and the relevant results should be abstracted onto purpose-designed forms and the validity of the studies evaluated as out-lined in Chapter 9. In an ideal world the appraisers should be blinded to the authors and the study results because this knowledge has been shown to influence judgements about validity. In practice this is not always possible, because the reviewers may already be too familiar with the literature. Rigorous systematic reviews like that described in Box 11.1 will often specify the need for multiple assessors to reduce the potential for bias.

A common approach to grading the quality of individual studies has been to classify study designs according to a hierarchy such that those at the top are considered to provide stronger evidence of an effect than those further down the scale (Table 11.1). You will notice that this ranking puts randomised trials at the top of the pile. While a classification of this type may be appropriate in the clinical context where RCTs are the norm, it is often not much help for an aetiological review. In 2003, the *British Medical Journal* published an entertaining systematic review of randomised controlled trials of 'parachute use to prevent death and major trauma related to gravitational challenge' (Smith and Pell, 2003). Not surprisingly, the authors failed to find any randomised trials for this particular preventive intervention. Despite the tongue-in-cheek nature of the report, the fact remains that not all interventions can be evaluated in RCTs and a lack of RCT evidence does not mean a lack of useful evidence for public health action. Even more important is the disregard for the quality of individual studies inherent in this approach. A well-designed and properly conducted cohort or case–control study could provide better

Table 11.1 A system commonly used to classify levels of evidence.

Level	Evidence
I	Evidence from at least one properly randomised controlled trial
II-1	Evidence from well-designed controlled trials without randomisation
II-2	Evidence from well-designed cohort or case–control studies, preferably from more than one centre or research group
II-3	Evidence from comparisons over time or between places with or without the intervention; dramatic results in uncontrolled experiments could also be regarded as this level of evidence
III	Opinions of respected authorities, based on clinical experience, descriptive studies and case reports, or reports of expert committees

(Harris *et al.*, 2001.)

evidence than a small or poorly conducted trial, but this rigid hierarchy would rate the evidence from the trial more highly. Box 11.2 considers the value of randomised and non-randomised designs in healthcare evaluation in more detail.

The need to move away from such a rigid approach has been well documented both for clinical research (Glasziou *et al.*, 2004) and for health services research in general (Black, 1996). A preferable approach, adopted by decision-making bodies around the world such as the US Preventive Services Task Force (USPSTF) and the Canadian Task Force on Preventive Health Care (CTFPHC), is not to classify studies purely on the basis of their *design* but also according to the *quality of the evidence* they provide. As its name suggests, the USPSTF regularly reviews the evidence for and against a wide range of preventive interventions. They rate studies according to specific criteria for that design (based on the key questions of subject selection and measurement that we discussed in Chapters 4 and 7). A 'good' study would generally meet all of the specified criteria, a 'fair' study does not meet them all but is judged not to have a fatal flaw that would invalidate the results, and a fatally flawed study is classified as 'poor' (Harris *et al.*, 2001). Another tool for assessing the quality of a study is the Cochrane 'Risk of bias' tool that we mentioned in Chapter 9 (Box 9.2) and was used by the authors of the review in Box 11.1.

Summarising the data

The next step in any review is to draw the data together to simplify their interpretation and to assist in drawing valid conclusions. It is important to look both for consistency of effects across studies (homogeneity) and for differences among studies (heterogeneity). Could differences be due to chance variation, or can they be explained by features of the studies or the populations they were conducted in? Graphs can be used to summarise the results of many studies in a simple format and in some situations the technique of **meta-analysis** can be used to combine the results from a number of different studies.

Graphical display of results

One way to display the results of a number of different studies is in a figure called a *forest plot*. Figure 11.1 shows a forest plot from a systematic review of the relation between weight/BMI and ovarian cancer risk (Purdie *et al.*, 2001). It shows the results of all 23 case–control studies whose authors had reported

Box 11.2 Randomisation versus observation

Most generic lists rank RCTs first in terms of study quality. For appropriate questions, i.e. about the effects of various interventions, this is reasonable, as you have seen. However, even for such questions caveats need to be applied. If a randomised trial is not competently conducted, or is too small, then its theoretical advantages disappear, and it can give misleading results (Schultz *et al.*, 1995). There are also many situations in which a trial would be unfeasible, unethical, undesirable or unnecessary (Black, 1996), and trials are generally irrelevant for questions related to frequency or measurement validation (e.g. of the performance of a screening or diagnostic test).

Estimates of the effects of treatment may differ between randomised and non-randomised studies, but when direct comparisons have been made neither method has consistently given a greater effect than the other (McKee *et al.*, 1999). Overall, it seems that dissimilarities between the participants in RCTs and non-randomised studies explain many of the differences; the two methods should therefore be compared only after patients not meeting the RCT eligibility criteria have also been excluded from the non-randomised study. Not surprisingly then, treatment effects measured in randomised and non-randomised studies are most similar when the exclusion criteria are the same and where potential prognostic factors are well understood and controlled for in the non-randomised setting. Taking this approach has helped reconcile some of the apparently major differences between the effects of menopausal hormone therapy (MHT) as found in RCTs (evidence of harm) and cohort studies (evidence of health benefits). Closer consideration of the details of the different studies suggests that differences in the ages at which women started taking MHT – around menopause (average age 51 years in the USA) in the cohort studies but at a mean age of more than 60 years in the trials – could explain many of the differences (Manson and Bassuk, 2007). It is also important to consider the precision of the RCT effect estimates – some are based on so few events (especially when death is the outcome of interest) that chance differences from the true underlying effect are quite likely. (For an example of these issues from studies comparing the effectiveness of various interventions to unblock coronary arteries see Britton *et al.*, 1998.)

The **generalisability** (see Chapters 7 and 9) of the results of RCTs can also be questionable, given the highly selected nature of the participants:

(*continued*)

Box 11.2 *(continued)*

patients excluded from randomised controlled trials tend to have a worse prognosis than those included (McKee *et al.*, 1999). When both randomised and non-randomised studies have been conducted and estimates of treatment effect are reasonably consistent for patients at similar risk, it allows more certain generalisation to the broader target populations of the non-randomised studies.

data on this association, ordered with the most recent study at the top and the oldest at the bottom. The odds ratio for each individual study is represented by the black square, with the size of the square indicating the size (or 'weight' – see 'Meta-analysis', below) of that particular study. The horizontal bar through each box shows the 95% confidence interval for the odds ratio and the vertical line indicates the point where there is 'no effect', i.e. an odds ratio of 1.0. When the confidence interval crosses this line (i.e. it includes the null value) it

Figure 11.1 Diagrammatic representation of the results of 23 case–control studies evaluating the relation between extremes of weight/BMI and risk of ovarian cancer (Purdie *et al.*, 2001).

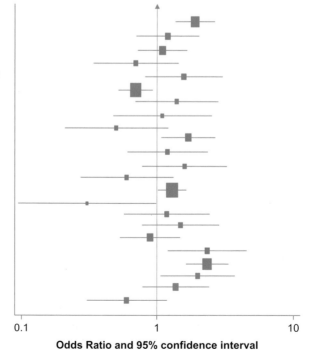

Odds Ratio and 95% confidence interval

indicates that the result is not statistically significant (i.e. $p \geq 0.05$). (Note the use of the logarithmic scale, which balances positive and inverse relative effects visually around the null; i.e. an OR of 2.0 would be the same distance from 1.0 as an OR of 0.5 in the opposite direction.)

Assessing heterogeneity

In this example the results of the 23 studies are scattered both sides of the line that marks an odds ratio of 1.0 (i.e. no effect), and they show no obvious pattern. The next step should be to evaluate this *heterogeneity* in more detail. Are there any differences between the studies that could explain some of the variation in their results?

One major methodological difference between the studies in this example is subject selection: some were population-based and others were hospital-based. We touched on some of the problems inherent in hospital-based studies in earlier chapters – could this difference explain any of the variation in the study results? Other possibilities to consider might include the geographical areas where the research was done – for example, separating high- and low-risk countries, and the ages of the participants. In this case, if we separate the hospital- and population-based studies (Figure 11.2) we start to see some regularity. In each of the 11 population-based studies at the bottom of Figure 11.2, the OR is greater than 1.0 (although many of the individual results are not statistically significant), suggesting that obesity/higher weight is associated with an increased risk of ovarian cancer. In contrast, the results of the hospital studies still vary widely. In this situation it was felt that using hospital-based controls might not be appropriate, as obese people are more likely to have other health problems and thus end up in hospital so their use could lead to overestimation of the prevalence of obesity in the population and thereby to underestimation of the obesity–cancer association.

> There are formal statistical tests to check for **heterogeneity** between the results of different studies. For example Cochran's Q-test and I^2 statistics.

Meta-analysis

Meta-analysis is a powerful technique that allows the results of a number of different studies to be combined. Each study is assigned a weight based on the amount of information it provides (e.g. the inverse of the standard error of the OR) and in general larger studies have greater weight. A weighted average of the individual study results can then be calculated. The assumption underlying this analysis is that all of the studies are estimating the same underlying effect and any variation between their results is due to chance. If their results

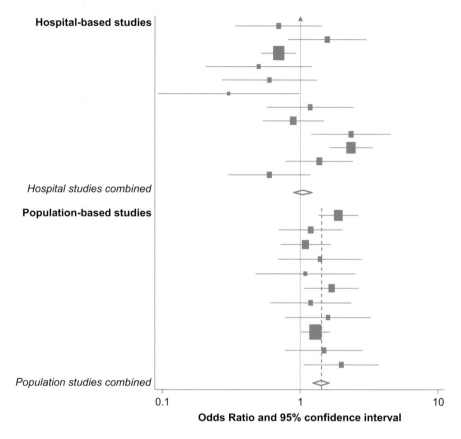

Figure 11.2 Diagrammatic representation of the results of 12 hospital-based and 11 population-based case–control studies evaluating the relation between extremes of weight/BMI and risk of ovarian cancer (Purdie *et al.*, 2001).

are very different (i.e. they are *heterogeneous*), as in the hospital-based studies of BMI above, then this assumption may not be true and it might not be appropriate to combine the results.

The diamond at the bottom of Figure 11.2 represents the combined odds ratio for the 11 population-based studies; the centre indicates the point estimate and the ends show the 95% confidence interval. In this case, it indicates that being overweight increases the risk of ovarian cancer by 40% (pooled OR = 1.4; 95% CI 1.2–1.6). Notice that the diamond does not overlap the 'no-effect' line (i.e. the confidence interval does not include 1.0), so the pooled OR is statistically significant. If we draw a dotted line vertically through the combined odds ratio, it passes through the 95% confidence interval of each of the individual studies. This is an indication that the results of the studies are fairly *homogeneous*, but it is certainly not definitive. In this case a formal statistical test for heterogeneity gives a *p*-value of 0.63. If *p* were < 0.05, this would suggest that differences between the results of the individual studies were unlikely to be due to chance; however, the observed p-value is well away from this, suggesting there is no significant heterogeneity and thus supporting the 'eyeball' finding that the results are all fairly similar.

In contrast, if we combine the results of the 12 hospital-based studies, we find a combined OR of 0.9 (95% CI 0.9–1.2), but a line through this point would not pass through the confidence intervals of the individual studies. This suggests that the results of the hospital-based studies are heterogeneous, and this is confirmed by a statistical test for heterogeneity, which gives $p < 0.001$, which is highly statistically significant. In this situation it is inappropriate to combine the results into a single estimate of effect.

Pooled analysis

An even more rigorous but much more time-consuming approach is known as a *pooled analysis* or re-analysis. Instead of combining the summary results (OR or RR) from a number of different studies, the investigator obtains copies of the raw data from the original studies and re-analyses them in a consistent way. An excellent example is the Oxford-based Collaborative Group on Hormonal Factors in Breast Cancer which, since the mid-1990s, has been producing reports based on analyses of over 50,000 women with breast cancer and 100,000 without, from data provided by more than 50 separate studies. The collaboration's first paper showed with great precision the very low absolute risk of breast cancer conferred by the majority of patterns of oral contraceptive pill use (Collaborative Group on Hormonal Factors in Breast Cancer, 1996). This report removed a great deal of the uncertainty that remained about this relation, despite many prior publications from individual studies.

Until recently, such pooled analyses were relatively uncommon: the effort required to obtain the original data, clean, recode and re-shape each data set to a common standard, conduct a new analysis and write the paper, all the while maintaining full approval of all contributing investigators, is monumental. However, the last few years have seen an explosion in the number of international consortia (and acronyms!) established specifically to bring together investigators from around the world to pool genetic and/or epidemiological data from different studies. This has been particularly true in the field of molecular epidemiology, where it seems likely that aside from a small number of 'high-risk' genes, such as the *BRCA1* and *BRCA2* genes identified for breast and ovarian cancer, the effects of any individual genetic variant on cancer risk are likely to be small and, as a result, very large numbers of individuals are needed to show an association with any certainty. Examples of these consortia include BCAC (Breast Cancer Association Consortium), OCAC (Ovarian Cancer Association Consortium), PANC4 (Pancreatic Cancer Case Control Consortium), E2C2 (Epidemiology of Endometrial Cancer

Consortium), BEACON (Barrett's and Esophageal Adenocarcinoma Consortium), DIAGRAM (DIAbetes Genetics Replication And Meta-analysis) Consortium ... the list is ever-growing.

A word of caution

Combining the results of a number of studies usually generates an estimate with narrow confidence limits, thereby giving a sense of precision and accuracy that may be illusory. However, the combined results of a meta-analysis will depend entirely on the studies selected for inclusion (or exclusion) and Box 11.3 gives an example of where two systematic reviews reached almost diametrically opposing conclusions due, at least in part, to the different sets of studies considered appropriate for inclusion. (Note, this is also another example of when simple descriptive data can be informative.)

Furthermore, as you saw in Chapters 7 and 8, there are numerous ways in which bias can occur and the old adage still holds true: 'rubbish in = rubbish out'. Combining results cannot get rid of bias or undetected confounding and, although a combined odds ratio from several poor studies may look good, it will not compensate for problems in the individual studies. Figure 11.3 shows the results of a pooled analysis of data from 32 studies looking at the relation between birth weight and subsequent risk of breast cancer (dos Santos Silva *et al.*, 2008). When the authors separated the studies according to the source of the birth weight information, they saw a clear trend towards increasing risk of breast cancer with increasing birth weight among the 16 studies where the information on birth weight came directly from birth records and was thus, presumably, most accurate. The association was much weaker in the one study where the information was provided by the women's mothers when the women themselves were children, and there was no association at all among the 11 studies that relied on the women reporting their own birth weight – almost certainly the least reliable source of information. (Note also that the results of the statistical tests for heterogeneity are all non-significant ($p > 0.05$), suggesting that the results of the various studies within each group are all quite consistent.) This is a striking example where error and subsequent non-differential misclassification (see Chapter 7) in the self-reported data has completely masked what appears to be quite a strong association based on the more accurate birth record information. If all of these studies had been pooled together, it is likely that this association would have been missed.

Drawing conclusions

Once a review is complete, the final challenge is to draw appropriate conclusions. Meta-analyses and pooled analyses that generate combined

Box 11.3 Do mobile telephones cause brain cancer?

Given the unprecedented growth in the use of mobile telephones over the last 25 years such that usage is now almost ubiquitous in many countries, a major question is whether exposure to the radiofrequency fields they generate causes brain cancer. This is both a highly controversial and highly emotive area as brain cancers often occur at younger ages than many other cancers and, because of their location, are often fatal. In mid-2009, two meta-analyses attempted to address this question.

The first study focussed on the long-term effects of mobile phone use and thus only included published studies where participants had used mobile phones for at least 10 years. Because the radiofrequency waves generated by mobile phones do not penetrate very far into the brain, they also restricted their review to studies with a 'laterality' analysis, i.e. that considered whether the cancer arose on the same side of the head preferred for phone use. A total of 11 studies met these criteria. They found that use of a mobile phone for 10 or more years approximately doubled the risk of being diagnosed with a brain tumour on the side of the head preferred for phone use, and that the association was statistically significant for two types of brain cancer: gliomas and acoustic neuromas. *They therefore concluded that there was adequate epidemiological evidence to suggest a link* (Khurana *et al.*, 2009).

The second group took a broader approach and included all published studies that had evaluated this association (>20 individual reports). They found that the current data did not show any increase in risk of brain cancer with up to 10 years of mobile phone use and concluded that the data *do not suggest a causal association between mobile phone use and fast-growing brain tumours such as gliomas* (Ahlbom *et al.*, 2009). The authors did, however, acknowledge that longer follow-up was needed before any conclusions could be drawn regarding longer-term use and the effects on slow-growing tumours.

So why did these two meta-analyses come to such different conclusions?

The individual studies included in the meta-analyses have given quite different results; some show a strong association and others see no effect. No-one has, as yet, been able to adequately explain the reasons for this, but it is likely that the different criteria used to determine which studies would be included/excluded from each of the reviews led to their differing conclusions. As to which is correct? It may be that only time and a longer follow-up period will tell, although it is worth noting that, as yet, there have been no overall increases in reported incidence or mortality rates of brain cancer since use of mobile phones has become widespread (Deltour *et al.*, 2009; Inskip *et al.*, 2010).

Figure 11.3 Relative risk of breast cancer (and 95% confidence intervals) associated with increasing birth weight, stratified by source of birth weight data (*from*: dos Santos Silva *et al.*, 2008).

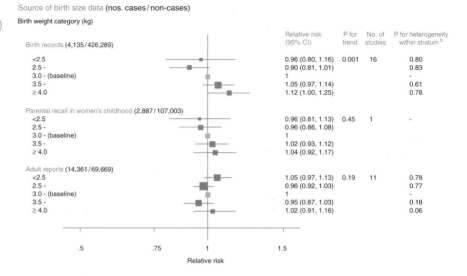

effect estimates across studies provide more precise summary measures of the *strength* of an association and sometimes of the *dose–response* relationship. The homogeneity (or otherwise) of study results addresses the concept of *consistency* – we do not require that effect estimates be near-identical across studies to meet this criterion, simply showing that most are positive (or negative) and reasonably similar with respect to their confidence intervals (i.e. the 95% CIs are overlapping) may suffice. Also, if more extreme heterogeneity can be shown to be due to differing methodology or degrees of study error, and results among the better studies are reasonably consistent, then the review still provides helpful causal information (Weed, 2000).

One system that was developed specifically to guide those reviewing evidence in order to establish clinical guidelines, but that is also more widely applicable, is 'GRADE' (Grading of Recommendations, Assessment, Development and Evaluation Guyatt *et al.*, 2008). This classifies the quality of evidence as high, moderate, low and very low. Evidence based on RCTs is initially considered as high quality, but this rating is downgraded if the trials have limitations, their results are inconsistent or imprecise, the evidence is indirect (it does not directly address the question of interest) or there are concerns about reporting bias. In contrast, evidence based on observational studies is initially considered low but this rating can be upgraded if the effects are very large, there is evidence of a dose–response relation or the likely effect of any bias would have been to underestimate the true effect. The Cochrane Collaboration has adopted the principles of the GRADE system for evaluating the quality of evidence from systematic reviews so this approach was used by the authors in Box 11.1.

Assessing the quality of a systematic review

A principal feature of a modern systematic review is that it must have a comprehensive methods section. As you saw in Box 11.1, the authors should have detailed their literature-searching strategy and the processes of study selection and appraisal and data extraction. Table 11.2 outlines a fairly comprehensive set of the key criteria for appraising the validity of a systematic review which summarises and extends the major points made above. As for reports from individual studies (Table 9.1), guidelines have been developed to improve the reporting of meta-analyses. The main focus of the 'Preferred Reporting Items for Systematic reviews and Meta-Analyses' or PRISMA statement (Liberati *et al.*, 2009, http://www.prisma-statement.org/) is on meta-analyses of randomised controlled trials, but it can also be used for other types of research, particularly evaluations of interventions. A parallel guide for meta-analyses of observational studies is the 'Meta-analysis Of Observational Studies in Epidemiology' or MOOSE statement (Stroup *et al.*, 2000). Omitted from some such lists, however, but always central to making a comprehensive judgement, is a consideration of the logic and insight of the review, especially its treatment of error, heterogeneity, causality and practical importance.

Making judgements in practice

Primary epidemiological data (from individual studies) and secondary data (from reviews) are not ends in themselves. They aim to tell us about the healthiness of populations, what we might need to change to improve their condition, and how we might go about this. The goal of the enterprise is to take action to improve health. This is not a modern phenomenon and, as you have seen, many advances in public health pre-dated epidemiology. The strong call to base action on good evidence (*evidence-based practice*) is, however, quite recent, and has spread rapidly from clinical medicine to public health. We will conclude this chapter with descriptions of how some influential national and international bodies conduct and use reviews to make judgements regarding causation to inform practice and policy.

> The **SUPPORT Tools** (SUPporting POlicy relevant Reviews and Trials) have been developed to guide the evaluation of research evidence for evidence-informed policymaking (see Lavis *et al.*, 2009).

The US Preventive Services Task Force (USPSTF)

The USPSTF was convened by the US Public Health Service in the 1980s to assess the merits of preventive activities in clinical practice

Table 11.2 Guidelines for appraising the validity of a systematic review.

Criteria	What to look for	Comments
Focused research question	The main research question should be clear from either the title or the abstract. The exposure, such as a risk factor or therapy, and the outcome(s) of interest should be expressed in terms of a simple relationship	If the review addresses multiple questions it is likely to be a general introduction to the area and may have limited sources of evidence for the conclusions drawn. Statements may be made with few citations and limited in-depth analysis of studies. Caution should be taken in accepting conclusions from this type of review
Inclusion and exclusion criteria	The eligibility criteria used to select studies should be stated and should specify the participants, exposures and outcomes of interest and in some cases the study design	If the eligibility criteria are not clearly stated you have no way of knowing whether studies were included (or excluded) solely on the basis of their results, which could bias the conclusions of the review
Comprehensiveness of search strategy	Detailed search strategy indicating that the authors have searched all the relevant bibliographic databases with a variety of appropriate search terms. Other strategies such as hand searching and snowballing^a may be used	It is only possible to evaluate the thoroughness of the search strategies if the methods used by the authors are made explicit. If there is no methods section then you should be cautious in accepting any of the results
Assessment of included studies	Statements that indicate whether individual included studies are scientifically sound as measured against established criteria	The criteria for appraising the individual studies should reflect the study design. For example, if the review was examining a treatment effect then the criteria should relate primarily to RCTs
Reproducibility of assessments^b	Statements that the appraisals were conducted independently by at least two reviewers and any differences resolved by consensus or by a third person	Because appraisal of studies involves judgement calls, decisions based on these appraisals are subject to random errors or mistakes and systematic errors or bias. Having two independent reviewers should minimise these
Similarity of results of included studies	Detailed reporting of the results of individual studies with some measure of the differences (heterogeneity) between them	If the results are very different it may not be appropriate to combine them in a meta-analysis. Instead there should be some exploration of the reasons for the differences (e.g. different populations, different study methods, etc.)
Overall logic and insight	Discussion of how error and heterogeneity have been handled, also causality and practical importance	These issues are central to making a comprehensive judgement

(Adapted from Oxman *et al.*, 1994.)

^{a} Snowballing refers to the iterative process of searching where the results of the initial search are used to identify missed papers through either a search of the reference list at the end of the identified paper or by using Science Citation Index to see who has cited the identified paper.

^{b} Multiple assessors are used in rigorous systematic reviews of clinical interventions such as those conducted through the Cochrane Collaboration, but this level of rigour is less commonly used for aetiologic reviews. This need not invalidate the results as long as the criteria used to include and exclude studies are clearly described.

(http://www.uspreventiveservicestaskforce.org/). It aims to provide simple practical guidelines for clinicians regarding the utility of preventive interventions that they might use in their practice (over 200 to date). Many of the interventions assessed relate to early detection of a wide range of conditions, counselling to change behaviour and primary chemoprevention (e.g. aspirin to prevent cardiovascular disease). Topic teams assigned by the task force prepare systematic reviews of the evidence according to a standard protocol. The evidence for a particular preventive service is classified as good, fair or poor and then combined with a judgement of the net benefit of the service (substantial, moderate, small or zero/negative). Notably, the public is invited to comment at all stages of the process from the draft research plan to the draft evidence review and recommendation statements. The USPSTF assesses the reviews centrally and then makes formal recommendations with specific ratings (AHRQ, 2004; Harris *et al.*, 2001), examples of which are given below. These recommendations translate into practice guidance for clinicians who are advised to offer or provide services with 'A' and 'B' recommendations to eligible patients; discourage the use of services with 'D' recommendations; offer or provide services with 'C' recommendations to selected patients depending on individual circumstances; and, for services with 'I' (insufficient evidence) statements, carefully read the Clinical Considerations section for guidance, and help patients understand the uncertainty surrounding these services.

A The USPSTF *recommends* that clinicians screen all pregnant women for HIV, including those who present in labour who are untested and whose HIV status is unknown. The net benefit of screening for HIV infection in pregnant women is *substantial* (April 2013).

B The USPSTF *recommends* offering or referring adults who are overweight or obese and have additional cardiovascular disease (CVD) risk factors to intensive behavioural counselling interventions to promote a healthful diet and physical activity for CVD prevention . . . The USPSTF *concludes with moderate certainty* that intensive behavioural counselling interventions to promote a healthful diet and physical activity have a *moderate net benefit* in adults who are overweight or obese and at increased risk for CVD (August 2014).

C The USPSTF recommends that clinicians selectively offer screening for abdominal aortic aneurysm in men ages 65–75 years who have never smoked rather than routinely screening all men in this group (June 2014).

D The USPSTF *recommends against* prostate-specific antigen (PSA)-based screening for prostate cancer . . . The benefits of PSA-based screening for prostate cancer do not outweigh the harms (May 2012).

I The USPSTF concludes that the *current evidence is insufficient to assess the balance of benefits and harms* of screening for vitamin D deficiency in asymptomatic adults (November, 2014).

Table 11.3 Some findings from the US Community Guide regarding community interventions.

Finding	Intervention	Date
Recommended	Combined diet and physical activity promotion programmes to prevent type-2 diabetes among people at increased risk	July 2014
	Universal motorbike helmet laws	August 2013
	Behavioural interventions that aim to reduce recreational sedentary screen time among children	August 2014
Insufficient evidence	Community-based interventions to encourage use of helmets, facemasks and mouthguards in contact sports	October 2013
	Internet-based smoking cessation interventions	December 2011
Recommended against	Policies facilitating the transfer of juveniles to adult justice systems	April 2003

A parallel activity for community prevention, the Community Guide, was established by the US Department of Health and Human Services in 1996 and is conducted by the Task Force on Community Preventive Services (http://www.thecommunityguide.org/index.html). Some typical findings are summarised in Table 11.3.

The International Agency for Research on Cancer (IARC): monographs programme

Three times a year the IARC convenes a working party of experts to review all of the literature relating a specific exposure or exposures to cancer. This process is one of the most comprehensive conducted anywhere; in addition to studies in humans, the working parties also include experts on the exposure itself (chemists, toxicologists, physicists, etc.), on animal studies and on molecular biology. The IARC secretariat performs comprehensive literature searches and sends the material to the individual scientists who are asked to summarise the literature in a particular area. During a week-long face-to-face meeting, subgroups of the working party (exposure data, human studies, animal studies and laboratory data) discuss and finalise the draft sections of the report and prepare a summary for their section. The full group then comes together to reach a final consensus. The human and animal data are first classified separately as providing *sufficient*, *limited* or *inadequate* evidence of carcinogenicity or, occasionally, evidence suggesting a lack of carcinogenicity. These data are then combined with the exposure data and molecular information to make a more formal assessment of causality, classifying agents as:

- carcinogenic to humans,
- *probably* carcinogenic to humans,
- *possibly* carcinogenic to humans,
- *not classifiable* regarding carcinogenicity to humans or
- *probably not* carcinogenic to humans (http://monographs.iarc.fr).

As at August 2016 they had classified 118 agents or mixtures as clear carcinogens with another 80 classified as probable and 289 as possible carcinogens, reflecting the general lack of certainty when dealing with evidence of this type. (Only one compound has been classified as probably not carcinogenic.) A further 502 agents were found to be not classifiable because there was insufficient evidence to make any judgement. (For further information see http://monographs.iarc.fr/.)

The World Cancer Research Fund and American Institute of Cancer Research

The aim of the World Cancer Research Fund (WCRF) International is to 'lead and unify a global network of cancer charities dedicated to the prevention and control of cancer by means of healthy food and nutrition, physical activity and weight management' (http://www.wcrf.org/index.php). In 1997, the WCRF joined forces with the American Institute for Cancer Research (AICR) to jointly publish a comprehensive review of the current state of knowledge regarding the relation between nutrition and cancer (WCRF and AICR, 1997). In 2007 the second edition of this report was published to incorporate new evidence that had accumulated since 1997 (WCRF and AICR, 2007) and since then updates for a number of cancer sites have been published via the 'Continuous Update Project'. The reviews are contracted out to international teams of experts and their detailed methodological plans for the review are critiqued by others and refined before the reviews are conducted and again before the results are published. While these reviews are not directly linked to policy, the aim is to provide good scientific evidence that can be used by policy makers, research scientists, health professionals and community groups around the world.

The end result

Once a cause-and-effect association has been established beyond any reasonable doubt, action can be taken to change public policy, legislation, health education, clinical practice or the direction of research. Thalidomide is no longer given to women during pregnancy because it causes birth defects; diethylstilboestrol is no longer prescribed to prevent miscarriage because it can cause vaginal cancer in the women's daughters; dietary advice and drugs are used to lower cholesterol levels to prevent heart disease; the hazards of smoking are publicised, and legislation restricting smoking in public has been enacted in many countries; seat-belt wearing is becoming ubiquitous internationally – the list goes on. It is, however, worth noting that it has taken a long time, decades even, to establish causality for some of these associations. This tension between the desire for full knowledge and the social need for action is a given in public health so policy makers and planners have to act despite this and make the best of what is available. As one of the seminal figures in health services research said:

The absence of excellent evidence does not make evidence-based decision making impossible; what is required is the best evidence available not the best evidence possible (Muir Gray, 1997).

We will end with a question that still causes controversy: should we recommend widespread mammographic screening for women under the age of 50 years (Box 11.4)? (Or, some would argue, should we recommend it at all? (Various, 2004).)

Box 11.4 Should women under the age of 50 be offered routine mammographic screening?

The debate surrounding this question highlights the difficulties of interpreting evidence. In 1993, an expert panel at the US National Cancer Institute (NCI) concluded that there was no evidence for a benefit of mammographic screening for women aged 40–49 years and the NCI withdrew their recommendation for screening in this age group. In response, the American Cancer Society reaffirmed their recommendation *for* screening, which was based on the view of a separate expert panel. The publication of additional data in 1996 opened up the question again and the NCI responded by convening a consensus conference in 1997. The independent experts at the conference again concluded that there was insufficient evidence to recommend routine mammography for women under the age of 50 years. This conclusion led to such a public outcry that the NCI was forced to reconsider their position. The question went back to the National Cancer Advisory Board, a presidentially appointed committee, who voted 17 to 1 in favour of recommending mammographic screening for younger women. Since then, the controversy has continued, with groups reaching opposing conclusions based on the same evidence.

(continued)

Box 11.4 *(continued)*

As you will see in Chapter 15, the evaluation of screening programmes is not simple, and in this particular instance there is still no clear consensus. In 2015, IARC convened a working group to assess the evidence and, although the overall conclusion was that the evidence for a benefit for women under 50 was *limited*, almost half of the group considered there was sufficient evidence of a benefit for women aged 45–49 (Lauby-Secretan *et al.*, 2015). In the same year, the USPSTF released their new draft recommendations for breast cancer screening concluding that 'The decision to start screening mammography in women before age 50 years should be an individual one. Women who place a higher value on the potential benefit than the potential harms may choose to begin screening between the ages of 40 and 49 years. (C recommendation)'. They also noted that 'A C grade is not a recommendation against screening. It means that the balance of benefits and harms for any individual woman is a delicate one. The Task Force recognizes mammograms can help women in their 40s reduce their risk of dying from breast cancer. Because the risk of developing breast cancer is lower in women under 50, the potential benefit of mammography for women under 50 is also smaller' (USPSTF, 2015). [Both groups recommended mammography for women aged 50–74 years (USPSTF B recommendation), but USPSTF concluded the current evidence was insufficient to assess the balance of benefits and harms of screening mammography in women 75 years and older (I statement).]

Conclusion

In the previous chapters we have discussed the practical 'nuts and bolts' of epidemiology. In Chapters 2–5 we considered the ways in which we can measure health and quantify associations between 'exposures' and health 'outcomes'. We then looked critically at how we interpret the results of individual studies in Chapters 6–9 and in Chapter 10 we started to think about how we can assess whether an association might be causal. In this chapter we have considered how we can bring together all of this information to inform decision-making. We will now move on to look at some practical applications of epidemiology that aim to reduce the burden of disease in a community: surveillance, outbreak management, prevention and screening. These will draw on the core concepts that you have learned so far and reinforce the epidemiological perspective – a mix of science and art that requires an open mind, attention to detail and the potential for error, a willingness to consider alternative explanations and, finally, the ability to be both constructively critical and pragmatic.

Questions

Additional questions

1. List three strategies you might use to identify relevant literature to include in a systematic review.
2. What is meant by the term 'grey literature' and why is it a good idea to search this to identify potentially relevant studies for a systematic review?
3. If early results from a trial were published after one year of follow-up and then a second paper with longer follow-up was published a few years later, is it appropriate to include both of these publications in a systematic review or meta-analysis of the topic? Why/why not?

REFERENCES

References

Ahlbom, A., Feychting, M., Green, A., *et al*. (2009). Epidemiologic evidence on mobile phones and tumor risk. A review. *Epidemiology*, 20: 639–652.

AHRQ. (2004). *Guide to Clinical Preventive Services, Third Edition: Periodic Updates*. AHRQ Publication No. 04-IP003, January 2004. Rockville, MD: Agency for Healthcare Research and Quality.

Black, N. (1996). Why we need observational studies to evaluate the effectiveness of health care. *British Medical Journal*, 312: 1215–1218.

Britton, A., McKee, M., Black, N., *et al*. (1998). Choosing between randomised and non-randomised studies: a systematic review. *Health Technology Assessment*, 2 (13): 1–124.

Collaborative Group on Hormonal Factors in Breast Cancer. (1996). Breast cancer and hormonal contraceptives: collaborative reanalysis of individual data on 53297 women with breast cancer and 100239 women without breast cancer from 54 epidemiological studies. *The Lancet*, 347: 1713–1727.

Deltour, I., Johansen, C., Auvinen, A., *et al*. (2009). Time trends in brain tumor incidence rates in Denmark, Finland, Norway, and Sweden, 1974–2003. *Journal of the National Cancer Institute*, 101: 1621–1724.

dos Santos Silva, I., de Stavola, B., McCormack, V. and Collaborative Group on Pre-Natal Risk Factors and Subsequent Risk of Breast Cancer. (2008). Birth size and breast cancer risk: re-analysis of individual participant data from 32 studies. *PLoS Medicine*, 5: e193.

Glasziou, P., Vandenbroucke, J. and Chalmers, I. (2004). Assessing the quality of research. *British Medical Journal*, 328: 39–41.

Guyatt, G. H., Oxman, A. D., Vist, G. E., *et al*. (2008). GRADE: what is "quality of evidence" and why is it important to clinicians? *British Medical Journal*, 336: 995–998.

Harris, R. P., Helfand, M., Woolf, S. H. *et al.* for the Methods Work Group Third US Preventive Services Task Force. (2001). Current methods of the US Preventive Services Task Force: a review of the process. *American Journal of Preventive Medicine*, 20 (3S): 21–35.

Inskip, P. D., Hoover, R. N. and Devesa, S. S. (2010). Brain cancer incidence trends in relation to cellular telephone use in the United States. *Neuro-Oncology*; 12: 1147–1151.

Khurana, V. G., Teo, C., Kundi, M., Hardell, L. and Carlberg, M. (2009). Cell phones and brain tumors: a review including the long-term epidemiologic data. *Surgical Neurology*, 72: 205–214.

Lauby-Secretan, B., Scoccianti, C., Loomis, D., *et al.* for the IARC Handbook Working Group. (2015). Breast-cancer screening – viewpoint of the IARC Working Group. *The New England Journal of Medicine*, 372: 2353–2358.

Lavis, J. N., Oxman, A. D., Lewin, S. and Frethein, A. (2009). SUPPORT Tools for evidence-informed health policymaking (STP). *Health Research Policy and Systems*, 7(Suppl I): II.

Liberati, A., Altman, D. G., Tetzlaff, J., *et al.* (2009). The PRISMA statement for reporting systematic reviews and meta-analyses of studies that evaluate healthcare interventions: explanation and elaboration. *British Medical Journal*, 339: b2700 doi: 10.1136/bmj.b2700.

Manson, J. E. and Bassuk, S. S. (2007). Invited commentary: Hormone therapy and risk of coronary heart disease – why renew the focus on the early years of menopause? *American Journal of Epidemiology*, 166: 511–517.

McKee, M., Britton, A., Black, N., *et al.* (1999). Interpreting the evidence: choosing between randomised and non-randomised studies. *British Medical Journal*, 319: 312–315.

Muir Gray, J. A. (1997). *Evidence-Based Health Care – How to Make Health Policy and Management Decisions*. Edinburgh: Churchill Livingstone.

Oxman, A. D., Cook, D. J. and Guyatt, G. H. (1994). Users' guides to the medical literature VI. How to use an overview. *Journal of the American Medical Association*, 272: 1367–1371.

Purdie, D. M., Bain, C. J., Webb, P. M., *et al.* (2001). Body size and ovarian cancer: case–control study and systematic review (Australia). *Cancer Causes Control*, 12: 855–863.

Reveiz, L. and Cardona, A. F. (2015). Antibiotics for acute laryngitis in adults. *Cochrane Database of Systematic Reviews*, Issue 5. Art. No.: CD004783. DOI: 10.1002/14651858.CD004783.pub5.

Schultz, K. F., Chalmers, I., Hayes, R. J. and Altman, D. G. (1995). Empirical evidence of bias. Dimensions of methodological quality associated with estimates of treatment effects in controlled trials. *Journal of the American Medical Association*, 273: 408–412.

Smith, G. C. S. and Pell, J. P. (2003). Parachute use to prevent death and major trauma related to gravitational challenge: systematic review of randomised controlled trials. *British Medical Journal*, 327: 1459–1461.

Stroup, D. F., Berlin, J. A., Morton, S. C., *et al.* (2000). Meta-analysis of observational studies in epidemiology. A proposal for reporting. *Journal of the American Medical Association*, 283: 2008–2012.

USPSTF (United States Preventive Services Task Force). (2015). *Draft Recommendation Statement: Breast Cancer: Screening*. U.S. Preventive Services Task Force. May 2015. http://www.uspreventiveservicestaskforce.org/Page/Document/UpdateSummaryFinal/breast-cancer-screening1, accessed 6 June 2015.

Various. (2004). Screening for breast cancer: point–counterpoint. *International Journal of Epidemiology*, 33: 43–74.

WCRF (World Cancer Research Fund) and AICR (American Institute for Cancer Research). (1997). *Food, Nutrition and the Prevention of Cancer: A Global Perspective*. Washington, DC: AICR.

WCRF (World Cancer Research Fund) and AICR (American Institute for Cancer Research). (2007). *Food, Nutrition, Physical Activity, and the Prevention of Cancer: A Global Perspective*. Washington, DC: AICR.

Weed, D. L. (2000). Interpreting epidemiological evidence: how meta-analysis and causal inference methods are related. *International Journal of Epidemiology*, 29: 387–390.

RECOMMENDED FOR FURTHER READING

- A thorough review of a tricky contemporary exposure:

  Ahlbom, A., Feychting, M., Green, A., *et al.* (2009). Epidemiologic evidence on mobile phones and tumor risk. A review. *Epidemiology*, 20: 639–652.
- A clear reminder of the need to consider all study types for inclusion in a review:

  Black, N. (1996). Why we need observational studies to evaluate the effectiveness of health care. *British Medical Journal*, 312: 1215–1218.

Surveillance: collecting health-related data for epidemiological intelligence and public health action

Martyn Kirk and Adrian Sleigh

Description
Chapters 2–3

Association
Chapters 4–5

Alternative
explanations
Chapters 6–8

Integration &
interpretation
Chapters 9–11

Practical
applications
Chapter 12:
Surveillance

Box 12.1 The Ebola virus outbreak, 2014–2015

Detection of the primary event: In March 2014, Guinea reported an outbreak of febrile illness among 49 people with a high case fatality rate (59%); it was later confirmed as Ebola virus. Epidemiological investigation of the reports identified that the primary case was likely to have been a two-year-old child who died in December 2013 (Baize *et al.*, 2014).

(*continued*)

Box 12.1 (*continued*)

International response: The international response to the outbreak initially seemed effective, but cases continued to spread in Guinea and to neighbouring countries, leading to Médecins Sans Frontières declaring that the outbreak was 'out of control' in June 2014. The World Health Organization (WHO) published a roadmap to control in August 2014 (WHO, 2014) and declared the outbreak a 'Public Health Emergency of International Concern'.

Controlling the outbreak: With support from international partner organisations, affected countries established programmes to identify cases, deaths and those who had been in contact with them. This required investigative teams to travel from house to house in very remote areas to track down contacts. The resulting information was entered into specialised databases and communicated through regional and country offices to WHO. The data were discussed at daily meetings and used to identify areas of high risk and those where the infection had been cleared. This 'surveillance' was vital for detecting new cases and outbreaks and for monitoring spread of infections to neighbouring countries.

Preparedness of unaffected countries: Despite the challenges, the WHO Africa region now advocates integrated surveillance of disease and, in response to this outbreak, international agencies have assisted neighbouring countries to strengthen their surveillance and control activities (WHO Ebola Response Team, 2014).

In the previous chapters we have considered the nuts and bolts of epidemiology. In this and the next few chapters we move on to look at how epidemiology is used in practice to improve public health. We start with 'surveillance' as, without the ability to gather timely information on emerging and changing health problems, public health can be paralysed or, at best, inefficient. In this chapter we discuss the design and use of surveillance systems that allow health officials to detect new risks and diseases such as Ebola promptly, track known diseases and generate data needed for effective health planning and resource allocation.

The scope of surveillance

Surveillance is a cornerstone of public health activities as it provides data and intelligence for development of policy, disease prevention programmes,

> ## Box 12.2 The role of epidemiology in surveillance
>
> Epidemiology has a fundamental role in public health surveillance:
>
> - epidemiology provides the tools to guide data collection, collation and analysis;
> - the concepts of rates of infection and analysis by subpopulations are key to analysis of surveillance data;
> - epidemiology provides a systematic framework for assessing potential biases that are inherent in surveillance data; and
> - surveillance provides much of the data essential to descriptive epidemiology (see Chapter 3).

estimation of disease burden, detection of outbreaks and applied research. It was originally applied primarily to infectious diseases, and we will mainly discuss surveillance in this context, but the approach, principles and practice have broadened to include chronic diseases, injuries, health system outcomes, risk factors and even potential hazards to human health. Surveillance is defined as the: 'systematic and continuous collection, analysis, and interpretation of data, closely integrated with the timely and coherent dissemination of the results and assessment to those who have the right to know so that action can be taken' (Porta, 2014). Ultimately, these data should be used to inform public health interventions and action to prevent human illness. The emphasis of this definition, and the feature that separates surveillance from the collection of data for monitoring purposes, is the dissemination of data for the purposes of public health action.

A good example of the importance of public health surveillance comes from the Ebola virus disease epidemic in West Africa in 2014–2015 – a crisis in international health (Box 12.1). The Ebola virus is spread by close contact with an infected person during the symptomatic phase of their illness, or contact with the body of someone who died from the disease. In the outbreak in West Africa, the international community focussed on controlling the outbreak rapidly, supported by establishment of surveillance for possible Ebola infections. This surveillance was critical to determine when disease activity had declined in a given regional area (WHO Ebola Response Team, 2014).

Why conduct surveillance?

Public health surveillance provides information on the changing nature of diseases in populations and, ideally, there is a clear link between the surveillance system outputs and control programmes or interventions, such as introduction of a vaccine or health promotion campaign. There are several reasons why it is important to conduct surveillance:

- *To inform public health policy.* For some diseases, such as influenza, information arising from surveillance of circulating strains in one hemisphere is used to inform decisions about vaccine composition for the next influenza season in the other hemisphere.
- *To detect clusters or outbreaks.* Diseases that are prone to occurring in clusters or outbreaks require surveillance to allow timely and effective investigation to identify a source. We will discuss this further in Chapter 13.
- *To monitor the effect of interventions.* Public health and other agencies may institute control measures that should reduce the incidence and prevalence of diseases; the effects of these can be observed in disease-specific surveillance data.
- *To monitor the introduction of new pharmaceutical drugs.* New drugs are often licensed before long-term safety data are available. Electronic databases now make it much simpler to link prescribing and health databases to identify unexpected safety concerns more rapidly than before.
- *To quantify the burden of disease.* Surveillance data can be critical to identifying the effects that diseases have on affected populations in terms of cases, hospitalisation, disability and deaths.
- *To support disease elimination and eradication.* Multiple modes of surveillance play a critical role during the phases of elimination and eradication of a disease (e.g. during the eradication of smallpox, see Box 1.5) and surveillance efforts are intensive due to the need to have highly sensitive systems for detecting cases.

Surveillance can provide dynamic data on population risks, morbidity and mortality – all key indicators for epidemiological intelligence on community health. However, given the limited resources of public health, it is important that only conditions of public health importance are considered for surveillance. Public health importance may be defined by a range of factors (we will discuss these further below) that should be well articulated before a condition is put under surveillance.

Surveillance essentials

To understand the basics of surveillance, we need to consider the exposure–disease–diagnosis pathway as this influences whether cases progress from exposure through to reporting to a surveillance system. Firstly, a person must be exposed to a hazard, such as another infectious person, and there will then be a latency or incubation period that depends on the agent. In some instances, there may be some other necessary cause, such as prior exposure to antibiotics or a comorbid illness, that will potentiate or result in the person moving on to develop disease. There are then other factors that predict whether a diseased person goes on to seek diagnosis and medical treatment. These include the proportion of people who develop symptoms, the severity of the major signs and symptoms and how communicable the disease is. Finally, for a case to be reported to a surveillance system, the health care provider making the diagnosis must recognise that it fits the criteria (whether these are specific tests for a clearly defined condition or the more general characteristics of a disease syndrome) for a reportable condition.

The steps in this pathway highlight many important criteria of surveillance, including timeliness of the data, the sensitivity of the system to detect a case, the representativeness of cases that are reported and, ultimately, the cost of the system. The key steps in surveillance are (1) collection of data, (2) collation and cleaning of data, (3) analysis and interpretation and (4) dissemination of data to those who can take action and, importantly, back to those who provided the data. Surveillance systems should have well-defined aims and objectives that are clearly communicated to stakeholders for surveillance to be successful.

It is likely that only a proportion of people with the disease under surveillance will present to a health care recorder, be tested and test positive for the disease in question. This is equivalent to the 'sensitivity' of the system (we will discuss this further in Chapter 15) and is the complement of 'undercount', the proportion of those with disease who are not counted. For diseases where some people may experience mild symptoms and not present for medical attention, such as *Salmonella* infections, the undercount may be substantial. In contrast, for a condition with a severe outcome, such as meningococcal meningitis where most of those affected are very ill and present to a hospital, there may only be a small degree of undercount inherent in surveillance. A system with low sensitivity may be acceptable if there is still a reasonable probability of identifying outbreaks. Undercount in surveillance is typically represented by a pyramid showing loss of cases through the system. Figure 12.1 shows the reporting pyramid for surveillance of a disease transmitted by contaminated foods where a person must visit a doctor and submit a specimen for testing in order to be counted as a case.

Depending on the nature of the disease and the aims of surveillance, the response to a single case will be different. For many diseases, health departments do not follow up all cases. However, they may interview all cases of diseases with epidemic potential, if there is a planned evaluation of an

Health care recorders are those who provide reports of cases or other details about disease. They include physicians in community clinics or microbiologists in a laboratory.

In the USA an estimated 29 *Salmonella* infections – a common cause of foodborne disease – occur in the community for every one that is reported to surveillance (Scallan *et al.*, 2011).

Figure 12.1 The surveillance pyramid for gastrointestinal illnesses.

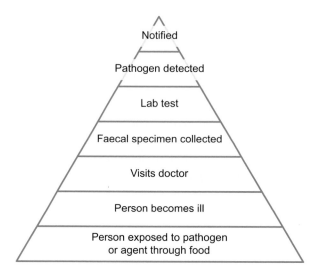

Figure 12.1 The surveillance pyramid for gastrointestinal illnesses.

intervention or where there is a requirement to provide prophylaxis. For example, the incidence and burden of hepatitis A has declined globally due to improvements in sanitation and hygiene (Franco *et al.*, 2012). It is routine for health department staff to contact and interview all cases of hepatitis A in high-income countries to determine if there is a need to offer hepatitis A immunoglobulin (prophylactic vaccination) to contacts, and to use their exposure histories to identify links between cases that might indicate an outbreak is occurring.

Defining a case for surveillance purposes

All forms of surveillance rely on some form of case definition which specifies elements of person, place and time. The case definition may be syndromic in nature and specify clinical signs and symptoms, or it may be more specific and require particular pathology, but it is important to recognise that what defines a case for surveillance purposes may differ from what a doctor might use to diagnose a condition in a patient. This is particularly true for surveillance during outbreak settings when there may be multiple case definitions representing greater degrees of certainty about whether a patient is a true case or not.

Where a case definition is based on a syndrome, it is called 'syndromic surveillance'. Syndromic surveillance can be much more sensitive as it picks up cases of illness that may be due to many different disease-causing agents, but it may not be very specific and may consequently be less useful for public

Box 12.3 Polio eradication – surveillance and progress in India

By 2001, polio had largely been limited to two states in India with only 268 new cases that year, but in 2002 there was a resurgence with 1600 new cases. In 2003, a network of 248 medical officers trained in surveillance assisted Indian health authorities with surveillance for acute flaccid paralysis (AFP), the critical clinical marker of polio. The WHO criteria for assessing the quality of polio surveillance require that

- *non-polio* AFP should be detected at a rate of $\geq$1 per 100,000 in the population aged <15 years (to ensure that 'background' AFP cases are being detected at a level showing the detection system is working) and
- adequate stool specimens are collected from $\geq$80% of people with AFP for polio diagnosis.

India had been meeting these criteria since 2000, but in 2003 the non-polio AFP rate was <1/100,000 in seven small states and stool specimens were inadequate in 11 states covering one-third of India's population. Investigation showed that during 2002, the proportion of infants aged <1 year who received three or more routine doses of oral poliovirus vaccine had fallen to only 21% in some states. Vaccination rates increased again in 2003 and only 225 wild poliovirus cases were reported that year (Anonymous, 2004). In February 2012, India was finally removed from the list of polio-endemic countries. This list now includes only six countries in the Eastern Mediterranean Region including Afghanistan and Iraq, and 23 African countries. Of these, all six Eastern Mediterranean countries but only 15 of the African countries (down from 20 in 2013) met both surveillance quality indicators in 2014 (Porter *et al.*, 2015).

health action. Syndromic surveillance is very useful for diseases where there is a need for a sensitive indicator of disease activity. Box 12.3 shows an example of this with surveillance for acute flaccid paralysis (AFP) – the syndrome potentially signalling the presence of cases of poliovirus in a community (Porter *et al.*, 2015).

Collection of surveillance data

Data collection for surveillance relies on a combination of reports on paper or electronically from recorders and supplementary information obtained from

Box 12.4 Using mobile phones for surveillance

In Papua New Guinea, mobile phones were trialled for surveillance of syndromes such as haemorrhagic fever, bloody diarrhoea, AFP and acute watery diarrhoea, which may indicate the occurrence of important illnesses of national and international significance. The objectives of the system were to rapidly identify outbreaks of illness and provide confirmation of events to complement other surveillance. The system was piloted in several sites where health workers in provinces sent weekly text messages to the central coordinating unit in the national Department of Health. The text messages reported the numbers of cases of different syndromes. For urgent conditions reports were sent immediately, and this proved very effective at identifying cases of AFP and dengue haemorrhagic fever. The pilot system was more timely, complete and sensitive than reporting through existing systems although it required development of software and a secure online database, along with the costs associated with preparation of investigational materials, mobile phones and field missions (Rosewell *et al.*, 2013).

interviews of case patients or next of kin. In low-resource settings, novel data collection strategies can be useful, such as short-messaging system (SMS) reporting of syndromic surveillance data via mobile phone to a central system (Box 12.4).

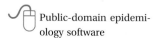 Public-domain epidemiology software

Surveillance data are entered or captured into computer-based databases which are usually built for this purpose. Simple databases for surveillance can be developed quickly and cheaply using free public-domain software and agencies have developed specific systems for certain diseases, such as those caused by organisms resistant to antibiotics. However, these databases may not be sufficient for sophisticated systems housing millions of records of data, and health agencies often commission the development of expensive systems for collecting and managing data.

Surveillance is commonly described in terms of whether managers of surveillance actively seek reports from recorders ('active surveillance') or wait for them to be sent in ('passive surveillance'). Many traditional notifiable disease systems are passive in that health departments do not actively seek reports from doctors or laboratories. This is in contrast to what may occur in an outbreak of a new infection. Active surveillance, such as that used for Ebola in Box 12.1, is based on specific collection of data from health care providers or institutions, both as a need arises and in the longer term. Active surveillance can produce more complete data of better quality than that provided by other systems. However, it is resource-intensive to maintain, especially to produce timely output of information. It is used, for example, during outbreaks of foodborne illness or measles when health care providers may be contacted and asked to provide details of any possible cases they have seen.

Analysis of surveillance data

Surveillance data are usually presented as numbers and rates per population at risk (see Chapter 2). It is vital that the analyses support the aims and objectives of the system, and that they are conducted in a timely fashion to identify changes. Data are often analysed to examine disease occurrence in high-risk groups, such as certain age groups, geographic regions and time periods. For comparison of different areas and populations, it may be necessary to standardise the resulting rates to remove the confounding effects of age and other factors. For routine notifiable disease systems, it is important that there is regular analysis of data to detect potential outbreaks, which can then be discussed at routine surveillance team meetings to identify whether case numbers represent more than would be expected historically and so require investigation.

Analysis of surveillance data to identify disease 'clusters', both temporal and geographical, is an important and specialised area of public health (we will discuss clusters further in Chapter 13). Analysis of clustering is aided by specific case definitions for a disease or characterisation of infectious agents into epidemiologically meaningful categories. A good example of this is the classical serotyping of *Salmonella enterica* – a bacterium causing gastroenteritis that often results in outbreaks from contaminated food. There are over 2000 different serotypes and an increase in the number of cases of a specific serotype in a defined geographic area above what is expected may indicate a cluster requiring investigation. Typing of many infectious agents is undergoing significant change with the ability to sequence whole genomes of organisms and this will dramatically improve surveillance and identification of clusters.

> Strains or **serotypes** of bacteria like *Salmonella* can be identified based on proteins measured in serum. Common serotypes can be further characterised by considering the appearance (*phenotype*) and/or genetic make-up (*genotype*) of the organism.

Evaluation of surveillance systems

It is important to regularly evaluate surveillance systems to ensure that they meet their objectives. It is unfortunately common for health agencies to establish surveillance for diseases and for the system to continue for many years without any changes, despite it being inefficient. There are several frameworks for evaluating surveillance, including those prepared by the

> It is almost as easy to be drowned in useless information as to be starved of essential elements.
> Sir Richard Doll
> (Doll, 1974, p 309).

Centers for Disease Control and Prevention (CDC) (see: www.cdc.gov/surveil lancepractice/). These frameworks direct evaluators to focus the nature of the evaluation, consult stakeholders about system performance, and evaluate system data against various criteria, including timeliness, sensitivity, representativeness and cost (McKerr *et al.*, 2015).

Sometimes surveillance information will indicate a public health problem but there is slow or no response or communication of results is suppressed. A combination of system failure and/or misguided political judgement can compromise the best surveillance systems. Response failures have been shown to lead to much avoidable morbidity and mortality for infections such as plague, cholera, Ebola haemorrhagic fever, West Nile virus and SARS (severe acute respiratory syndrome). It is even worse when the infection spreads to multiple countries, or around the world. Early responses to outbreaks of serious transmissible infections, or to diseases caused by new exposures to environmental toxins, may save many lives. However, it is challenging for public health officials to exercise good judgement to balance the scale of the response against the risk. Once an emergency is declared, trade, travel, schools and many facets of normal life and the economy may be disrupted.

Types of surveillance

There are several different types of surveillance that can be divided into two main categories: **indicator-based surveillance** where selected 'indicator' conditions are under surveillance for specific purposes, such as evaluating an intervention or detecting outbreaks, and **event-based surveillance** where the main focus is to identify events of public health significance.[1]

Indicator-based surveillance

Examples of indicator-based surveillance include traditional reporting of cancer diagnoses to a cancer registry, or pathology laboratories reporting cases of notifiable diseases such as tuberculosis to a health department. It relies on recorders, such as a doctor or laboratory, reporting details about each case. The level of relevant detail about cases can be extensive and sophisticated systems may incorporate molecular information as well as, for example, more traditional pathology data. Many systems for infectious diseases and cancer now rely on automated reporting from pathology systems and this has

---

[1] Active and passive surveillance are often described as types of surveillance but, as discussed above, these are really characteristics of the data collection which is just one component of a surveillance programme.

greatly improved the timeliness and completeness of the data collected, although the amount of information available may be more limited.

Notifiable disease reporting refers to the process, usually enabled by public health legislation, whereby physicians, laboratories and other responsible bodies report diagnoses of specific types of diseases to a health department. The legislation allows reporting of confidential and private data about patients for the purposes of surveillance, and the interrelated activities of follow-up and investigation. For many years, notifiable disease surveillance has been a key focus of health departments in preventing and controlling many diseases, particularly those of an infectious nature. In high-income countries, there may be between 50 and 100 different infectious conditions that it is mandatory for physicians or laboratories to report. These conditions range from those that are very rare, such as botulism, through to those that are very common, such as salmonellosis and pertussis.

Similarly, reporting is mandatory for a number of non-communicable diseases (NCDs) such as different forms of cancer. For mesotheliomas, which are cancers caused almost exclusively by exposure to asbestos, there is a need to conduct surveillance to identify if there are changes in the epidemiology of disease that might result from novel exposures in a community, and to monitor the incidence over time. While cases of mesothelioma are reported to cancer registries, extra information is usually sought from the treating doctor, patients and the next of kin about likely exposure to asbestos for public health surveillance purposes. The resulting actions for chronic diseases such as this differ from the response to an infectious disease as there is no obvious requirement to search for a source of disease in a rapid fashion and the focus may be more on development of public health policies to prevent further cases of disease.

Health departments consider the overall public health importance of a disease when deciding to make it notifiable under public health law. Public health importance is determined by several factors, including:

- the incidence or prevalence of the condition in the community;
- the severity of the illness in terms of hospitalisations, deaths and sequelae;
- whether the disease manifests in clusters or outbreaks;
- the societal costs and disease burden using metrics such as DALYs;
- the presence of an intervention, such as a publicly funded vaccine; and
- if there are specific vulnerable subpopulations that are affected.

In addition, there can be substantial pressure from the public, the media and politicians to make diseases notifiable, although this may not represent a good use of public health resources. Most importantly, health departments must be able to do something about reported cases.

Some diseases may not initially be considered of sufficient public health importance to be made notifiable, but it may become important for health departments to institute surveillance at a later stage. A good example of this is the case of chicken pox and herpes zoster infections. Chicken pox due to the varicella-zoster virus is a highly infectious illness common in childhood. The infection used to be so common that it was not considered necessary to have it under surveillance. In recent decades, many countries have introduced vaccines for varicella-zoster viruses into childhood immunisation programmes, and this led to a need for data on pre-vaccine levels of disease, both for chicken pox and zoster infections. In this case, surveillance has become more manageable with the reduced levels of disease, and is more important for identifying the age of infection and evaluating the impact that the vaccine programmes have had on reports of zoster infections. It can, however, be difficult to conduct surveillance for diseases such as measles when a country is close to eliminating indigenous transmission, as the system must be extremely sensitive or many false positive cases may be reported.

Event-based surveillance

In event-based surveillance the specific aim is to detect events of public health concern such as potential outbreaks of disease (WHO, 2008a). It is a distinct form of surveillance in that it usually relies on reports of groups of cases, i.e. one report for multiple patients, such that individual patient details are not transmitted to the system. It often has loose or non-existent case definitions to ensure the system is highly sensitive and all possible outbreaks are reported. It is not concerned about who reports an event, it may rely on reports from health clinics or regional public health units about disease clusters that require verification and investigation, or if there are multiple reports regarding the same event. The emphasis is on detecting events that affect many people rather than all individual cases; it is therefore important that there is a system to verify reports of cases or outbreaks to confirm or deny common sources. Once a report of an outbreak or event is received, surveillance system managers must try to gather other information to confirm that the event is occurring and make a decision about whether to investigate further.

The importance of event-based surveillance was dramatically highlighted during the outbreak of SARS in 2003 where the disease had a high case–fatality ratio (10% overall), mysterious origins and cause, apparent rapidity of long-distance spread and the consequences for the travel industry were severe. Although there were only 8096 cases worldwide, 1706 (21%) of those affected were health care workers and in some areas (like Hong Kong and Canada) the case–fatality ratio was as high as 17%. Initially, reports about the outbreak were patchy or non-existent from some countries. To capture information about disease occurrence, WHO established 'rumour surveillance' by technical officers monitoring media reports and email list server sources, such as Promed – an electronic mailing list of disease outbreaks run by the International Society for Infectious Diseases. The SARS outbreak led many countries to make SARS a notifiable disease, but event-based surveillance was very important for obtaining information from countries with weak or non-existent surveillance systems. The rumour surveillance was further developed for surveillance of H5N1 avian influenza in Asia in 2005 (Samaan *et al.*, 2005).

The experience with SARS and H5N1 influenza helped strengthen the global surveillance and notification system. In 2007, WHO member states adopted new International Health Regulations (WHO, 2008b). The regulations include a decision-making algorithm (Figure 12.2) to identify events that might indicate a 'Public Health Emergency of International Concern' (PHEIC) and countries are required to report these to WHO. Under the regulations, countries are required to nominate a focal point – a national centre that is accessible 24 hours a day and 365 days per year – for reporting PHEIC, including events that are not infectious in nature. The revised regulations include a smaller number of diseases where every case is reportable to WHO and the focus has shifted to event-based surveillance based on guidance to member states. The appearance of a new low-virulence variant of pandemic influenza (H1N1) in 2009 tested the new regulations in ways that had not been anticipated as WHO had to balance well-prepared responses against a public heath impact that was less severe than expected. One impact of the International Health Regulations is that there is now a well-developed surveillance system for countries reporting outbreaks to WHO (Heymann *et al.*, 2013).

Digital surveillance – a new era for event-based surveillance

Digital surveillance refers to the use of the Internet to detect events or outbreaks. The email list server Promed – an initiative of the International Society for Infectious Diseases – started in the 1990s and was one of the earliest digital forms of surveillance (Brownstein *et al.*, 2009). Promed relies on web-based trawling and information submitted by subscribers to identify reports about emerging infectious disease threats from public domain reports and technical specialists in the field. This information is then circulated to Promed subscribers. Reports to Promed are moderated by infectious disease specialists who oversee what is posted and provide commentary about the agent or event.

An explosion of the use of the Internet in the early 2000s made it possible for health investigators to use it identify events, such as outbreaks of respiratory illness, gastroenteritis or other possible emerging events. Investigators have

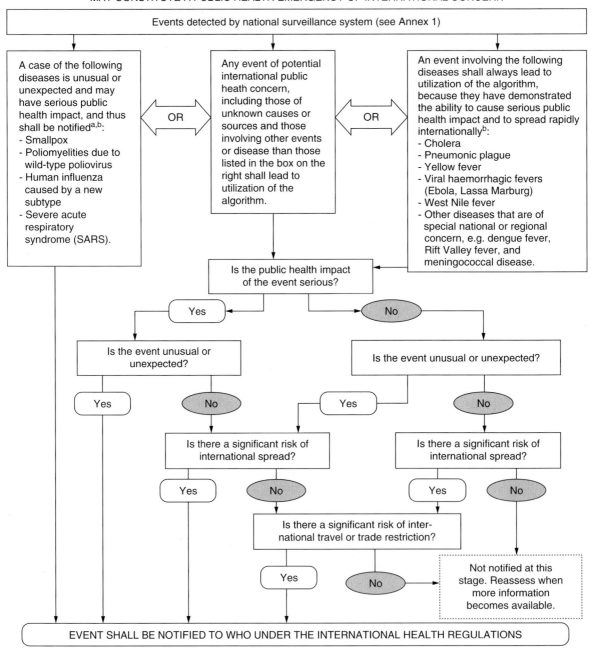

ANNEX 2
DECISION INSTRUMENT FOR THE ASSESSMENT AND NOTIFICATION OF EVENTS THAT
MAY CONSTITUTE A PUBLIC HEALTH EMERGENCY OF INTERNATIONAL CONCERN

Events detected by national surveillance system (see Annex 1)

A case of the following diseases is unusual or unexpected and may have serious public health impact, and thus shall be notified[a,b]:
- Smallpox
- Poliomyelities due to wild-type poliovirus
- Human influenza caused by a new subtype
- Severe acute respiratory syndrome (SARS).

OR

Any event of potential international public heath concern, including those of unknown causes or sources and those involving other events or disease than those listed in the box on the right shall lead to utilization of the algorithm.

OR

An event involving the following diseases shall always lead to utilization of the algorithm, because they have demonstrated the ability to cause serious public health impact and to spread rapidly internationally[b]:
- Cholera
- Pneumonic plague
- Yellow fever
- Viral haemorrhagic fevers (Ebola, Lassa Marburg)
- West Nile fever
- Other diseases that are of special national or regional concern, e.g. dengue fever, Rift Valley fever, and meningococcal disease.

Is the public health impact of the event serious?

Yes   No

Is the event unusual or unexpected?

Yes   No

Is the event unusual or unexpected?

Yes   No

Is there a significant risk of international spread?

Yes   No

Is there a significant risk of international spread?

Yes   No

Is there a significant risk of international travel or trade restriction?

Yes   No

Not notified at this stage. Reassess when more information becomes available.

EVENT SHALL BE NOTIFIED TO WHO UNDER THE INTERNATIONAL HEALTH REGULATIONS

[a] As per WHO case definitions.
[b] The disease list shall be used only for the purposes of these Regulations.

Figure 12.2 WHO decision-making algorithm to identify events that might indicate a 'Public Health Emergency of International Concern' (*from*: WHO, 2008b reproduced with permission).

used public domain social networks, such as Twitter, to trawl for key words about illness, or restaurant rating sites to look for multiple reports about gastroenteritis (Aslam *et al.*, 2014). Currently, health departments use this form of surveillance as an adjunct to traditional methods, and it has gained a lot of attention from researchers, defence and security agencies, and the non-government sector.

Digital surveillance can be very effective at detecting events, particularly in low-resource settings. For example, the surveillance network HealthMap (www.healthmap.org) detected the first cases of an unexplained illness in Guinea in 2013 that was later confirmed to be Ebola virus disease that affected several West African countries (Stevens and Pfeiffer, 2015). There is no doubt that there will be more use of digital disease detection in the future and it will become integrated into routine public health practice.

Mass gathering surveillance

Surveillance has a special use in settings such as major religious, musical and sporting events (e.g. the Olympics) where large numbers of people gather together and this is sometimes called 'mass gathering surveillance'. Surveillance at these events requires substantial additional resources and relies on multiple sources of data (McCloskey *et al.*, 2014). Although in practice the risk of major outbreaks of disease is likely to be low at mass gatherings, it is vitally important that the public are reassured about the absence of problems.

Sentinel surveillance – the health status of sentinels

Sentinel surveillance refers to the concept of monitoring the health of specific regional sites in a population as 'sentinels' for the health of the larger or target population. Sentinel surveillance often relies on sentinel clinics within a population that report the number of diagnoses of specific conditions, often with simple case definitions. Health departments in many countries have used physician clinics for sentinel surveillance for influenza to determine when the flu season has begun and to collect specimens for confirmation of circulating strains. Sentinel surveillance may also be used in resource-poor settings where it is desirable to know about various conditions, but it is impractical to have every clinic in the country report cases.

Typically, these sentinel surveillance programmes collect quite limited information, but there are also much more sophisticated systems that have enhanced surveillance in sentinel sites to provide information about potential disease incidence and changes in the whole population. A good example is the FoodNet system of active surveillance for various foodborne diseases that occurs in 10 geographically distinct sites across the USA as sentinels for the rest of the country (http://www.cdc.gov/foodnet/). FoodNet sentinel sites contact all pathology laboratories within their region each week to gather information about specific infections that may be foodborne (Henao *et al.*, 2010). The data are used for detecting events, describing the epidemiology of foodborne infections, applied research and planning for public health response. The high-quality FoodNet system has provided rich insights into the epidemiology of foodborne diseases that are relevant both in the USA and globally.

Other forms of surveillance

There are several other types of surveillance that are important, including that for risk factors; post-marketing for adverse events from medical devices, medications and vaccines (see Box 12.5); and hazards, such as poor water quality. Many health agencies now conduct surveillance for risk factors using repeat cross-sectional surveys. The most well-known of these systems is the Behavioural Risk Factor Surveillance System (BRFSS) in the USA (http://www.cdc.gov/brfss/). The BRFSS is a national computer-assisted telephone interview survey of over 400,000 people each year that captures vital information about health-related risk behaviours, chronic health conditions and preventive health measures, such as intake of fruit and vegetables (Moore *et al.*, 2015).

In practice, many diseases such as influenza require information from multiple surveillance data streams. For example, in high-income countries, influenza surveillance may rely on a combination of surveillance of absenteeism in workplaces, surveillance of patients hospitalised with influenza-like illness, and phone calls to health advice centres, in addition to information obtained from notifiable disease systems and sentinel surveillance (Budgell *et al.*, 2015; Dawood, *et al.*, 2010). This allows health agencies to develop a more complete picture of incidence, health impact and strains that are circulating in the community in a given influenza season.

Summary

Information and data arising from surveillance systems represent a cornerstone for public health action. There are two main types of surveillance: indicator-based surveillance and event-based surveillance. Surveillance systems are changing to make greater use of electronic data streams, such as electronic reporting from laboratories and searching information posted on social media. Many health agencies around the world conduct routine surveillance of notifiable diseases and regularly report results. The objectives of surveillance for a specific disease or risk factor should dictate the system attributes, such as timeliness, sensitivity and representativeness, and surveillance managers should regularly evaluate systems to ensure that they are efficient and continue to fulfil important public health functions. Then, once a potential problem has been identified, the next challenge is to identify the likely causes and to implement control measures and we will go on to discuss these issues in the next chapter.

Questions

1. An increasing trend in surveillance data for a given disease can be accounted for by:
   (a) An increase in the incidence of a disease
   (b) Less testing of true cases
   (c) Use of a new database system
   (d) Use of statistical analysis tools for trend analysis
   (e) All of the above

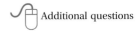 Additional questions

2. For surveillance data, undercount is best defined as:
   (a) Cases recorded by local health department, but not referred onto the national surveillance system
   (b) Cases not reported by a laboratory
   (c) The ratio of cases occurring in the community to cases reported to surveillance system
   (d) People who are infected but asymptomatic
   (e) All of the above
3. Briefly define event-based surveillance and describe some of the potential advantages and disadvantages of such systems.
4. Name two purposes of indicator-based surveillance.

REFERENCES

 References

Anonymous. (2004). Progress toward poliomyelitis eradication – India, 2003. *Morbidity and Mortality Weekly Report*, 53: 238–241.

Aslam, A. A., Tsou, M. H., Spitzberg, B. H., *et al.* (2014). The reliability of tweets as a supplementary method of seasonal influenza surveillance. *Journal of Medical Internet Research*, 14: e250.

Baize, S., Pannetier, D., Oestereich, L., *et al.* (2014). Emergence of Zaire Ebola virus disease in Guinea. *New England Journal of Medicine*, 371: 1418–1425.

Brownstein, J. S., Freifeld, C. C. and Madoff, L. C. (2009). Digital Disease Detection – harnessing the web for public health surveillance. *New England Journal of Medicine*, 360: 2153–2157.

Budgell, E., Cohen, A. L., McAnerney, J., *et al.* (2015). Evaluation of two influenza surveillance systems in South Africa. *PLoS ONE*, 10: e0120226.

Dawood, F. S., Hope, K. G., Durrheim, D. N., *et al.* (2010). Estimating the disease burden of pandemic (H1N1) 2009 virus infection in Hunter New England, Northern New South Wales, Australia, 2009. *PLoS ONE*, 5: e9880.

Doll, R. (1974). Surveillance and monitoring. *International Journal of Epidemiology*, 3: 305–313.

ECDC (European Centre for Disease Prevention and Control). (2012). *Narcolepsy in Association with Pandemic Influenza Vaccination (A Multi-country European Epidemiological Investigation)*. Stockholm: ECDC. ecdc.europa.eu/en/publications/Publications/Vaesco%20in%20brief%20final.pdf, accessed 31 May 2015.

Franco, E., Meleleo, C., Serino, L., Sorbara, D. and Zaratti, L. (2012). Hepatitis A: epidemiology and prevention in developing countries. *World Journal of Hepatology*, 4: 68–73.

Henao, O. L., Scallan, E., Mahon, B. and Hoekstra, R. M. (2010). Methods for monitoring trends in the incidence of foodborne diseases: Foodborne Diseases Active Surveillance Network 1996–2008. *Foodborne Pathogens and Disease*, 7: 1421–1426.

Heymann, D. L., Mackenzie, J. S. and Peiris, M. (2013). SARS legacy: outbreak reporting is expected and respected. *Lancet*, 381: 779–781.

McCloskey, B., Endericks, T., Catchpole, M. A., *et al.* (2014). London 2012 Olympic and Paralympic Games: public health surveillance and epidemiology. *Lancet*, 383: 2083–2089.

McKerr, C., Lo, Y. C., Edeghere, O. and Bracebridge, S. (2015). Evaluation of the national notifiable diseases surveillance system for dengue fever in Taiwan, 2010–2012. *PLoS Neglected Tropical Diseases*, 9: e0003639.

Moore, L. V., Dodd, K. W., Thompson, F. E., *et al.* (2015). Using behavioral risk factor surveillance system data to estimate the percentage of the population meeting US Department of Agriculture food patterns fruit and vegetable intake recommendations. *American Journal of Epidemiology*, 181: 979–988.

Nohynek, H., Jokinen, J., Partinen, M., *et al.* (2012). AS03 adjuvanted AH1N1 vaccine associated with an abrupt increase in the incidence of childhood narcolepsy in Finland. *PLoS ONE*, 7(3): e33536.

Porta, M. (ed.) (2014). *A Dictionary of Epidemiology*, 6th edn. New York, NY: Oxford University Press.

Porter, K. A., Diop, O. M., Burns, C. C., Tangermann, R. H. and Wassilak, S. G. (2015). Tracking progress toward polio eradication – worldwide, 2013–2014. *Morbidity and Mortality Weekly Report*, 64: 415–420. http://www.cdc.gov/mmwr/preview/mmwrhtml/mm6415a4.htm

Rosewell, A., Ropa, B., Randall, H., *et al.* (2013). Mobile phone-based syndromic surveillance system, Papua New Guinea. *Emerging Infectious Diseases*, 19: 1811–1818.

Samaan, G., Patel, M., Olowokure, B., Roces, M. C. and Oshitani, H. (2005). World Health Organization Outbreak Response Team. Rumor surveillance and avian influenza H5N1. *Emerging Infectious Diseases*, 11: 463–466.

Scallan, E., Hoekstra, R. M., Angulo, F. J., *et al.* (2011). Foodborne illness acquired in the United States – major pathogens. *Emerging Infectious Diseases*, 17: 7–15.

Scallan, E., Kirk, M. and Griffin, P. (2013). Estimates of disease burden associated with contaminated food in the United States and globally. In Morris, J. G. and Potter, M. E. (eds), *Foodborne Infections and Intoxications*. New York, NY: Elsevier Inc., pp. 3–18.

Stevens, K. B. and Pfeiffer, D. U. (2015). Sources of spatial animal and human health data: casting the net wide to deal more effectively with increasingly complex disease problems. *Spatial and Spatio-temporal Epidemiology*, 13: 15–29.

WHO (World Health Organization) Western Pacific Region. (2008a). *A Guide to Establishing Event-based Surveillance*. Geneva: World Health Organization. www.wpro.who.int/emerging_diseases/documents/docs/eventbasedsurv.pdf, accessed 19 May 2015.

WHO (World Health Organization). (2008b). *International Health Regulations (2005) Second Edition.* Geneva: World Health Organization.

WHO (World Health Organization). (2014). *Ebola Response Roadmap.* WHO. http://www.who.int/csr/resources/publications/ebola/response-roadmap/en/, accessed 31 May 2015.

WHO Ebola Response Team. (2014). Ebola virus disease in West Africa – the first 9 months of the epidemic and forward projections. *New England Journal of Medicine,* 371: 1481–1495.

RECOMMENDED FOR FURTHER READING

• A special case of surveillance that is of interest:

McCloskey, B., Endericks, T., Catchpole, M. A., *et al.* (2014). London 2012 Olympic and Paralympic Games: public health surveillance and epidemiology. *Lancet,* 383: 2083–2089.

Outbreaks, epidemics and clusters

Martyn Kirk and Adrian Sleigh

Description Chapters 2–3	Association Chapters 4–5	Alternative explanations Chapters 6–8	Integration & interpretation Chapters 9–11	Practical applications Chapter 13: Outbreaks

Box 13.1 A massive outbreak of haemolytic uraemic syndrome

Detection of event: A local health department requested assistance from the German federal government with investigation of 3 cases of haemolytic uraemic syndrome (HUS, a rare condition that affects the kidneys) in northern Germany on 19 May 2011. On investigation, it became obvious that the outbreak had started weeks earlier and the number of cases of gastroenteritis and HUS peaked on 22 May 2011.

Descriptive epidemiology: In total, 3816 cases were reported in Germany. The majority of patients had bloody diarrhoea with 22% progressing to

(continued)

Box 13.1 *(continued)*

develop HUS and 36 (4.2%) died. The rates of infection were highest in northern Germany and most of those affected were adults (median age 42 years) and women (68%). The estimated incubation period was 8 days from exposure to illness. Cases also occurred in several other countries in Europe and North America, but the majority of these had acquired their infection while visiting Germany.

Investigation: The investigating teams conducted multiple studies to understand the source of infection, including: explorative hypothesis-generating interviews, 30 cohort studies, several case–control studies, testing of potentially contaminated foods and microbiological studies. Initial interviews of patients did not reveal the food causing the outbreak – contaminated fenugreek seed sprouts – as they were difficult to remember. The particular strain of *Escherichia coli* responsible – serotype O104:H4 – had not been seen in animals previously and was rare in humans; importantly, it showed characteristics of multiple pathogenic types of *E. coli* and resulted in an unusually high proportion of people developing HUS.

Containment: The outbreak was rapidly brought under control once sprouts were identified as the food vehicle. The fenugreek seeds originated from Egypt and were sprouted at a small farm in northern Germany. Once the vehicle was identified and removed from the food supply the only new cases were due to secondary transmission within households.

Implications: The outbreak resulted in significant societal concern and had major implications for trade of food and agricultural produce. Early reports suggested the outbreak was linked to Spanish cucumbers. These were later shown to be false, but costs to agriculture were estimated to be hundreds of millions of Euro.

(Frank *et al.*, 2011)

The distribution of infectious diseases often occurs in a non-random fashion leading to what may be referred to as *clusters*, *outbreaks* or *epidemics*. Investigation of outbreaks like that described in Box 13.1 is part of the core business of field epidemiology and it relies on multidisciplinary approaches to identifying and controlling disease. The outbreak of toxigenic *E. coli* O104:H4 is a dramatic example of the seriousness of contamination in the food supply, and

Box 13.2 The role of epidemiology in outbreak investigation

Epidemiology is central to investigating and correctly managing outbreaks of disease. In particular, epidemiology is used to:

- detect clustering in surveillance data that may represent an increase in cases of disease warranting investigation
- identify and count cases that may be related to an outbreak or cluster
- develop and conduct cohort or case–control studies to identify sources of illness during or after an outbreak has occurred
- characterise the risks to populations potentially exposed to a source of illness
- monitor the effectiveness of risk communication in outbreak settings

how spread of infectious diseases can be controlled through rapid investigation and intervention.

Historically, the study of epidemic infections helped develop methods for epidemiology, especially retrospective cohort and case–control studies, and, as shown in Box 13.2, epidemiology still plays a central role in outbreak investigation. Investigations of outbreaks still have a high public profile today, particularly because of the globalisation of trade and increasing ease of international travel. Emerging and re-emerging infections have become prominent over the last two to three decades and the threat of global epidemics, or pandemics, has mobilised resources to plan for, detect and combat such catastrophes. Many examples earlier in this book focussed on 'chronic' or 'non-communicable' diseases. Now we will discuss infectious diseases, although not exclusively, because other agents such as toxins and chemicals can also result in 'outbreaks' of non-communicable intoxications, injuries and cancer.

Outbreaks, epidemics and clusters

What do we mean by an epidemic or an outbreak? The two terms are often used interchangeably, although they are perceived differently in the media and by the public. **Epidemic** comes from the Greek words *epi* (upon) and *dēmos* (the people) and means an increase in disease in a region or time period that is clearly above what would normally be expected. Most diseases are **endemic**, in that they are commonly present at a baseline level in a given geographic area or population group. Increases above the endemic baseline or incursions of diseases into new areas may signal the occurrence of an epidemic.

An **outbreak** is defined as 'an epidemic limited to a localised increase in the incidence of a disease, e.g. in a village, town or closed institution' (Porta, 2014, p. 206). Outbreak may also be used to refer to a small epidemic arising in an area that has had no cases for a long time. In general, outbreaks include two or more cases, but a single case of a rare disease, such as botulism, could represent an outbreak.

When a disease affects a large number of people and crosses international boundaries it is called a **pandemic**. Historically, pandemics have caused great loss of human populations, notably plague in the late middle ages and 'Spanish' influenza at the end of World War I. The organism causing the most recent pandemic as declared by the World Health Organization (WHO) under the International Health Regulations – H1N1 influenza virus – first appeared in Mexico in April 2009 and quickly spread to over 200 countries by the end of the year. H1N1 infections resulted in less-severe disease than health departments had planned for, but did result in more serious outcomes in young adults and pregnant women.

Finally, it is important to understand the use of the word **cluster**, which is an aggregation 'of relatively uncommon events or diseases in space and/or time in amounts that are believed or perceived to be greater than could be expected by chance' (Porta, 2014, p. 47). Health agencies often use this term where there is no obvious source of disease identified, and it may be used for both infectious and non-communicable diseases, such as cancer.

Epidemiology of infectious diseases

Infectious disease epidemiology is often presented as a different discipline from the epidemiology we have been describing, but the fundamental principles are similar and causal reasoning is conceptually simpler for infectious diseases where the agent or 'pathogen' is a necessary cause of the disease. The major difference for most infectious conditions, and other outbreaks we discuss here, is the urgency with which investigations take place and the direct link to management activities. This is often extreme and demands robust, practical methods for identifying people who are exposed and infected, along with a constant focus on controlling the outbreak before all information has been gathered.

Infectious or communicable diseases are defined as 'An illness due to a specific infectious agent or its toxic products that arises through transmission of that agent or its products from an infected person, animal or reservoir to a susceptible host, either directly or indirectly through an intermediate plant or animal host, vector, or the inanimate environment' (Porta, 2014, p. 51). The burden of infectious diseases in terms of incidence and mortality in industrialised countries has declined dramatically since the

1950s when the use of powerful antibiotics, vaccines and other interventions became routine (van Panhuis *et al.*, 2013). In low-income countries, there is still an ongoing epidemiological transition from a pattern of high mortality rates due to infectious diseases of childhood to one of non-communicable diseases later in life (Dye, 2014; GBD 2013 Mortality and Causes of Death Collaborators, 2015). Despite these major changes in burden of disease, infectious diseases remain highly prevalent and important in all countries of the world. Some of the major concerns with infectious diseases globally include:

- the threat of antimicrobial resistance leading to untreatable infections;
- the emergence of new highly pathogenic and virulent strains;
- the resurgence of diseases once thought controlled because of lowered vaccination rates;
- the opportunity to eliminate, and potentially eradicate diseases such as smallpox, Guinea worm, polio and measles;
- the regular occurrence of high-profile outbreaks of infectious diseases that threaten community health, trade and security; and
- the synergistic effects of infectious diseases on the burden of non-communicable diseases.

Acute infections affect all sectors of society and the public health impacts are substantial. Even common infections, such as gastroenteritis and respiratory infections, result in considerable lost productivity. Periodically, epidemics of vaccine-preventable diseases recur, even in countries with very high vaccine coverage; for example, pertussis (whooping cough), rubella and measles. There are also many infections that have recently emerged or re-emerged and for some we have made little headway with prevention or treatment, for example Hendra virus transmitted from horses and bats in Australia, novel coronaviruses in the Middle East, and varicella-zoster infection, which causes shingles and is common among the elderly.

Many of these emerging infections are zoonotic in origin, in that they have reservoirs in animal populations (Jones *et al.*, 2008), and a high proportion are due to pathogenic viruses, such as rapidly evolving RNA viruses including those that cause AIDS, SARS and influenza. Emergence is based on many factors including population growth, expanding trade and travel, mass-produced food, intensive livestock production, environmental change, resistance to antimicrobial drugs, human encroachment on wilderness and forest, and global warming (Sleigh *et al.*, 2006). The SARS multicountry epidemic of 2003 was an example of a global threat due to emergence of a new infectious disease that had origins in live animal markets in Asia, which were also subsequently identified as a potential risk for transmission of highly pathogenic H5N1 influenza (Samaan *et al.*, 2011).

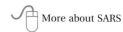 More about SARS

In addition, infectious diseases are a particular problem for vulnerable populations, such as the very young, the elderly or those who are immuno-compromised due to disease or medical treatment. In some instances, those who are vulnerable may be predisposed to infection or, when infected, they may experience worse outcomes. Many people in these categories are regular visitors to the hospital environment where they are at risk of opportunistic infections, some of which have become highly resistant to antimicrobial agents. WHO (2015) has declared the emergence of antimicrobial resistance a global health concern resulting in many countries developing plans for antibiotic stewardship, monitoring of usage and surveillance of antibiotic resistant organisms.

The public health impacts of infectious diseases are substantial: *epidemics* capture the public and media attention, but the majority of burden arises from infections that are *endemic*. Sometimes outbreak alerts trigger worldwide alarm and politically complex national and international responses, as has been noted recently with Ebola virus in West Africa and Middle East Respiratory Syndrome (MERS) caused by a novel coronavirus. Increasingly, small or large outbreaks threaten economically important industries, as seen with Hendra virus in Australia in 1994 that had impacts on the horse racing industry, Nipah virus in Malaysia in 1998–1999 affecting pig farming, SARS in Hong Kong and Canada in 2003 affecting services and tourism, and regular outbreaks of food-borne disease affecting various food businesses.

A causal model

Simple ecological models of the 'agent–host–environment' interplay have served infectious disease epidemiology well, providing a neat structure for linking the variety of factors that determine whether disease occurs. Figure 13.1 shows the interaction between an infectious agent and its potential host, the transmission process (how the disease is spread) and how all of these may be influenced by the environment. The relationship between the agent, host and environment are largely understood by laboratory testing, epidemiology and environmental surveys, respectively.

The infectious agent

There are many different types of infectious agent: bacteria, viruses, fungi, protozoa, helminths (parasitic worms), etc. In almost every natural habitat there will be agents potentially infectious to humans. Animal contact is particularly important in the genesis of human infections and many (perhaps most) infections afflicting us have been traced back to the beginnings of agriculture and animal farming.

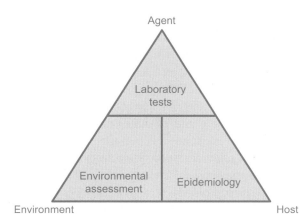

Figure 13.1 The relationships among agent, host and environment and the methods used to evaluate these.

Infection is the entry of a microbial agent into a higher-order host and its multiplication within the host. When a lower organism lives on an external surface of another organism it is called an **infestation** rather than an infection; for example, lice and scabies. Infections do not necessarily lead to overt disease and the principal characteristics of microbial agents that influence their ability to cause disease are defined below.

Infectivity is the ability of an organism to invade and multiply in a host and is assessed by the proportion of exposures that result in infection. One measure of infectivity is the **secondary attack rate**, which measures the number of cases of infection that develop among susceptible contacts of an infected case. Polio virus is a highly infectious agent infecting most susceptible people who are exposed, but only a small proportion will develop symptoms or chronic sequelae from their infection. Its **pathogenicity**, the power of an organism to produce overt illness, measured as the proportion of those infected who develop clinical or overt illness, is therefore relatively low. Measles virus is highly infectious like polio, but is much more pathogenic in that most people infected develop symptoms. **Virulence**, the ability of an organism to produce serious disease, is measured by the proportion of those infected who develop severe disease. If death is a criterion of severity, this can be measured by the case–fatality ratio (CFR, see Chapter 2). The **intensity** of an infection, the number of organisms infecting an individual, is especially important for parasitic infections, such as hookworms or schistosomes, where the burden of parasites often predicts the severity of disease.

The natural habitat of the agent is known as its **reservoir** and this may be human, animal or in the environment. Agents with human reservoirs include the pertussis bacterium, the malarial parasite and the roundworm. For some agents such as *Vibrio cholera*, the cause of cholera, it is unclear what the reservoir is between epidemics. The source of an infectious agent is the person, animal or object from which the host acquires the infection. If human, this may be someone who is sick or convalescent, or a long-term carrier of infection who was never clinically sick themselves, as can happen with hepatitis B, typhoid and HIV.

Laboratory testing (chemical, microbiological, serological or genetic) is a critical element in understanding the agent. A detailed discussion is beyond the scope of this book, but it is important to realise that, combined with epidemiology, new genomic testing of infectious agents has revealed striking new insights into their transmission as the genetic code of the agent from the putative source can now be compared with that of the infected humans. In investigations of acute outbreaks, laboratory testing of foods and water, animals, humans and the environment is critical to identify the source of infection.

> In a study of typhoid in Nepal, the diversity of typhoid genotypes revealed that while human-to-human transmission occurred, this was overwhelmed by indirect transmission, possibly via contaminated water (Baker *et al.*, 2011).

The host

The host is a human or animal that an agent enters and in which it multiplies. A host's reaction to infection can be extremely variable, depending on the interplay between the characteristics of the agent, including the dose received, and the immune status of the host. The immune response of the very young and the old may not be as protective as that of a young healthy adult. If the host has been exposed to the agent before there may be natural immunity, or immunity may be induced artificially by vaccination. A person who is not immune to a particular agent is often referred to simply as a 'susceptible'. These factors, and others to do with the biology, maturation and replication of the agent, influence the **incubation period** which is the time between initial infection and the onset of clinical disease as shown by signs and symptoms. For control of infectious diseases it is also important to know the **latent period**, the time from entry into the host until the onset of infectiousness, which may be longer or shorter than the incubation period. If it is shorter, then infected persons may pass on the infection before they become ill, as with hepatitis A, and if it is longer they will be ill before they are very infectious, as for SARS. These features are known for the majority of infectious diseases and are an important determinant of infection dynamics. They are useful tools in the investigation and control of epidemics and are always the focus of attention for new emerging infectious diseases. Infections transmitted before someone becomes ill, or by someone who does not become ill, are the most difficult to control and the most likely to cause explosive epidemics in susceptible populations.

Transmission

Transmission of an agent is its spread from a reservoir or source to a new host by one or more of three possible routes: direct, indirect or airborne. For example, SARS is usually transmitted by (large) respiratory droplets reaching

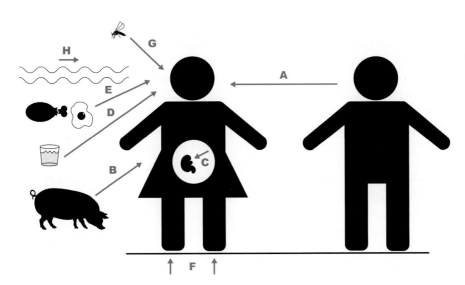

Figure 13.2 Patterns of spread for infectious agents showing (A) person-to-person, (B) zoonotic, (C) vertical, (D) waterborne, (E) food-borne, (F) soil-transmitted, (G) vectorborne and (H) airborne modes of transmission.

close contacts, but some cases have spread infection to scores of persons with whom they had little or no direct contact (Li *et al.*, 2004). The mode of transmission has a profound effect on how infectious diseases are managed, both in the clinical setting and in the community. As an example, ordinary masks and gloves are used in hospitals as precautions against heavy respiratory droplets, but are inadequate against airborne infections which require fitted masks or respirators, eye shields and negative-pressure ventilation. Some modes of transmission are shown in Figure 13.2 and discussed in more detail below.

Direct transmission arises from 'close personal contact' by touching infectious secretions or excreta from another person (A) or animal (B). This includes touching or inhaling the large (10–100 µm) respiratory droplets produced by a person suffering from a respiratory infection sneezing, coughing or talking. These heavy droplets contain mostly water and pass through the air to fall on surrounding objects within 1 metre of the source (Fernstrom and Goldblatt, 2013). Examples of direct transmission include sexual, skin, eye, congenital and most respiratory infections, including measles and influenza. Sometimes **vertical transmission** (as opposed to the usual **horizontal transmission** (A)) occurs directly from mother to unborn child (C) for diseases such as listeriosis where serious bacterial meningitis or septicaemia can result from eating contaminated foods.

Indirect transmission always involves a vehicle, which may be inanimate, such as bedding, clothes or utensils (collectively called 'fomites'), water (D) or food (E), or the soil (F). Alternatively, the infection may be transmitted via a vector (G), such as a mosquito responsible for malaria or dengue.

Airborne transmission (H) became an outmoded concept in the nineteenth century after Snow had shown that London cholera was waterborne, disproving the prevailing theory of an infectious airborne 'miasma' rising from the river. Later, Pasteur and others demonstrated the existence of germs and showed that they could be transmitted directly through the air. In the 1930s, the laboratory production of 'bioaerosols' of tiny infectious droplet nuclei that could be inhaled, as well as careful epidemiological studies on TB and Q fever in the 1940s and 1950s, eventually resurrected the concept of airborne infection as an important mode of transmission (Langmuir, 1961). Bioaerosols may also be produced in abattoirs when cutting open the body cavities of infected animals, in air-conditioning cooling towers, or by germ warfare. WHO uses a particle size of <5 μm in diameter to define particles that may be airborne and infectious over large distances. These include pathogens such as *Mycobacterium tuberculosis*, for which this mode is *obligate* (it is transmitted only in this way), and pathogens that can infect by multiple routes but are mostly transmitted by droplet nuclei (their preferential pathway), such as measles and chickenpox (Fernstrom and Goldblatt, 2013).

The environment

The environment has a critical influence on the transmission of infectious diseases as it affects the survival of pathogens, vectors and of vertebrate hosts. The physical environment or climate has obvious influences, sometimes for reasons we do not understand well. Many infectious diseases exhibit strong seasonality. For example, in temperate zones, influenza and other respiratory infections appear in the colder winter months, times of close human contact. On the other hand, Ross River fever usually occurs in hot humid months, reflecting the importance of an abundance of mosquitoes for the transmission of that disease.

Other environmental influences on infectious disease dynamics include levels of sanitation, air pollution, water quality, human and livestock population density, overcrowding, poverty, housing conditions and food availability. Human behaviour itself often creates environments suitable for infections, such as warm, well-aerated water in cooling towers that is suitable for proliferation of *Legionella pneumophila* – the bacterium responsible for the pneumonia named Legionnaires' disease. Often, infections are the result of ecological conditions directly stemming from poverty, such as the transmission of cholera in settings where sanitation and hygiene are inadequate. It can also be due to necessity, such as wet-rice farming to produce a crucial food staple that also creates breeding sites for the intermediate host snails of schistosome infections.

Figure 13.3 summarises the key aspects that influence the occurrence of an outbreak, picking up on the key attributes of the agent, host and environment that we discussed above.

Legionnaires' disease acquired its name in 1976 when an outbreak of pneumonia occurred among people attending a convention of the American Legion at a Philadelphia hotel. Of the 221 reported cases, 34 died. The causative agent was a previously unknown bacterium, subsequently named *Legionella pneumophila*.

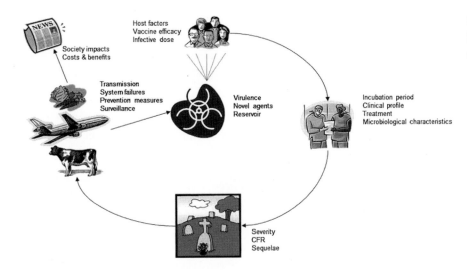

Figure 13.3 Key elements that influence the development of an outbreak.

Non-infectious clusters and outbreaks

Clusters in space and time of rare chronic diseases, injuries and birth defects, and especially cancer, are often reported by members of the community and public awareness of environmental hazards has increased demand for public health authorities to investigate them. Any apparently unusual frequency of any disease will now attract attention and this causes great difficulty for health officials who are asked to respond to the problem. Rare diseases will inevitably be distributed in small numbers and their frequency will fluctuate widely. In a country like the USA with a large population and a large area it is inevitable that numerous small-area clusters will arise for rare diseases – for example, several of the cases in a large state may just happen to occur in one corner of that state by chance. Community members are likely to note the cluster and then to look for possible causes, including any nearby environmental contamination. Investigating such clusters rarely leads to conclusive evidence as to the cause and usually reveals that the cluster is most probably a chance effect due to the variation of small expected numbers. This might not be considered a satisfactory answer, especially if people have formed their own hypotheses as to the cause.

When a decision is made to investigate a cluster formally, it needs to be recognised from the outset that it can be extremely challenging given the latency between exposure and development of disease may be several decades and the aetiology may be unclear or multifactorial. Investigation of these clusters should take an epidemiological approach potentially including:

- rapid case ascertainment, and subsequent refinements of case definition (possibly using novel molecular or other biomarkers);
- obtaining residential, occupational and other pertinent history;

One of the best-known cancer clusters, involving 33 cases of mesothelioma (a rare cancer of the lining of the chest), emerged in South Africa in the late 1950s. Researchers identified that 32 of those affected had worked with asbestos and exposure to asbestos is now known to be the major risk factor for mesothelioma (Wagner *et al.*, 1960).

The US Centers for Disease Control (CDC) have issued guidelines for investigating clusters (http://www.cdc.gov/nceh/clusters).

- analysis of case distributions by place, time and personal characteristics;
- reviewing registry and other available electronic data;
- assessing the environment for possible causes, including approaches where the totality of environmental exposures is taken into account; and
- investigating possible infectious causes.

For an example of a very thorough and expensive investigation into a cluster of cancer that yielded far more striking results than usual, see Box 13.3.

Box 13.3 Investigating a cluster of breast cancer cases at the Toowong Australian Broadcasting Commission (ABC) worksite, Queensland, Australia

Nature of event: Between January 1994 and June 2006, 13 women who had worked at an ABC site, many in the newsroom, were diagnosed with breast cancer. The staff expressed concerns that this was related to working at the ABC.

Epidemiological assessment: Investigators examined rates of cancer in the ABC workforce. Ten women were diagnosed with invasive breast cancer while working at the ABC and this was significantly higher than the expected number of 1.6 based on rates in all Queensland women (Standardised Incidence Ratio 6.25; 95% CI 3.0–11.5, $p < 0.001$), although the *p*-value increased to 0.04 after adjusting for multiple comparisons. There was a statistically significant increasing trend in breast cancer risk of 12% (95% CI 2–23%) per year of employment at the ABC. Detailed environmental assessments detected no current or historical evidence of contamination or exposure to known or suspected carcinogens on the site, nor was there any unusual pattern of personal risk factors among the affected women.

Interpretation: The investigators concluded that there was a statistically significant increase in the risk of cancer in female ABC employees in the newsroom. It was, however, considered highly unlikely that this increase was caused by exposure while working at the site, although the exact cause of the cluster of breast cancer cases could not be explained. A record linkage-based cohort study of 5969 women working at other comparable ABC sites showed no excess risk at any site other than Brisbane. Thus, despite the strong association and dose–response effect present in the Brisbane cluster, its origin is likely to be due to chance.

Bottom line: Despite the scientific reassurances, the ABC studio moved premises and sold the building in question.

(Armstrong *et al.*, 2007; Sitas *et al.*, 2010)

However, many epidemiologists remain concerned that the resources consumed by the investigation of rare disease clusters, especially if political pressure is applied, may far exceed the benefits gained. Such expenditure may deprive the community of public funds needed for other activities, including environmental clean-ups that should be done anyway. Ultimately, the final public health decisions are often based on expert opinion and prudent judgements and do not depend on *p*-values and associated mathematical models (Coory, 2008).

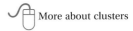 More about clusters

Chemicals and toxins can also result in clusters of disease that fit the definition of an outbreak, particularly where there is a putative common source. A classic example of a non-infectious outbreak is ciguatera, where those affected experience neurological symptoms such as blurry vision, nausea, vomiting, diarrhoea, cramps, excessive sweating, headaches and muscle aches along with unusual taste sensations after consuming tropical reef fish contaminated with algal toxins. Outbreaks and small clusters of ciguatera are common, as groups of people usually eat larger fish together and these larger fish have a higher concentration of ciguatoxin resulting in multiple cases of illness within 6–12 hours. These non-communicable disease outbreaks can be investigated using an identical framework to infectious diseases, as outlined below.

Outbreak management and investigation

As we noted above, a key feature of nearly all outbreak and epidemic investigations is that they must occur rapidly to limit spread. In addition, there is much to be learned about the nature and epidemiology of disease from outbreaks. They are 'natural experiments' and can provide new insights into the natural history, clinical features, outcomes, modes of transmission and societal impacts of disease as well as into the specific pathogen or agent itself.

Management of outbreaks

Managing outbreaks is a complex task, as it involves many different agencies and may require social mobilisation to limit spread of infection. Furthermore, there are often public and legal inquiries following outbreaks that focus on 'who knew what and when'. In large complex outbreaks, the agency responsible for managing the overarching response may not be the health department. Depending on the nature and scale of the outbreak, the development of an appropriate and measured response may require input from aid agencies, clinicians, emergency services, customs, agriculture, environment, industry and the public.

The communication of risk is a vital and specialised component of managing an outbreak or epidemic and it is important that stakeholders and those affected are aware of the need for and process of investigating and managing outbreaks. For many outbreaks, rapid communication can allay community concern and direct possible cases to seek attention to assist authorities. In the 2014 Ebola virus outbreak in West Africa, the Firestone rubber company provided a robust risk management and communication strategy to their employees and the surrounding population in response to a case within the Firestone plantation. This increased awareness about spread of the disease appeared to limit spread (Reaves *et al.*, 2014).

WHO has developed a risk assessment tool to assist countries to manage outbreaks and public health incidents, independent of the type of agent responsible (WHO, 2012). The risk assessment process encourages a systematic approach involving examining information about the hazard, the means and context of exposure, and characterisation of level of risk, which helps focus the different options available to manage an outbreak or epidemic, even in the early phases. At the end of any outbreak or epidemic there should also be an audit of activities, or a debrief to ensure that any insights for management of the outbreak are incorporated into future responses (Dalton *et al.*, 2009).

International United Nations agencies, such as WHO, the Food and Agriculture Organization and World Organization for Animal Health, also have significant roles in outbreak management where there is the potential for multicountry spread. Under the International Health Regulations (IHR) (2005) (WHO, 2008), WHO maintains a surveillance system for Public Health Events of International Concern (PHEIC), which includes significant outbreaks occurring in member states. The IHR (2005) allow countries to be alerted to outbreaks and epidemics in other countries, along with potential events that could result in serious outbreaks. In addition, many non-government organisations, such as Médecins Sans Frontières and the International Red Cross, are important players in understanding and responding to epidemic disease. In light of the Ebola virus outbreak of 2014–2015, there has been significant debate about the strength and capacity of the international health system to effectively manage large-scale epidemics (Gates, 2015).

Finally, it is important to have a well-trained workforce. The Centers for Disease Control and Prevention (CDC) established the Epidemic Intelligence Service (EIS) programme in the USA in the 1950s and this has served as a model programme for many other countries, including Australia, Canada, Europe, Thailand, Malaysia and China. The Training Programmes in Epidemiology and Public Health Interventions Network (http://www.tephinet.org/) now links over 50 Field Epidemiology Training Programmes around the world.

Investigating outbreaks

The CDC prescribe 10 recognised steps of investigation for infectious disease outbreaks (Gregg, 2008). These steps, which are accepted world best practice, are as follows.

1. Determine the existence of an outbreak.
2. Confirm the diagnosis of the disease in question.
3. Define and count cases of human infection.
4. Orient the data collected in terms of time, place, person – i.e. when, where and who have been infected.
5. Identify people who are specifically at risk of the disease.
6. Develop and test hypotheses relating to the cause of the outbreak.
7. Compare hypotheses with current facts.
8. Plan more systematic study.
9. Prepare a written a report.
10. Execute control and prevention activities.

Steps 1–5 represent the 'identification phase' of any investigation and are important to establishing that an outbreak has actually occurred and describing its key features. Steps 6 and 7 represent the 'hypothesis-generation and testing phase' of the investigation, while steps 8–10 are the 'confirmation phase' where public health action takes place. The whole framework represents the piecing together of disparate information to identify a cause for the outbreak.

More about investigating outbreaks

The identification phase

Health authorities are the main agencies responsible for detection of outbreaks which are then investigated under public health legislation. Health agencies detect outbreaks using public health surveillance (see Chapter 12), or reports from alert clinicians, the media or the public. It is vital that neighbouring agencies communicate about investigations, as it is possible that one or more agencies (nationally or internationally) may be investigating the same outbreak without realising it. It is important that investigators identify the agent responsible for an outbreak early, as this knowledge will guide control efforts. It is important that the agent is identified using standardised and reliable tests. There are many examples of misdiagnosis due to poorly performing test kits or contamination occurring during testing of clinical samples.

Investigation of an apparent increase in human samples testing positive for *Salmonella* showed this was likely due to use of contaminated media (Thiolet *et al.*, 2011).

Epidemiologists define cases using the traditional '*person, place* and *time*' to decide who is part of an outbreak for investigative purposes. This case definition may involve different levels of certainty about case status and may change during the course of an outbreak as more information comes to light.

The use of highly specific laboratory tests, such as whole genome sequencing, is starting to rapidly improve recognition of the true scale and nature of outbreaks from common sources.

Analysis of case data follows traditional descriptive epidemiology. In particular, it is important to present data with regards to spatial and temporal orientation. Traditionally, epidemiologists have put pins in maps, but with new geographical information systems, sophisticated mapping allows for excellent visualisation of the geographical distribution of cases. Free software for epidemiological investigation, such as Epi Info™ from the CDC, now incorporates simple mapping tools.

⌐ Public domain epidemiology software

During an investigation, it is normal to produce a graphical representation of the outbreak in the form of an 'epidemic curve' which identifies when cases first developed symptoms. The epidemic curve can give critical clues to the nature of the outbreak, such as whether it originated from a single source or is propagated from person to person. Figure 13.4 shows a typical epidemic curve for a **point-** or **common-source outbreak** which occurs when many people are suddenly exposed to the same source of infection, leading to a clear increase in incidence of disease. Here the average incubation period was between 12 and 13 hours, which is typical for an outbreak of food poisoning such as salmonellosis where illness usually occurs within 6–48 hours of eating contaminated food. Figure 1.3 showed an actual point-source epidemic that you met in Chapter 1.

Figure 13.5 shows the pattern typical of an epidemic which arose from the introduction of an infection into a susceptible population (sometimes called a **propagative epidemic**). On 12 May there was a single case and 8–11 days later we see another cluster of cases, sometimes referred to as secondary cases, which arose from the primary case by person-to-person transmission. A further 8–13 days later there is a third generation of cases, serially infected by the secondary cases.

Figure 13.4 The epidemic curve for a point-source epidemic.

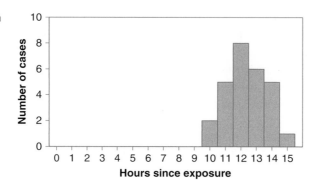

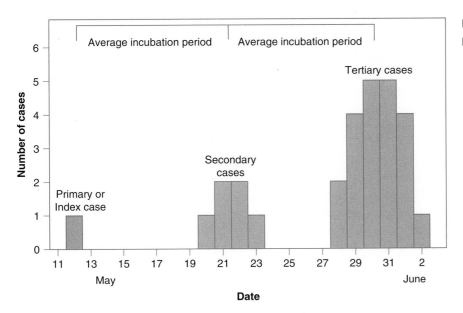

Figure 13.5 The epidemic curve for a propagative epidemic.

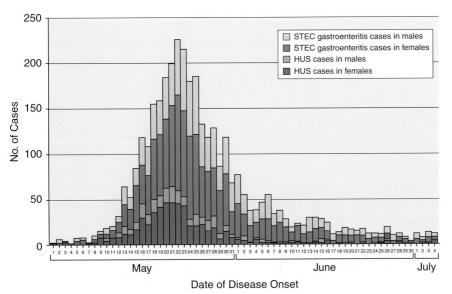

Figure 13.6 Epidemic curve of *E. coli* 01014:H4 outbreak in Germany, 2011, showing the numbers of cases of haemolytic uraemic syndrome (HUS) and Shiga-toxin–producing *E. coli* (STEC) gastroenteritis by sex (*from*: Frank *et al., New Engl J Med*, 2011; 365: 1771–1780, with permission).

It is normal for the epidemic curve to be refreshed at least daily during the outbreak. Figure 13.6 shows the epidemic curve for the outbreak of *E. coli* O104 infections and haemolytic uraemic syndrome associated with fenugreek sprouts from Box 13.1. It shows that numbers of patients in the outbreak started to grow dramatically on 8 May 2011 and peaked on 21–22 May 2011.

The hypothesis-generation and testing phase

During the outbreak, investigators develop hypotheses regarding the likely cause through interviews of cases, inspection of the environment and testing of samples of food, water and other environmental specimens. Interviewing cases with standardised questionnaires to examine clinical features of the infection or disease and potential exposures to develop ideas about a common cause is an important but difficult task, as many people find it hard to recall what they did prior to becoming ill. These interviews are often conducted over the telephone or face to face and can take some time to fully explore all important issues.

Although most outbreak investigations are carried out retrospectively after the event has occurred, in some instances investigators may prospectively recruit cases. If it is possible to identify the entire population at risk of developing the disease then it may be possible to conduct a cohort study in order to compare the risk of disease amongst those who are exposed compared to the unexposed. The advantage of this type of study is that the resulting relative risk is easy to interpret. If it is not possible to enumerate the study population, investigators will conduct a case–control study that will test hypotheses about different exposures. This allows calculation of an odds ratio to estimate the association between the source and disease in the usual way (see Chapter 5). Increasingly, investigators are using online tools to collect epidemiological data from people affected by an outbreak, thereby speeding up the data collection process.

The confirmation phase

The final phase in an investigation of an outbreak relates to documentation and control activities. In reality, taking action to control the spread of a disease occurs prior to many of the preceding steps. However, proper epidemiological investigation can provide focus for risk management and intervention activities. Outbreaks are exceedingly common and not all outbreaks are worth documenting in peer review literature. There are in excess of 1500 outbreaks of gastroenteritis reported in Australia annually (OzFoodNet Working Group, 2012); however, it is important for public accountability that brief summaries are included in reports. These summaries can then be used to quantify the burden of human food-borne illness attributable to specific sources in order to prioritise food safety interventions (Pires et al., 2010).

Evidence for causation

Identifying whether a specific exposure caused an outbreak can be complex, particularly where there are multiple potential modes of transmission. Several streams of evidence are important for developing control and interventions. Epidemiological information, in terms of persons at risk and measures of association, is a key determinant. Other forms of information include test results from foods, waters, environments and animals; tracing of movements of foods and animals; and contact tracing between infected persons and subsequent cases.

For complex outbreaks, it is necessary to specifically collect these forms of information to take action. Box 13.4 shows an example, in this case a multinational food-borne outbreak of hepatitis A. There have been situations where outbreaks that were initially thought to be due to one cause were subsequently shown to be due to another vehicle, for example an extremely large and complex outbreak of *Salmonella* Saintpaul gastroenteritis in the USA that initially implicated tomatoes, but was subsequently linked to chile peppers (Barton Behravesh *et al.*, 2008). In practice, to attribute causation in these

---

Box 13.4 A large, multistate outbreak of hepatitis a associated with semi-dried tomatoes, Australia, 2009

Detection of outbreak: An initial increase of locally acquired hepatitis A infections occurred in two Australian States in March 2009 and subsequently spread to other jurisdictions. A multijurisdictional investigation team was formed to identify the potential source of the outbreak.

Nature of investigation: The team conducted several investigations of cases, foods and supply chains to identify a source for the outbreak. A case–control study identified that cases were significantly more likely to have eaten semi-dried tomatoes during their incubation period than controls (odds ratio 3.0, 95% CI 1.4–6.7); however, the food supply chain could not identify a specific brand or ingredient. The outbreak then declined in June 2009 before resurging in October 2009, particularly in the state of Victoria. A second case–control study also showed a strong association between illness and consuming semi-dried tomatoes (OR = 10.3; 95% CI, 4.7–22.7). This time, hepatitis A virus was detected in semi-dried tomatoes and the supply chain linked the contaminated product back to the country of Turkey. Related outbreaks were detected in the France, the Netherlands and the United Kingdom.

Weight of evidence: This was strong in this outbreak with epidemiological evidence implicating semi-dried tomatoes, related outbreaks occurring in other countries, foods positive for a viral sequence that was

(*continued*)

Box 13.4 *(continued)*

indistinguishable from the virus infecting cases, and traceback implicating a common source.

Implications: This was a serious outbreak with >560 cases of hepatitis A reported to the national surveillance system in Australia during the outbreak period. Approximately 45% of locally acquired cases were hospitalised during the outbreak, with one fatality. Due to the potential for international spread, the outbreak was reported to WHO under the International Health Regulations (2005).

(Donnan *et al.*, 2012)

widely distributed outbreaks requires coherent evidence from at least two of: epidemiology, microbiology, and traceback of implicated foods from consumers to a common source of supply.

There is extreme time pressure on public health investigators to gather these streams of evidence and intervene at the same time. This often occurs before all of the relevant information has been gathered, analysed and interpreted. In complex outbreaks, it is vital that health departments and other agencies conduct multiple smaller investigations to develop a sensible picture of the cause of the outbreak. This is a time-consuming and labour-intensive process, but it is vital to ensure that the process is thoroughly and meticulously investigated, while constantly revising the interventions in light of new knowledge.

Summary

Outbreak and cluster investigation are an important function of public health and should follow well-defined frameworks. There has been rapid change in the nature of outbreak investigation as a result of improved microbiological tests and greater availability of online data. Increasingly, health agencies are becoming connected during outbreak investigations due to rapid spread of agents via air travel, food and infected animals. It is not only infectious agents that can present in clusters, but also other diseases, such as birth defects, injuries and cancers. These non-communicable clusters are challenging to investigate due to the often long latency and multifactorial disease causation. Outbreaks and epidemics are challenging to investigate due to the complex nature of information, and the need for information in a timely fashion to take effective public health action.

Questions

1. List three categories of information that should be collected in a hypothesis-generating interview of a patient involved in an outbreak. 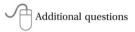 Additional questions

2. The following odds ratios were calculated for different foods eaten by patrons at a restaurant buffet which was later connected with an outbreak of *Clostridium perfringens*. Which one of the following measures of association most strongly suggests that there is a true association between food and illness?
   a. OR = 1.3 (95% CI = 0.61–2.45)
   b. OR = 0.4 (95% CI = 0.25–0.56)
   c. OR = 5.4 (95% CI = 0.92–13.97)
   d. OR = 3.6 (95% CI = 1.00–6.45)

3. Three inmates in a prison have been diagnosed with acute hepatitis B – an acute infection of the liver transmitted by blood-borne and sexually transmitted routes – in the previous month. With reference to the modes of transmission, suggest three possible measures that could be used to stop this potential outbreak of infection.

4. See also the TB Case-Study online for additional questions (and answers). 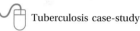 Tuberculosis case-study

REFERENCES

 References

Armstrong, B., Aitken, J., Sim, M. and Swan, N. (2007). Breast Cancer at the ABC Toowong Queensland. Final Report of the Independent Review and Scientific Investigation Panel. Available at: http://about.abc.net.au/wp-content/uploads/2013/04/BreastCancerABCToowongQLDFinalReportJune2007.pdf, accessed 15 May 2015.

Baker, S., Holt, K. E., Clements, A. C., *et al.* (2011). Combined high-resolution genotyping and geospatial analysis reveals modes of endemic urban typhoid fever transmission. *Open Biology*, 1(2):110008.

Barton Behravesh, C., Mody, R. K., Jungk, J., *et al.* (2011). 2008 outbreak of *Salmonella* Saintpaul infections associated with raw produce. *New England Journal of Medicine*, 364: 918–927.

Coory, M. (2008). Statistical inference is overemphasised in cluster investigations: the case of the cluster of breast cancers at the Australian Broadcasting Corporation studios in Brisbane, Australia. *Internal Medicine Journal*, 38: 288–291.

Dalton, C. B., Merritt, T. D., Durrheim, D. N., Munnoch, S. A. and Kirk, M. D. (2009). A structured framework for improving outbreak investigation audits. *BMC Public Health*, 9: 472. doi: 10.1186/1471-2458-9-472.

Donnan, E. J., Fielding, J. E., Gregory, J. E., *et al.* (2012). A multistate outbreak of hepatitis A associated with semidried tomatoes in Australia. *Clinical Infectious Diseases*, 54: 775–781.

Dye, C. (2014). After 2015: infectious diseases in a new era of health and development. *Philosophical Transactions of the Royal Society B*, 369: 20130426.

Fernstrom, A. and Goldblatt, M. (2013). Aerobiology and its role in the transmission of infectious diseases. *Journal of Pathogens*, 2013, Article ID 493960, doi:10.1155/2013/493960.

Frank, C., Werber, D., Cramer, J. P., *et al.* (2011). Epidemic profile of Shiga-toxin-producing *Escherichia coli* O104:H4 outbreak in Germany. *New England Journal of Medicine*, 365(19): 1771–1780.

Gates, B. (2015). The next epidemic – lessons from Ebola. *New England Journal of Medicine*, 372(15): 1381–1384.

GBD 2013 Mortality and Causes of Death Collaborators. (2013). Global, regional, and national age-sex specific all-cause and cause-specific mortality for 240 causes of death, 1990–2013: a systematic analysis for the Global Burden of Disease Study. *Lancet*, 385(9963): 117–171.

Gregg, M. B. (ed.) (2008). *Field Epidemiology*. New York, NY: Oxford University Press.

Jones, K. E., Patel, N. G., Levy, M. A., *et al.* (2008). Global trends in emerging infectious diseases. *Nature*, 451(7181): 990–993.

Langmuir, A. D. (1961). Keynote address. Epidemiology of airborne infections. *Bacteriological Reviews*, 25: 173–181.

Li, Y., Yu, I. T. S., Xu, P., *et al.* (2004). Predicting super spreading events during the 2003 severe acute respiratory syndrome epidemics in Hong Kong and Singapore. *American Journal of Epidemiology*, 160: 719–728.

OzFoodNet Working Group. (2012). Monitoring the incidence and causes of diseases potentially transmitted by food in Australia: annual report of the OzFoodNet network, 2010. *Communicable Diseases Intelligence Quarterly Report*, 36(3): E213–241.

Pires, S. M., Vigre, H., Makela, P. and Hald, T. (2010). Using outbreak data for source attribution of human salmonellosis and campylobacteriosis in Europe. *Foodborne Pathogens and Disease*, 7(11): 1351–1361.

Porta, M. (ed.) (2014). *A Dictionary of Epidemiology*, 6th edn. New York, NY: Oxford University Press.

Reaves, E. J., Mabande, L. G., Thoroughman, D. A., Arwady, M. A. and Montgomery, J. M. (2014). Control of Ebola virus disease – Firestone district, Liberia. *Morbidity and Mortality Weekly Reports*, 63(42): 959–965.

Samaan, G., Gultom, A., Indriani, R., Lokuge, K. and Kelly, P. M. (2011). Critical control points for avian influenza A H5N1 in live bird markets in low resource settings. *Preventive Veterinary Medicine*, 100(1): 71–78.

Sitas, F., O'Connell, D. L., van Kemenade, C. H., Short, M. W. and Zhao, K. (2010). Breast cancer risk among female employees of the Australian Broadcasting Corporation in Australia. *Medical Journal of Australia*, 192: 651–654.

Sleigh, A. C., Chee, H. L., Yeoh, B. S. A., Phua, K. H. and Safman, R. (2006). *Population Dynamics and Infectious Diseases in Asia*. London: World Scientific.

Thiolet, J. M., Jourdan-Da Silva, N., Reggiani, A., *et al*. (2011). Nationwide pseudo-outbreak of *Salmonella enterica* ssp. *diarizonae*, France. *Clinical Microbiology and Infection*, 17(6): 915–918.

van Panhuis, W. G., Grefenstette, J., Jung, S. Y., *et al*. (2013). Contagious diseases in the United States from 1888 to the present. *New England Journal of Medicine*, 369(22): 2152–2158.

Wagner, J. C., Sleggs, C. A. and Marchand, P. (1960). Diffuse pleural mesothelioma and asbestos exposure in the North Western Cape Province. *British Journal of Industrial Medicine*, 17: 260–271.

WHO (World Health Organization). (2008). *International Health Regulations (2005)*, 2nd edn. Geneva: WHO.

WHO (World Health Organization). (2012). *Rapid Risk Assessment of Acute Public Health Events*. Geneva: WHO. http://whqlibdoc.who.int/hq/2012/WHO_HSE_GAR_ARO_2012.1_eng.pdf?ua=1, accessed 27 May 2015.

WHO (World Health Organization). (2015). *Worldwide Country Situation Analysis: Response to Antimicrobial Resistance*. Geneva: WHO. http://www.who.int/drugresistance/en/, accessed 27 May 2015.

RECOMMENDED FOR FURTHER READING

- A good example of the complexity of investigating cancer clusters:
  Armstrong, B., Aitken, J., Sim, M. and Swan, N. (2007). Breast Cancer at the ABC Toowong Queensland. Final Report of the Independent Review and Scientific Investigation Panel. Available at: http://about.abc.net.au/wp-content/uploads/2013/04/BreastCancerABCToowongQLDFinalReportJune2007.pdf, accessed 15 May 2015.

14

Prevention: better than cure?

Prevention is so much better than healing, because it saves the labour of being sick.

(Adams, 1618)

We can happily agree with Adams; where possible, prevention should be a central element of any disease control strategy and epidemiology plays a key role in its development, implementation and evaluation (see Box 14.1). When we speak of prevention in the context of public health, we usually think of what is sometimes called **primary prevention** which aims to prevent disease from occurring in the first place, i.e. to reduce the incidence of disease. Vaccination against childhood infectious diseases is a good example of primary prevention, as is the use of sunscreen to prevent the development of skin cancer. However, somewhat confusingly, the term prevention is also used to describe other strategies to control disease. One of these is the use of screening to advance diagnosis to a point where intervention is more effective, often described as *secondary prevention*, and we will discuss this in the next chapter. What is sometimes called *tertiary prevention* is even more remote from the everyday concept of prevention, usually implying limiting disease

> ## Box 14.1 The role of epidemiology in disease prevention
>
> Epidemiology underpins much of our work in the area of prevention:
>
> - it is central to identifying modifiable causes of disease through the various analytic study designs you have encountered, ideally the results of these would be summarised in a systematic review or meta-analysis;
> - it provides quantitative measures of relative and absolute risk and summary measures of disease burden such as PAF, PIF (potential impact fractions) and DALYs that help identify areas where realistic benefits might be achieved;
> - it informs the design of studies, often RCTs but sometimes non-randomised comparisons, to evaluate the potential for an intervention to prevent disease in practice;
> - together with other disciplines (e.g. statistics, anthropology and economics), it contributes to development of policy to introduce an overall intervention strategy; and, once the strategy has been put in place, it guides the use of appropriate descriptive data to evaluate whether the intervention actually delivers on its promise.

progression or providing better rehabilitation to enhance quality of life in the longer term. In terms of *disease control* it seems more useful to emphasise the fundamental distinction between primary prevention, the focus of this chapter, and all other actions that lead to improved clinical outcomes once disease occurs. The former lowers disease incidence and hence limits the clinical burden from a disease while, as you will see in the next chapter, the latter (e.g. screening) can actually lead to large increases in clinical activity to bring about additional reductions in morbidity and mortality.

Disease prevention in public health

Figure 14.1 shows tuberculosis (TB) mortality over time in England and Wales. This is a disease that had all but disappeared from developed countries but is now re-emerging as a worldwide scourge.

Considering the figure, how important do you think the BCG vaccine and new therapy were in promoting the decline in TB mortality?

Figure 14.1 Age-standardised death rates from tuberculosis in England and Wales, 1840–1968. (Republished with permission of Princeton University Press and Wiley *from*: McKeown, *The Role of Medicine. Dream, Mirage or Nemesis?* (1979).)

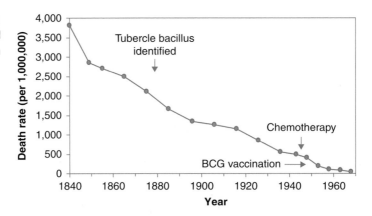

Figure 14.1 and other historical trends make it clear that major health gains were made before the advent of any sophisticated medical therapies and preventive measures. Social and cultural changes such as improved housing, sanitation, general hygiene and nutrition have had a major influence on TB mortality, presumably both by reducing incidence and by increasing survival. The effects of such 'upstream' effects on disease incidence are sometimes termed *primordial prevention*, because they are remote from the more proximal causes that medicine and (conventionally) public health usually deal with. Our view is that the upstream and proximal causes are inter-related and in practice it can be difficult to distinguish the two; any intervention that lowers incidence is thus sensibly termed *primary prevention*.

So, should we dismiss the value of the proximal strategies for TB control? On the absolute scale of Figure 14.1 their contribution does seem marginal. But would mortality have declined less quickly if there had been no BCG vaccine and no chemotherapy? Consider Figure 14.2, which shows the same information plotted on a log scale so that a 50% reduction in mortality looks the same regardless of whether the drop is from a death rate of 4000 to 2000 per million or from 40 to 20 per million, i.e. Figure 14.2 depicts the *rate of change*. We now see a slow and steady fall in mortality across the first 80 years that quickens slightly around 1920. The slope steepens just after the introduction of chemotherapy and continues to fall following the introduction of BCG vaccination. These are hardly definitive evaluations of the benefits of these advances, but the acceleration of the fall in mortality around 1950 implies that something has changed, and the introductions of vaccination and treatment are the best candidates. And here, as elsewhere, when evaluating the 'big-picture' population effects of interventions we have to realise that such apparently simple descriptive data are often going to be the principal basis on which our judgements rest.

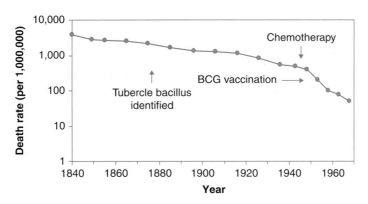

Figure 14.2 Age-standardised death rates from tuberculosis in England and Wales, 1840–1968, plotted on a logarithmic scale.

While the principal goal of public health should first and foremost be primary prevention, for many diseases we do not have enough information (biological and/or epidemiological) to mount such a programme effectively (or cost-effectively). Even when we do have the knowledge, the barriers to implementation may be substantial (e.g. financial, cultural, social, ethical). For example, we already know that ensuring everyone has access to clean water would prevent a large proportion of infectious disease, but for many countries the practical and financial implications are enormous. Similarly, by persuading more people to stop smoking, stay out of the sun, lose weight, exercise more and eat better we could prevent much of our present burden of chronic disease, but changing behaviour remains a major challenge.

Additional strategies are therefore required in order to enhance disease control and decisions as to the most appropriate approach need to be disease-specific: less disease is most desirable, but might not be attainable if causal knowledge is limited, or if causes are not readily modifiable. Screening may be a good second choice in some circumstances if advancing diagnosis really does produce better outcomes (not as straightforward as it might seem, as you will see in the next chapter). Finally, improvements in treatment remain an important avenue for enhancing survival and quality of life for affected individuals. Table 14.1 contrasts two cancers with markedly different control profiles.

The solution to the lung cancer epidemic is obvious (given a PAF of at least 80% for a single, modifiable cause), and concerted multilevel efforts to reduce smoking rates (including banning advertising, legislating for smoke-free public space, and plain paper packaging) have made big inroads on lung cancer rates in many countries (see Figures 3.6 and 3.7). Nonetheless, it remains a common disease, so efforts to improve clinical outcomes through early detection and better treatments are also important, although their yield to date has been limited. Other valuable benefits have come from smoking control

Table 14.1 The role of epidemiological knowledge in disease control: a case of two cancers.

Intervention	Accepted utility for widescale use	
	Lung cancer	Breast cancer
Prevention	YES. Smoking cigarettes is *the* strong risk factor (PAF[a] > 80%); and exposure is modifiable by actions at personal and community levels	NO. Many weak risk factors, most not readily modifiable (although limiting alcohol intake (PAF ~6%) and, post-menopause, weight control (PAF ~8%) and limiting use of hormone therapy (PAF ~3%) are possibilities)
Screening	NO. Even the newest tests (computed-tomography lung scans) yield very limited survival benefits	YES. Substantial good evidence (from RCTs) of lower mortality due to population screening programmes for over 50s
Improved treatment	NO. Minor survival improvements only with newer treatments	YES. Results from RCTs show that a survival advantage can be achieved with appropriate chemotherapy/radiotherapy

[a] PAF, population attributable fractions (from Parkin *et al.*, 2011 and Whiteman *et al.*, 2015).

programmes as noted in Box 14.2, but the other examples there point to the need to consider the balance of *all* effects – positive and negative – of any intervention before deciding if it should be introduced widely.

With breast cancer we see the reverse situation. Quite a lot is known about its aetiology, but there is no strong established causal factor that offers a basis for widespread intervention although reductions in use of postmenopausal hormones have probably lowered incidence in a number of countries (Parkin, 2009). Reducing alcohol intake and, in postmenopausal women, weight control could also yield some preventive benefits, but the PAFs of only 6–8% for alcohol and overweight/obesity (Parkin *et al.*, 2011; Whiteman *et al.*, 2015) show the more limited potential for prevention at present. Fortunately, dual approaches to decreasing morbidity and mortality, namely population screening by mammography to detect early lesions and more effective non-surgical treatments, have paid off. Despite incidence rates that have, until recently, been constant or even increasing, there have been downturns in mortality from breast cancer in a number of countries from the early 1990s, with examples from the USA and UK shown in Figure 14.3. This suggests that the improved outcomes predicted by tightly controlled clinical trials have transferred reasonably effectively to the community setting. Note again the use of routine descriptive data to evaluate the effects of interventions in the community; but also that this alone cannot separate out the relative contributions of early diagnosis and improved treatment. However, as this is important knowledge for setting the cancer control agenda,

Box 14.2 Choosing a preventive strategy: the whole story

An important aside to the lung cancer story is that anti-smoking campaigns have also greatly reduced incidence of other respiratory disease and heart disease. While much causal research is disease-specific, preventive interventions manipulate exposures that may have many consequences. Thus we need good information on the full array of effects of any exposure we plan on modifying. Even immunisation campaigns against infectious diseases have consequences beyond the clear preventive benefits, as they have lowered incidence so dramatically that fewer lives are now saved and the occasional severe side effects of immunisation start to take a more prominent place on the balance sheet. Although virtually every consequence of decreased exposure to cigarettes is positive and thus the total benefit-to-cost ratio is huge, counter-examples abound where complexity is the rule. For example, moderate alcohol consumption is linked to *lower* heart disease but *higher* breast cancer rates and, at high intakes, it is associated with an array of other health and social problems. While the oral contraceptive pill clearly prevents cancers of the ovary and uterus, it has an array of secondary effects which influence whether it is prescribed, and it also increases risks of clotting disorders and breast cancer. And so on.

How do we combine the different effects on morbidity and mortality for various diseases? Does the benefit of avoiding one non-fatal stroke obtained by long-term aspirin use outweigh the risk of three new life-threatening gastric bleeds? Measures such as the DALYs and QALYs that you met in Chapter 2 provide a more quantitative method of doing this and are increasingly reported by health agencies.

there have been a number of attempts to address the question by comparing disease characteristics and survival in eras with different screening and treatment interventions (Webb *et al.*, 2004) and statistical modelling (Morrell *et al.*, 2012).

We will not consider clinical contributions to disease control any further here; instead, our discussion will focus largely on the applications of both epidemiological data and epidemiological thinking to disease prevention and screening. In relation to disease prevention, we will concentrate on the conceptual underpinnings of the preventive approach and some current practical concerns and challenges as well as looking at the utility of using population attributable fractions (PAFs) to target potential 'high-yield' interventions. In

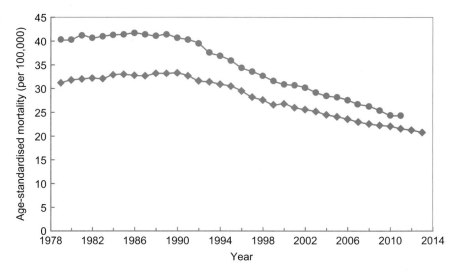

Figure 14.3 Age-standardised breast cancer mortality rates per 100,000/year for women in the UK, 1979–2011 (circles) and USA, 1979–2013 (diamonds). (*Drawn from:* CDC Wonder (CDC) and ONS, 2011.)

Chapter 15 we will go on to consider screening in terms of its underlying logic, and the major challenges to evaluating its contributions to the control of a given disease.

The scope for preventive medicine

Our earlier examples of disease variation by person, place and time have shown that there are large differences between groups, suggesting that much disease should be preventable if only we could lower everyone's risk to that of the lower-risk populations. Another striking example comes from an investigation seeking an explanation for the threefold excess of cardio-vascular disease (CVD) mortality in Finland compared with China. Surveys carried out in rural villages in the two countries over the same time period revealed quite different profiles of CVD risk factors (Table 14.2). The first three factors, all more prevalent in Finland, could be taken as related to overnutrition, and possibly to the fat content of the diet. Given China's history of major famines in the mid twentieth century it is not surprising that differences remain so profound, at least in rural populations. Countries undergoing the *health transition* away from a predominance of infectious diseases and problems of marginal nutrition are, in principle, well placed for intervention to prevent the emergence of Western lifestyle diseases, many of which are related to overconsumption and inactivity. However, social engin-eering is challenging, and the pace of development and industrialisation in China coupled with dramatic reductions in rates of most infectious diseases

Table 14.2 A comparison of prevalence of CVD risk factors between Finnish and Chinese village populations aged 20–64 years.[a]

Risk factor	Men		Women	
	Finns (%)	Chinese (%)	Finns (%)	Chinese (%)
Being overweight	63	21	61	24
Obesity	19	2	24	5
Hypercholesterolaemia	34	3	28	6
Hypertension	49	32	35	28
Smoking	26	73	7	37

[a] All differences were statistically significant ($p < 0.001$, except $p < 0.05$ for hypertension among women) (Hu *et al.*, 2001).

(except HIV/AIDS) and increases in rates of chronic diseases including cancer and cardiovascular disease (Yang *et al.*, 2013) suggest that the risk-factor profiles have already shifted towards those seen in the West. This is also true for other countries in transition, as can be seen in Thailand, where more frequent consumption of sugar-sweetened beverages in 2005 was associated with greater weight gain over the next four years (Lim *et al.*, 2014). Table 14.2 also reflects different attitudes to control of smoking, with the consequences of China's high rates now seen in the rising lung cancer and CVD rates there.

Population versus individual risk

There is a tendency in medicine and epidemiology to try to divide people into two groups – those who have a high risk of developing a particular disease and those at low risk. For instance, a woman of child-bearing age with high blood pressure who smokes and has a family history of blood clotting would be considered at high risk of complications if she took the oral contraceptive pill and this would not be prescribed. In population terms, however, the benefits of the pill outweigh the harms, and it is widely prescribed, although not primarily for the prevention of disease.

So, how should we think about preventing ill health? Should we devote most of our attention to the high-risk groups? This has been the basis of the vast improvements in occupational health and safety since the industrial revolution, and remains an appropriate approach for specifically disadvantaged or exposed groups, including many indigenous peoples. However, in the general population there are few well-defined natural borders between clearly

Risks and benefits of oral contraceptives: Ovarian and uterine cancer rates would be 20–30% higher if women did not use the pill, but breast and cervical cancer rates would be slightly lower. However, the number of cancers prevented by the pill in Australia in 2010 (~1340) greatly outweighs the number it potentially caused (Jordan *et al.*, 2015).

different levels of risk. As an example, consider the relationship between blood pressure and risk of fatal cardiovascular disease. We can see in data from the Whitehall cohort study of British public servants (Rose, 1992) that the age-adjusted risk of dying from CVD over 18 years of follow-up increases with increasing blood pressure (Figure 14.4). Clearly, reducing blood pressure levels is likely to reduce the CVD mortality rate. However, when we look at Figure 14.5, we see that individuals do not fall into obviously separate groups with low and high blood pressure and, therefore, clear-cut 'low' or 'high' risk of heart disease.

Figure 14.4 The relationship between systolic blood pressure and risk of fatal coronary heart disease or stroke over 18 years of follow-up. (*From*: *The Strategy of Preventive Medicine*, G. Rose (1992) figure 2.2, by permission of Oxford University Press.)

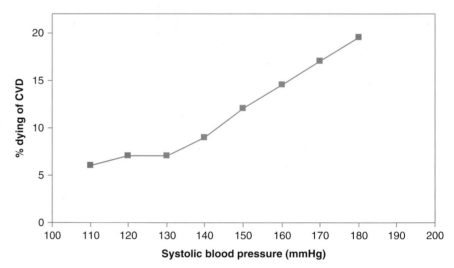

Figure 14.5 Distribution of systolic blood pressure in a population of middle-aged men. (*Adapted from*: *The Strategy of Preventive Medicine*, G. Rose (1992) figure 2.1, by permission of Oxford University Press.)

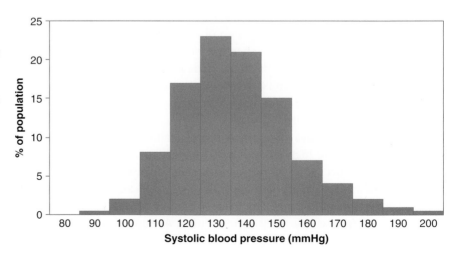

In Figure 14.4, is there any level of systolic blood pressure that is not 'riskier' than the one below it?

Looking at Figures 14.4 and 14.5, how many men in a population of 10,000 would have a systolic blood pressure of 150 mmHg? What is the risk (incidence proportion) of dying from CVD in this group?

So how many men with a blood pressure of 150 mmHg will die from CVD? What about those with a blood pressure of 170 mmHg?

From Figure 14.4 we can infer that the risk of dying from CVD at any level of blood pressure is greater than that at the level below. The risk increases slowly up to 130 mmHg and then increases more sharply and linearly from there. From Figure 14.5 we can estimate that 15% or 1500 of a population of 10,000 men would have a blood pressure around 150 mmHg, and from Figure 14.4 the risk of dying of CVD in this group is 12% over the 18 years of follow-up. We would, therefore, expect about 12% × 1500 = 180 CVD deaths in this group. Similarly, 4% or 400 of the population would have a blood pressure of 170 mmHg and they have a 17% risk of dying of CVD. We would therefore expect about 17% × 400 = 68 CVD deaths in this group. Thus, although the risk of dying of CVD is greater for those with very high blood pressure, over twice as many actual CVD deaths will occur among the much larger number of people with intermediate blood pressure. Targeting prevention at only those with very high blood pressure will not, therefore, address the majority of deaths (but see Box 14.3 for a clinical perspective).

Figure 14.6 shows a concrete example of the close overlap in risk-factor distributions (in this case serum cholesterol level) between those who did and did not subsequently die from ischaemic heart disease (IHD; if the disease terminology here is becoming confusing, check back to Box 2.6, page 52). The whole curve for those who died from IHD is clearly shifted to the right compared with those who did not die, but the two overlap considerably and the cut-off point identifying the extreme upper 5% of the 'healthy' cohort identifies only 15% of those who will develop IHD. So again, identifying and treating individuals with very high cholesterol level is not a good preventive strategy for the whole population.

Strategies for prevention

Choosing the best way to intervene in order to lower disease risk in a specific population will often be a challenge. We present below some brief comments on the theoretical extremes of practice, the *high-risk* and the *mass* or population strategies. Although we have seen why the mass strategy is widely considered to be preferable, it might not always be practical. We also show a

Box 14.3 A clinical perspective

The example in the text shows the population perspective on prevention: at the *community level* more CVD deaths would be prevented by focussing on the larger numbers of people at intermediate risk than on the few at high risk. However, let us focus on the individual for a moment. Lowering an individual's blood pressure from 150 to 120 mmHg would reduce their risk of CVD from 12% to about 7%, an absolute risk reduction of 5%. Similarly, lowering an individual's blood pressure from 170 to 120 mmHg would reduce their risk of dying from CVD from 17% to about 7%, an absolute risk reduction of 10%. At the *individual level*, therefore, the benefits are greatest for those at highest risk, so a clinical decision to identify and treat such individuals, despite potentially harmful side effects, can make sense and complement population strategies such as lowering the salt content of foods.

Note, from a health system perspective, these reductions translate to a number needed to treat (NNT) of 20 (1 ÷ 0.05) in order to prevent one CVD death among those with blood pressure 150 mmHg compared to NNT = 10 for those with blood pressure of 170 mmHg.

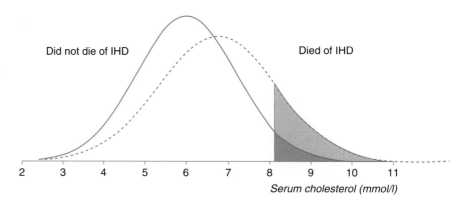

Figure 14.6 Relative distributions of serum cholesterol levels in men who subsequently died of ischaemic heart disease and men who did not. The shaded areas indicate the proportions of the population above a cut-point that identifies the top 5% of the healthy cohort. (*Reproduced from*: Wald and Law, *BMJ*, 2003; **326**: 1419–1425, with permission from BMJ Publishing Group Ltd.)

'middle path' showing the value of considering detailed patterns of risk factor–disease associations to guide intervention targets and strategies.

The high-risk strategy

Classically, preventive medicine takes a high-risk approach. First, those individuals in special need are identified (e.g. intravenous drug users). The preventive process then takes the form of controlling the level of exposure to a cause (e.g. introduction of a needle-exchange programme) or providing protection against the consequences of the exposure (e.g. vaccination against hepatitis B) in this high-risk group.

Another example can be found in the blood pressure problem we discussed earlier. We might decide that high-risk patients are those with a systolic blood pressure over 160 mmHg. The high-risk strategy would then involve screening out those individuals with high blood pressure, followed by intervention to bring their blood pressure down. This remains a common approach in clinical practice and, if fully applied, might lead to a population blood pressure distribution like that in Figure 14.7. If we compare this graph with Figure 14.5, we can see that those who were in the upper tail have lowered their blood pressure, and thus presumably their CVD risk, but the main group (among whom most cases will occur) is unaffected.

High-risk strategies appeal for a number of reasons. The intervention is well matched to individuals and their concerns (e.g. a needle-exchange programme is a specific and tailored response to a tightly defined group), and thus should also improve the benefit-to-risk and benefit-to-cost ratios. Furthermore, avoiding interference with the non-needy group and adopting a 'magic bullet' approach to the target group are readily accommodated within the ethos of the medical care system.

So, can the high-risk strategy play a useful preventive role? Of course, it remains highly appropriate and desirable in clinical practice, and can also be appropriate at the community level if a problem is confined to an identifiable minority and can be successfully controlled in isolation. This includes the well-documented benefits of targeting various occupational groups, for example, hepatitis vaccination for those who work with blood products, and

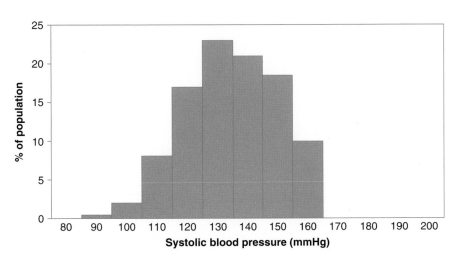

Figure 14.7 The hypothetical distribution of systolic blood pressure in middle-aged men after applying a 'high-risk' screening strategy. (*Adapted from*: The Strategy of Preventive Medicine, G. Rose (1992), figure 4.1, by permission of Oxford University Press.)

early treatment and targeted vaccination of contacts of infected persons can be a very effective way to control outbreaks of infectious diseases. However, we need to be cautious in claiming that a risk really is sufficiently limited to the so-called high-risk group. For example, screening only older pregnant women, who are known to be at highest risk of conceiving a child with Down's syndrome, will miss the majority of afflicted foetuses, which are conceived by younger women, in whom most pregnancies occur.

The mass strategy

In the case of a common disease or widespread cause, the extreme alternative approach is the mass or population strategy advocated by Geoffrey Rose (1992). This starts with the recognition that the occurrence of common diseases and exposures reflects the behaviour and circumstances of society as a whole. The mass strategy thus aims to reduce the health risks of the entire population.

Using the blood pressure data again we can illustrate a mass-strategy approach to this problem. Instead of targeting only those people with the highest blood pressure, we would aim to reduce everybody's blood pressure by a smaller amount. This would shift both the blood pressure and the CVD risk of the population to a lower level (Figure 14.8). This is a much healthier situation for the whole group (although perhaps not for some highest-risk individuals) than the truncated distribution we saw in Figure 14.7.

Other examples of the mass strategy are immunisation programmes, water fluoridation, fortification of common foods such as bread with vitamins

Figure 14.8 The distribution of systolic blood pressure in a population of middle-aged men before and after a hypothetical intervention. (*From*: *The Strategy of Preventive Medicine*, G. Rose (1992), figure 6.5, by permission of Oxford University Press.)

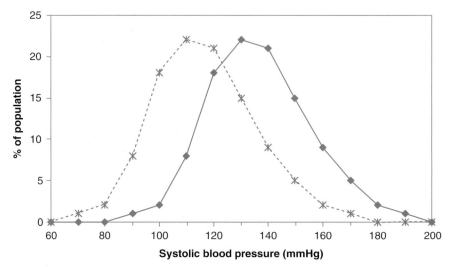

(e.g. folic acid), legislating use of seat belts (together with effective enforce-ment, as without this a number of countries have failed to realise the true benefits from introducing seat belt laws) and extensive legislative restrictions on cigarette advertising and on smoking in public. Implementation of effective preventive strategies for the current challenges of obesity is even more daunting, given the complex causal web leading to weight gain. Here, as for other preventive interventions, online motivational tools have been developed to assist individuals to lower their risks.

In Box 14.4 we show an example of a 'middle-road' approach that sits somewhere between the mass and high-risk approaches, reminding us of the need to test our presumptions and prejudices against the known data before proceeding with a particular approach to implementing a prevention programme. Indeed, Rose made it clear that careful attention must be paid to the patterns of association between risk factors and disease (e.g. a linear increase in risk versus an exponential one – see Box 14.4 for example). The prevalence of the high-risk exposures is also important, as seen for blood pressure and CVD above, and it is for this reason that the PAF that you met in Chapter 5 can be useful in identifying optimal preventive interventions. We will look at this further in the next section.

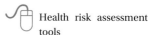 Health risk assessment tools

Prevention in practice: We have had sufficient evidence of the causal role of smoking in disease for more than 50 years (Office of the US Surgeon General, 1964) yet although mass prevention programmes have substantially decreased smoking rates in some countries, they remain high in many parts of the world.

Box 14.4 Weight and diabetes: a 'middle-road' strategy

Brown and colleagues (2007) used data from the Australian Longitudinal Study on Women's Health to model the effects of different patterns of weight reduction on risk of hypertension and diabetes. As predicted, for hypertension they found a larger benefit for a mass approach than for a targeted high-risk approach (Table 14.3). However, the pattern was

Table 14.3 Effects of different intervention approaches on risk of hypertension and diabetes in an Australian population.

Approach	Intervention	Risk reduction	
		Hypertension	Diabetes
Mass	Modest reduction in weight (1 BMI unit) across whole population	10%	13%
High-risk	Larger reduction in weight (3 BMI units) in heaviest 20% of the population	7%	17%
Middle-road	Moderate reduction in weight (2 BMI units) in heaviest 50% of the population	12%	23%

(Data source: Brown *et al.*, 2007.)

(*continued*)

Box 14.4 (*continued*)

somewhat different for diabetes where the high-risk approach was more effective, largely because unlike risks of hypertension which increase linearly with increasing BMI, the risks of diabetes are more concentrated at the higher end of the distribution. But for both outcomes, a 'middle-road' approach aiming for a moderate reduction in weight in the top half of the population gave the greatest reductions in risk. Ultimately, though, the predicted benefits have to be balanced against the costs and acceptability of each approach. For example, while targeting only a fifth of the population via a high-risk strategy may save money initially, achieving and maintaining the greater weight loss required to deliver the full benefit may prove impractical in the longer term and aiming for a more modest weight loss in a greater proportion of the population may be more cost-effective.

The population attributable fraction as a guide to prevention

As you saw in Chapter 5, one useful way to estimate the burden of disease in a population that can be attributed to a particular risk factor is to calculate the *population attributable fraction* (PAF)[1]:

$$PAF = P_{e(cases)} \frac{(RR - 1)}{RR}$$

where P_e is the prevalence of exposure to the risk factor of interest *in those with disease* and RR is the relative risk of disease for the exposure of interest. The PAF also represents the maximum percentage reduction in the burden of disease (or death) that might be expected if we could remove the exposure completely.

However, this formula assumes that exposure is dichotomous: people are either exposed to a risk factor or they are not. For instance, if we are interested in the PAF of CHD or stroke due to high blood pressure we could set a cut-off point at 140 mmHg to define 'high blood pressure'. However, we know that while the highest risks of CHD and stroke are seen at blood pressures above 140 mmHg, there is also some increase in risk between 110 and 140 mmHg (Figure 14.4).

---

[1] As you saw in Chapter 5, there are several different formulae for calculating the PAF. This version is the most flexible as it is still valid when we need to use adjusted relative risks to allow for confounding; however, it may not be the most useful in practice, as P_e may not be known and for this reason formula 5.18 (page 160) is often used.

We also know that most of the population have values below 140 mmHg (Figure 14.5), so using that simple cutpoint would underestimate the total amount of disease due to elevated blood pressure. Moreover, if we uniformly apply one average value of RR for the effects of having any systolic blood pressure over 140 mmHg, we ignore the dramatic increases in risk above that level. Despite these limitations, this approach still gives a reasonable quantitative appreciation of the potential benefits from improving population blood pressure distributions in most situations. However, it can be an issue if we want to compare populations with very different prevalences of high and very high blood pressures.

This was a particular challenge for the World Health Organization when it set out to estimate cross-national burdens of disease due to a range of risk factors as a basis for identifying preventive strategies (the *Comparative Risk Assessment* study). Their practical solution was to develop an approach which could account for several different levels of a risk factor by summing the effects across these levels to produce an overall PAF (Murray *et al.*, 2003).

Attributable and avoidable disease

A second challenge for WHO was to determine what the unexposed or *reference* level should be for a particular risk factor to allow sensible comparisons to be made between risk factors and preventive strategies. For risk factors with an obvious zero exposure level (e.g. smoking, air pollution) it makes intuitive sense to use that level as the reference. However, for risk factors such as blood pressure, body mass and serum cholesterol there is no zero exposure so, for these factors, the reference value was taken to be that level of exposure which would give the minimum disease/injury burden (Murray and Lopez, 1999). The **attributable burden** of disease due to a risk factor is thus *the absolute amount of disease in the population due to levels of exposure above the defined reference level* and the population attributable fraction[2] is the *proportion of that disease which can be so attributed.*

To gain the maximum future benefit from a preventive intervention we would have to reduce exposures to their reference level, e.g. by eliminating smoking or air pollution completely. This of course is infeasible, particularly for an exposure like smoking, because once someone has smoked they can never return to being a never smoker, so more realistic estimates are needed. A *plausible minimum* for tobacco exposure might be the low smoking prevalence in Sweden (16%); however, even this might not be realistic for the near

---

[2] Note that Murray and Lopez (1999) use the term attributable fraction to describe what we have called the population attributable fraction.

Figure 14.9 Attributable and avoidable burden. (*Adapted from*: Murray *et al.*, 2003.)

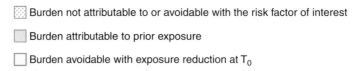

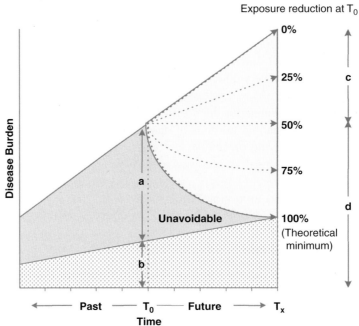

Potential impact fraction (PIF): this is another measure that can be used to assess the future impact of a reduction in exposure. It is similar to the PAF, but instead of estimating the fraction of disease that might be prevented by complete elimination of an exposure, it estimates the fraction of disease potentially preventable if exposure is reduced to a new lower level.

future and a more *feasible* target might be to reduce smoking prevalence by 5%, say from 25% to 20%.

Figure 14.9 shows the hypothetical effects of reducing levels of current exposure (at time T_0) on the future burden of disease (time T_x). The darker blue area represents the burden of disease *attributable* to prior exposure; at time T_0 this is equal to 'a' and the population attributable fraction at T_0 is therefore a ÷ (a + b). The dashed arrows represent the effects on the *future* burden of disease of different reductions in exposure at T_0: 0% (no change), 25%, 50%, 75% or 100% (complete elimination). Thus if we were to reduce the prevalence of exposure by 50% at time T_0 the amount of disease avoided at time T_x, the **avoidable burden**, would be that indicated 'c' and the **avoidable fraction** of disease in the population is c ÷ (c + d). Note that the burden of disease *not* attributable to the risk factor of interest (the spotted area) may be decreasing, constant or increasing (as shown in the figure) over time.

For a real-life example, see Figure 14.10. This shows standardised lung cancer mortality rates for men and women in Australia from 1979 to 2001, with projections to 2021. The lightest blue area shows the unavoidable burden

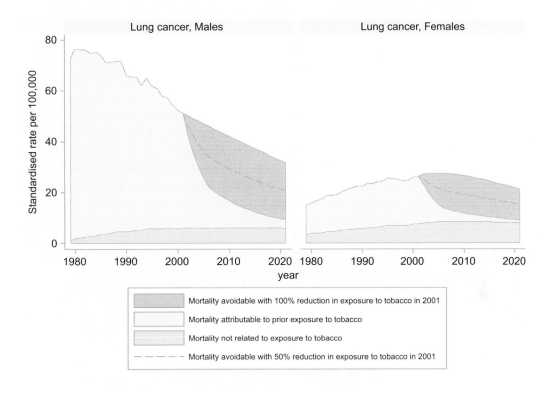

Figure 14.10 Attributable and avoidable lung cancer mortality due to tobacco (age-standardised rates), Australia 1979 to 2021. (*Source*: Stephen Begg, Queensland Health, reproduced with permission.)

of lung cancer attributable to past smoking, the dark blue area predicts the amount of future disease that would potentially be prevented if smoking levels had dropped to zero in 2001, and the area above the dashed line shows the effects of a 50% reduction in smoking in 2001. Of course, we must always keep in mind the uncertainty of all such forward projections as they are highly dependent on all of the other factors that affect population behaviours.

Prevention in practice

Box 14.5 describes an innovative population-wide suicide-prevention programme that was developed explicitly from Rose's ideal model of population change.

How highly would you rate this study design for evaluating such a programme?

Box 14.5 Flying higher: the US Air Force suicide prevention programme

Suicide rates in the US Air Force increased notably in the early 1990s, leading to a concerted effort by senior staff to halt and reverse this trend. A multilayered population-based prevention programme was introduced in 1996 to reduce risk factors and enhance protective factors among the more than 5 million personnel. The intervention focussed on removing the stigma from mental health problems, enhancing understanding of mental health, and changing policies and social norms. Strong and continuing endorsement of the initiative by senior leaders was a critical element. The approach adopted was explicitly a population-oriented risk-reduction approach. Its effectiveness was measured by comparison of suicide rates among US Air Force personnel before and after the intervention: overall suicide was reduced by 33% (Figure 14.11) (Knox et al., 2003). Further follow-up in 2008 found that suicide rates had remained at the new lower level since 2003 with the exception of a spike in incidence in 2004, which was found to coincide with a period when the programme was implemented less rigorously (Knox et al., 2010).

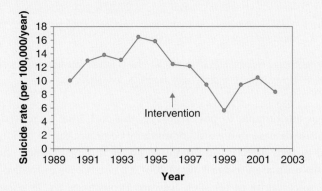

Figure 14.11 Suicide rates in the US Air Force before and after the population-based intervention in 1996–1997. (*Data source:* Knox et al., 2003.)

How easily can we generalise from these findings to, say, the US population as a whole?

The actual study design used is a simple pre–post-intervention comparison of suicide rates (i.e. very straightforward descriptive data). It would be nice to have RCT data on this issue but, for pretty obvious reasons, it is very difficult to conduct such a trial on this scale. Furthermore, because the interventions have to be applied to an entire community, not just to individuals, it would have to be a cluster randomised trial with only a few large groups and so would miss out on the core benefits of individual randomisation. A trial would, however, avoid the possible confounding of pre–post studies when there are underlying time trends in suicide rates that are independent of any intervention. (In this particular situation the unexposed and exposed cohorts, pre- and post-intervention, are likely to have been quite similar with regard to potential confounders among individuals, although external factors which might change over time, such as new wars and total population size, could influence suicide rates.) While the summary figures indicate the programme's likely benefit, we can see from Figure 14.11 that the pattern of change for suicide is not simple to interpret. More recent data which extend both the pre- and post-intervention periods for the study support a genuine benefit of the intervention (Knox *et al.*, 2010).

Generalising the specific findings to the whole population is more problematic, not the least because air force personnel and the air force environment are likely to be very different from the general US population; however, the underlying theories may well be generally applicable. Taken at face value, these results suggest that the mass strategy is capable of addressing the underlying social, economic and political determinants of ill health in a population, and need not be restricted to immediate causes. It is also a desirable approach to intervention because it aims to change not only the risk factors, but also the context in which they are embedded: it is easier to seek help for a problem, or give up smoking, for example, if the rest of the population is supportive.

Naturally, simpler solutions to preventive interventions are appealing – immunisations for infectious diseases and some cancers (HPV for cervical cancer, hepatitis B for liver cancer) are notable and valuable examples. However, the search for other 'magic bullets' continues; the editor of the *British Medical Journal* speculated that the 28 June 2003 edition might be 'The most

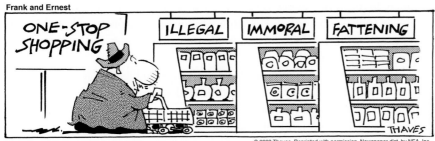

Frank and Ernest

© 2003 Thaves. Reprinted with permission. Newspaper dist. by NEA, Inc.

important *BMJ* for 50 years' (Smith, 2003). He referred to an article by Wald and Law (2003) proposing the 'Polypill', a six-drugs-in-one cardiovascular panacea that might prevent 80% of all vascular morbidity and mortality beyond the age of 55 by reducing blood pressure (a three-drug cocktail), serum levels of LDL cholesterol (a statin) and homocysteine (folate), and clotting tendency (aspirin). Their quantification of the benefits and risks of such a pill was based on combining relevant evidence from RCTs and long-term cohort studies drawn from a series of systematic reviews and meta-analyses. They recommended implementing a population strategy aimed to shift the whole cardiovascular 'risk curve' well to the left, exactly the sort of outcome of which Rose would have approved. This achieves the same preventive end as the Air Force suicide intervention programme by moderating whole-of-population risk, but the onus on achieving the goal is shifted from society to the individual, from primary structural and behavioural change to life-long pill taking (and if compliance is not high the benefits shrink rapidly). Whether this 'medicalisation' of a society is desirable or acceptable is contentious, and the paper engendered debate. A series of trials of variants of the polypill have now been published demonstrating the feasibility of the approach and showing good compliance; larger-scale interventions currently underway should yield direct measures of the polypill's preventive potential (Castellano *et al.*, 2014).

Evaluation of preventive interventions in practice

The first reasonably strong evidence that intervention (adding or removing an exposure) might decrease disease incidence often comes from observational epidemiology, i.e. case–control or cohort studies. If, as this evidence accumulates, a causal relationship between exposure and disease seems likely, and if the potential for practical change exists, then this preventive potential can be tested in randomised controlled trials. You have already seen some of these, for example the trial of polio vaccine (Box 9.4) and the Physicians' Health Study which tested aspirin for preventing coronary heart disease and beta-carotene to prevent cancer (Box 4.2). The utility (polio immunisation) or otherwise (beta-carotene) of these interventions as demonstrated by the trials directly underpinned decisions to implement the former but not the latter preventive programme.

However, once the programme has been shown to be feasible in a trial, and is rolled out to the wider population, it is no longer operating with the close overview that characterises most experimental research, and so it cannot automatically be assumed that it will be as effective as in the RCT setting. It now needs 'real-world' monitoring and evaluation and in the first instance this information usually comes from the 'routine' data sources that we discussed in Chapter 3, especially trends in disease-specific mortality. You have met a number of examples of this already, including the US Airforce suicide prevention programme, and in figures showing mortality declines from lung cancer (Figure 1.1), heart attacks (Figure 1.7), tuberculosis (Figure 14.1) and breast cancer (Figure 14.3). Interpretation of the falling lung cancer mortality among men in the USA is fairly straightforward from consideration of Table 14.1 and Figure 3.7, and the additional knowledge that the incidence of this cancer is also falling. The multiple strategies applied to induce falling smoking rates have produced effective primary prevention of this fatal cancer, although it is hard to know exactly which elements of the anti-smoking campaigns have had most effect. And the reduction in smoking is just one of many factors that have contributed to the massive declines in CHD deaths among Australian men (see Figure 14.12). We have discussed factors behind the mortality changes for TB and breast cancer above, and in the next chapter will consider the contributions of screening to controlling breast cancer in more detail.

These examples all underline the critical importance of having good mortality data (we discussed some of the challenges in getting this in Chapter 3) to monitor the effectiveness of disease control programmes whether they are attempting primary prevention or to improve treatment outcomes.

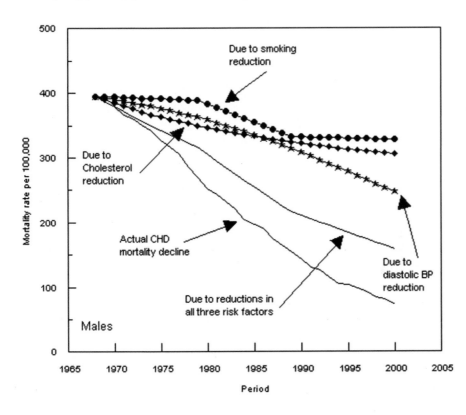

Figure 14.12 Contribution of changes in risk factors to decline in coronary heart disease (CHD) mortality rate in Australian men aged 35–64 years 1968–2000. (*From*: Taylor *et al.*, *Eur. J. Cardiovasc. Prev. Rehabil.*, 2006; 13: 760–768, with permission.)

A final (cautionary) word

There are inevitably limitations to the mass strategy, especially the difficulties of effective implementation. It is quite hard to persuade the public that a health problem is a matter for concerted public action rather than simply the responsibility of the few affected individuals. If everyone wants to smoke or drive cars fast then it is not easy to stop them (the enforced changes in views on drink-driving in many societies are, however, encouraging). Population-level interventions such as water fluoridation or fortification of flour products with folate are also highly controversial as they effectively remove an individual's choice as to whether they want to receive the intervention or not. Even if we know what is desirable and the public is on side, it can still be difficult to effect a change (e.g. to reduce poverty). All change involves costs, and change on a large scale involves large-scale costs. Finally, population change is made more difficult because of what Rose dubbed the *prevention paradox*: 'a preventive measure which brings much benefit to the community offers little to each participating individual' (Rose, 1981). We all have to change our risk profile (by wearing seat belts, changing our behaviour, etc.), but the only people who really benefit are the unidentifiable minority among us whose seat belt will save them in an accident or who would have died from CVD if they had not reduced their blood pressure. In practice we often fall short of fully informing the public of the very limited individual benefits that result from mass prevention programmes (and from screening programmes; see Chapter 15).

In the next chapter we will move from primary prevention to *secondary prevention* or screening, and will apply an epidemiological perspective to the use of population screening as a public health intervention. It often seems to be a given that early detection of disease must be a good thing but, as you will see, this is not always the case, and thus this assumption should never be allowed to go untested.

Questions

Additional questions

1. Comment on the utility of relative and absolute measures of effect in assessing the benefits a community will get from a prevention programme.
2. Refer back to Table 5.4. What are the implications of the data shown for the benefits an effective anti-smoking campaign could deliver?

REFERENCES

References

Adams, T. (1618). *Happiness of Church*; p. 146.
Brown, W. J., Hockey, R. and Dobson, A. (2007). Rose revisited: a "middle road" prevention strategy to reduce noncommunicable chronic disease risk. *Bulletin of the World Health Organization*, 85: 886–887.

Castellano, J. M., Sanz, G., Ortiz, A. F., *et al.* (2014). A polypill strategy to improve global secondary cardiovascular prevention. From concept to reality. *Journal of the American College of Cardiology*, 64: 614–621.

CDC (Centers for Disease Control and Prevention), National Center for Health Statistics. Multiple Cause of Death 1999–2013 on CDC WONDER Online Database, released 2015. Data are from the Multiple Cause of Death Files, 1999–2013, as compiled from data provided by the 57 vital statistics jurisdictions through the Vital Statistics Cooperative Program. http://wonder.cdc.gov/mcd-icd10.html, accessed 13 March 2015.

Hu, G., Pekkarinen, H., Halonen, P., *et al.* (2001). Different worlds, different tasks for health promotion: comparisons of health risk profiles in Chinese and Finnish rural people. *Health Promotion International*, 16: 315–320.

Jordan, S. J., Wilson, L., Nagle, C. M., *et al.* (2015). Cancers in Australia in 2010 attributable to and prevented by the use of combined oral contraceptives. *Australian and New Zealand Journal of Public Health*, 39: 441–445.

Knox, K. L., Litts, D. A., Talcott, G. W., Feig, J. C. and Caine, E. D. (2003). Risk of suicide and related adverse outcomes after exposure to a suicide prevention programme in the US Air Force: a cohort study. *British Medical Journal*, 327: 1376–1380.

Knox, K. L., Pflanz, S., Talcott, G. W., *et al.* (2010). The US air force suicide prevention program: implications for public health policy. *American Journal of Public Health*, 100: 2457–2463.

Lim, L., Banwell, C., Bain, C., *et al.* (2014). Sugar sweetened beverages and weight gain over 4 years in a Thai national cohort – a prospective analysis. *PloS ONE*, 9: e95309-e95309.

Morrell, S., Taylor, R., Roder, D. and Dobson, A. (2012). Mammography screening and breast cancer mortality in Australia: an aggregate cohort study. *Journal of Medical Screening*, 19: 26–34.

Murray, C. J. L., Ezzati, M., Lopez, A. D., Rodgers, A. and Vander Hoorn, S. (2003). Comparative quantification of health risks: conceptual framework and methodological issues. *Population Health Metrics*, 1(1): 1.

Murray, C. J. L. and Lopez, A. D. (1999). On the quantification of health risks: lessons from the Global Burden of Disease Study. *Epidemiology*, 10: 594–605.

Office of the Surgeon General. (1964) *Smoking and Health*. Public Health Service Publication No. 1103. United States. Public Health Service. Office of the Surgeon General.

ONS (Office for National Statistics). (2011). *Breast Cancer Incidence, Mortality and Survival, England, 1971–2011*. Cancer Statistics Registrations, England (Series MB1), No. 42, 2011 Release.

Parkin, D. M. (2009). Is the recent fall in post-menopausal breast cancer in UK related to changes in use of hormone replacement therapy? *European Journal of Cancer*, 45: 1649–1653.

Parkin, D. M., Boyd, L. and Walker, L. C. (2011). The fraction of cancer attributable to lifestyle and environmental factors in the UK in 2010: summary and conclusions. *British Journal of Cancer*, 105: S77–S81.

Rose, G. (1981). Strategy of prevention: lessons from cardiovascular disease. *British Medical Journal*, 282: 1847–1851.

Rose, G. (1992). *The Strategy of Preventive Medicine.* London: Oxford University Press.

Smith, R. (2003). The most important BMJ for 50 years? *British Medical Journal*, 326: un-numbered pages at the beginning of issue 7404.

Wald, N. J. and Law, M. R. (2003). A strategy to reduce cardiovascular disease by more than 80%. *British Medical Journal*, 326: 1419–1425.

Webb, P. M., Cummings, M. C. ,Bain, C. J. and Furnival, C. M. (2004). Changes in survival after breast cancer: improvements in diagnosis or treatment? *Breast*, 13: 7–14.

Whiteman, D. C., Webb, P. M., Green, A. C., *et al.* (2015). Cancers in Australia in 2010 attributable to modifiable factors: summary and conclusions. *Australian and New Zealand Journal of Public Health*, 39: 477–484.

Yang, G., Wang, Y., Zeng, Y., *et al.* (2013). Rapid health transition in China, 1990–2010: findings from the Global Burden of Disease Study 2010. *Lancet*, 381: 1987–2015.

RECOMMENDED FOR FURTHER READING

- Rose's classic and very readable paper describing the high-risk and mass approaches to prevention:

  Rose, G. (1981). Strategy of prevention: lessons from cardiovascular disease. *British Medical Journal*, 282: 1847–1851.

- A useful discussion of the issues involved when assessing the contributions of risk factors to disease and the potential for prevention in populations (includes some mathematics):

  Murray, C. J. L., Ezzati, M., Lopez, A. D., Rodgers, A. and Vander Hoorn, S. (2003). Comparative quantification of health risks: conceptual framework and methodological issues. *Population Health Metrics*, 1(1): 1.

- A practical example of the high-risk and mass strategies and a third 'middle road' approach:

  Brown, W. J., Hockey, R. and Dobson, A. (2007). Rose revisited: a "middle road" prevention strategy to reduce noncommunicable chronic disease risk. *Bulletin of the World Health Organization*, 85: 886–887.

Early detection: what benefits at what cost?

| Description Chapters 2–3 | Association Chapters 4–5 | Alternative explanations Chapters 6–8 | Integration & interpretation Chapters 9–11 | Practical applications Chapter 15: Screening |

Up to this point we have mainly focussed on the issues of how we can quantify health (or ill health) and how to identify factors that might be causing ill health, with a view to preventing it in the future. In the previous chapter we alluded to what is sometimes called 'secondary' prevention, where instead of

> ### Box 15.1 Just because screening should work doesn't mean it will
>
> In the 1960s, public health practitioners were seduced by the concept of early diagnosis – give people regular health checks to identify and treat disease early. It seemed so obvious it would work that initiatives of this type started springing up in the USA and the UK. The UK Ministry of Health realised that the cost implications were enormous, so between 1967 and 1976 a trial was conducted in London to evaluate the benefits of multiphasic screening of middle-aged adults in general practice. Approximately 7000 participants were randomly allocated to receive either two screening checks two years apart or no screening and all participants then underwent a health survey. The investigators did not find any significant differences between the two groups in terms of their morbidity, hospital admissions, absence from work for sickness, or mortality. The only outcome appeared to be the increased costs of healthcare – approximately £142 million to screen the entire middle-aged UK population (and that was at 1976 prices). (The South-East London Screening Study Group, 1977; reprinted in 2001 with a series of commentaries, Various, 2001.)

trying to prevent disease from occurring, we try to detect it earlier in the hope that this will allow more effective treatment and thus improved health outcomes. This is an aspect of public health that has great intuitive appeal, especially for serious conditions such as cancer where the options for primary prevention can be very limited. However, screening programmes are usually very costly exercises and they do not always deliver the expected benefits in terms of improved health outcomes (see Box 15.1). In this chapter we will introduce you to the requirements for implementing a successful screening programme and to some of the problems that we encounter when trying to determine whether such a programme is actually beneficial in practice. Box 15.2 summarises the various stages in this process and the central role of epidemiology in all of these.

Why screen?

It has been known for some time that infection with human papillomavirus (HPV) is a major and probably necessary cause of cervical cancer (see Chapter 10), but until the development of HPV vaccines in recent years we could not prevent people from becoming infected, other than through encouraging condom use. As uptake of these vaccines becomes widespread,

Box 15.2 The role of epidemiology in screening

Epidemiology has multiple roles to play in screening, from the initial decision-making on whether or not to use screening to help control a disease through to assessment of whether the screening works in practice. Elements of this (and the relevant study designs) include:

- identifying whether a disease has an appropriate 'natural history' to make screening an option (descriptive case series);
- considering if it conveys a significant burden (estimates of incidence, prevalence, mortality and overall burden e.g. in the form of DALYs);
- measuring test quality and estimating how it might perform in the population (cross-sectional studies);
- assessing the potential of a screening programme to improve outcomes while dealing with special forms of selection bias (RCTs); and finally
- evaluating the performance of the programme in practice (long-term descriptive and ecological coverage of regions and nations).

This dependence on the sound design and interpretation of a broad mix of epidemiological studies to determine the quality and practical utility of a screening programme emphasises the central role of epidemiology in health services assessment and policy evaluation.

they may eventually replace the current screening programmes as the preferred method for control of this disease. However, the screening programmes have shown that in the absence of primary preventives like vaccines, detecting disease before the usual time of diagnosis can provide an effective 'second level' of public health intervention.

When used as a public health measure for disease control, screening implies the widespread use of a simple test for disease in an apparently healthy (asymptomatic) population. A screening test will often not diagnose the presence of disease directly, but will instead separate people who are more likely to have the disease from those who are less likely to have it. Those who may have the disease (i.e. those who screen positive) can then undergo further diagnostic tests and treatment if necessary. The improved public health outcomes we seek through screening are reduced morbidity, mortality and/or disability. The benefits of public health screening are primarily for those people who are actually screened, and generally even among this group only very few will benefit directly, but there may also be wider social benefits if overall health costs are reduced.

Screening is also used, in a slightly different fashion, to protect the general population from exposure to disease. As an example, immigrants to a number of countries are screened for HIV and hepatitis B infection; and travellers from regions with epidemic acute infectious diseases, such as Ebola, SARS (severe acute respiratory syndrome) or H1N1 influenza, have been subjected to screening using health declaration cards to identify symptoms and sometimes thermal scanning to detect signs of infection at airports. The primary aim of this type of screening is not to benefit the individual who is screened, but to protect the local population from these viruses. Similarly, some occupations require regular screening; for example, airline pilots have regular medical checks in an attempt to ensure that they will not have a heart attack while flying. Insurance companies often require people to undergo health checks and screening before they offer them a life insurance policy. Here the 'screening' is done for purely financial reasons, because insurance companies charge higher premiums for people at higher risk.

The disease process

The first we know of the existence of a disease in a person is when it is diagnosed. This is usually some time after it first produces the symptoms which cause the person to seek medical care. The actual onset of disease will of course be earlier than this – how much earlier depends on the disease concerned. Figure 15.1 illustrates this point.

At some stage between the biological onset of disease and the time of usual clinical diagnosis there may come a time when early signs of disease are there, if only we could detect them. The position of this point will vary depending on

Figure 15.1 The natural history of a disease (*adapted from*: Sackett *et al.*, 1991).

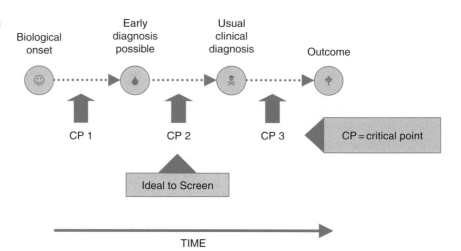

the disease, perhaps occurring many years before the appearance of clinical disease (e.g. high blood pressure, some cancers), or only shortly before symptoms appear (e.g. acute infectious diseases).

At some stage during the disease process there is also likely to be a **critical point**, after which the disease process is irreversible and treatment will confer little or no benefit. An example is the point at which a cancer starts spreading to other tissues (known as metastasis). If this 'point of no return' occurs before it is possible to detect the disease (CP 1 in Figure 15.1), then advancing the time of detection will simply mean that the person knows about their disease for longer but their outcome will not be improved. Similarly, if this point occurs after the time of usual clinical diagnosis (CP 3) there is no need to detect the disease any earlier, given that treatment following usual diagnosis will be effective.

Screening, then, is of greatest potential benefit when the critical point occurs between the time of first possible detection and the usual time of diagnosis (CP2). In this situation it may be that picking up the disease early would improve outcomes, and this is the aim of a **screening programme**. Unfortunately, we currently have too little knowledge of the progress of most diseases for this to have much practical value in planning screening programmes.

Screening versus case-finding

There is considerable debate about the best way to implement early detection of disease. Should the focus be on large-scale mass population screening, or are we better off pursuing opportunistic early detection or '**case-finding**' when someone comes into contact with the health system for another reason? There are some parallels here with the mass versus high-risk approach to primary prevention that we discussed in the previous chapter. The terms 'screening' and 'case-finding' can also have quite different meanings to different practitioners. We think it is most useful, and best accepted, to use the term 'screening' for organised population-wide approaches and 'case-finding' for more opportunistic attempts at early detection. If systematically applied, case-finding can nonetheless form the basis for quite good population coverage. For example, if a large proportion of the people visit a primary care physician every year or two, this contact could permit early detection of risks (e.g. from cigarette smoking, high blood pressure) in a setting that allows good follow-up.

The requirements of a screening programme

Screening differs from diagnostic testing in that it is performed *before* the development of clinical disease. Thus, those who undergo screening are free, or appear to be free, of the disease of interest. They are not seeking care because they are sick, but are instead persuaded to be screened by the health service. The requirements of a screening test are therefore somewhat different from those of a **diagnostic test**, which is performed only when someone is suspected to have a disease. While both should be as accurate as possible (see below), the screening test will often sacrifice some accuracy as it also has to be relatively cheap, very safe, and acceptable to someone who has no symptoms. Critically, though, an accurate test for a disease is not sufficient to justify a community screening programme. The suitability of a *disease* for screening has to be considered explicitly before all else and, finally, the whole *programme* must be shown to confer a net benefit to the community.

The disease

We need to consider the following characteristics of a disease before deciding whether screening for it may be desirable.

- The disease should be severe, relatively common and perceived as a public health problem by the community.
- We must understand the natural history of the disease sufficiently well that we can be reasonably sure that earlier detection will give a better outcome.

Prostate cancer shows us the importance of this. It appears to occur in a number of biological forms that we cannot tell apart, and it is probable that many men in whom a cancer could be detected by screening (e.g. with a prostate-specific antigen (PSA) test) would never develop symptoms or suffer from the disease (and therefore would not otherwise be diagnosed). This has been clearly seen in a number of studies of autopsies showing that many men who died of other diseases had microscopic cancers present in their prostate glands (Martin, 2007). To detect and treat these men would be wholly harmful and, largely for this reason, screening for prostate cancer is generally not recommended, even though there are tests that could be used (and which are used quite widely in some countries, e.g. the USA, on an ad-hoc case-finding basis). Research is under way in a number of countries in an attempt to shed light on this dilemma to allow a more informed judgement to be made.

- In general, there should be a high prevalence of pre-clinical (early-stage) disease.

This criterion becomes less important as the severity of the disease increases. For example, it may be of benefit to screen for a fairly uncommon disease if not treating it has severe consequences – an example is the use of screening for phenylketonuria (PKU) in newborns. Babies born with this condition lack an enzyme that metabolises the amino acid phenylalanine. When they eat proteins containing this amino acid, the end-products accumulate in the brain, leading to severe mental retardation. By simply restricting the phenylalanine in their diet this can be prevented. Although only about one in 15,000 babies is born with this condition, the availability of a simple, accurate and inexpensive test makes it worthwhile to screen all newborn babies (Wilcken *et al.*, 2003).

- Screening is likely to be more effective if there is a long period between the first detectable signs of disease and the overt symptoms that normally lead to diagnosis (the **lead time**).

If a disease progresses rapidly from the pre-clinical to clinical stages, i.e. the interval between the point when early diagnosis is theoretically possible and when clinical diagnosis would usually occur (see Figure 15.1) is short, then it is much harder to detect the disease by screening because this would have to occur within this narrow time window to have any benefit. (Clearly, metabolic conditions of early life, such as PKU, are exceptions to this because screening can be done at birth.)

The screening test

The next requirement for a worthwhile screening programme is that we have a test that will enable us to detect the disease before the usual time of diagnosis. Any such test must meet the following criteria.

- *Firstly it should be accurate.*

As discussed in Chapter 7, accuracy reflects the degree to which the results of the test correspond to the true state of the phenomenon being measured. In practice, accuracy can be influenced by the standardisation or calibration of the testing apparatus and by the skill of the person conducting or interpreting the test. Maintaining high standards of testing in a service setting is thus crucial for a screening programme to reach its full potential.

So what should we expect of a screening test in relation to its accuracy? We would expect it to be:

sensitive – ideally it would identify *all* people with the disease; in practice, it should identify *most* of these people;

specific – ideally it would identify *only* those with that particular disease and those without the disease should test negative; in practice, *most* of those without the disease should test negative.

The measures of **sensitivity** and **specificity** are also used to determine the accuracy of a diagnostic test (see Box 15.3).

• *It must be safe and acceptable to the population being screened.*

Because we are advising apparently well people to undergo screening, we should not offer them a test that might adversely affect their health. The only exception might be for those at very high risk of developing a serious disease, when a slight risk from screening might be outweighed by a large benefit of early diagnosis (e.g. regular colonoscopy for people with ulcerative colitis, who develop large bowel cancer at a high rate). Social and cultural acceptability are separate issues and are seldom related to the safety of the screening test. For example, the requirement to take a sample of their faeces to test for blood as an early indicator of colon cancer is unpalatable to many. Likewise, cervical cancer screening is not immediately appealing in many societies and in some it may be prohibited, particularly if the health professional is male.

• *It should be simple and cheap.*

If we wish to screen a large proportion of the population any test used should be relatively cheap to administer and simple to perform or it would be too costly to perform large-scale screening.

Mammography is neither simple nor cheap. Why then do you think that mammographic screening to detect early breast cancer is recommended?

Although mammography is neither simple nor cheap, breast cancer is a severe disease of substantial concern to many communities. It occurs relatively commonly and, if detected early, is usually highly treatable, with better outcomes than when treated later.

Test quality: sensitivity and specificity

We can evaluate the performance of a test by comparing the results with a 'gold standard' method that ideally would give 100% correct results (but more commonly is just the best test available). This standard might be a more costly or time-consuming test, or perhaps a combination of investigations performed in hospital that is reliable for diagnosis but unsuitable for routine use in screening.

For example, children in many countries undergo a simple hearing test in their first year at school. Any who fail this screening test are retested at a later date and/or referred to a hearing clinic for further, more extensive tests to identify whether they have a real hearing problem. Imagine that in a group of 500 children, 50 have a genuine hearing problem. Of these, 45 fail the school hearing test, as do 30 of the children with normal hearing (perhaps they had a cold on the day of the test).

Summarise the results of the test in a table, including labels for the rows and columns.

Your table should look something like Table 15.1.

Table 15.1 Hypothetical results from a school hearing test programme.

School hearing test	True hearing status		
	Hearing problem	Normal	Total
Fail (positive test result)	45	30	75
Pass (negative test result)	5	420	425
Total	50	450	500

Disease Status

		Positive	Negative
Test Result	Positive	True Positives *a*	False Positives *b*
	Negative	False Negatives *c*	True Negatives *d*

Figure 15.2 Possible outcomes from a screening test.

There are four possible outcomes for a child, as shown in Figure 15.2. A child with a real hearing problem may either fail the screening test (**true positive**; group '*a*' in Figure 15.2) or pass the test, suggesting falsely that they do not have a problem (**false negative**; group '*c*'). Similarly, a child without a problem may pass the test (**true negative**; group '*d*') or fail, falsely implying that they do have a problem (**false positive**; group '*b*').

For a test to be accurate it should produce few false positive and false negative results. So how good is the school hearing test? There are two issues to consider: how well has the test identified the children who do have a problem; and how well has it classified the normal children as normal?

What percentage of children with a real hearing problem failed the school test?

What percentage of children with normal hearing passed the school test?

Looking at Table 15.1, we see that 90% (45 ÷ 50) of children with a hearing problem failed the school test and 93% (420 ÷ 450) of children with normal hearing passed the test. These measures of a test are known, respectively, as its **sensitivity** and **specificity**.

The *sensitivity* of a test measures how well it classifies people with the condition as 'sick'. It is the *percentage of people with the condition who test positive* (90% in the example above). It is calculated by dividing the number of true positive results (*a*) by the total number of people with the condition $(a + c)$ from Figure 15.2:

$$\text{Sensitivity (\%)} = \frac{\text{True Positives}}{\text{All with Disease}} \times 100$$

$$= \frac{a}{(a + c)} \times 100 \tag{15.1}$$

The *specificity* of a test measures how well it classifies people without the condition as 'healthy'. It is the *percentage of people without the condition who test negative* (93% in the above example). To calculate it, we divide the number of true negative results (*d*) by the total number of people without disease $(b + d)$:

$$\text{Specificity (\%)} = \frac{\text{True Negatives}}{\text{All without Disease}} \times 100$$

$$= \frac{d}{(b + d)} \times 100 \tag{15.2}$$

A combination of high sensitivity and high specificity is essential for a good screening test – in this regard, the school hearing test works quite well.

Note that it is necessary to do a special (cross-sectional) study, as discussed in 'Diagnostic studies' in Chapter 4 (Box 4.7), to assess the sensitivity and specificity of a test. In the service setting, usually only those who test positive (groups '*a*' and '*b*' from Figure 15.2) will be followed up with formal diagnostic testing to determine the true positives. Those who test negative are not normally followed up, so the proportion of false negatives is not known and we cannot measure either the sensitivity or the specificity of the test.

Test performance in practice: positive and negative predictive values

Two other measures tell us how well a test performs in a given population. In practice we do not know at the point of testing whether a child does have a real hearing problem – we have to predict this from the screening test result. We therefore need to know how well a positive test result (i.e. failing the hearing test) predicts that a child really does have a hearing problem and, conversely, how well a negative test result (i.e. passing the hearing test) predicts that their hearing is normal.

What percentage of children who failed the school hearing test had a real hearing problem?

What percentage of children who passed the school hearing test really did have normal hearing?

Out of 75 children who failed the school hearing test, 45 (60%) had a real hearing problem. Out of 425 children who passed the school test, 420 (99%) really did have normal hearing.

These measures are known respectively as the **positive** and **negative predictive values** (PPV and NPV) of the test *in that situation*. Unlike the sensitivity and specificity, they are not fixed properties of the test because, as you will see below, they also depend on the prevalence of the condition in the population being tested.

The *positive predictive value* (PPV) tells us how likely it is that a positive test result indicates the presence of the condition. It is the *percentage of all people who test positive who really have the condition* (60% in the example). It is calculated by dividing the number of true positive results (a) by the total number of positive results ($a + b$):

$$\text{Positive Predictive Value } (\%) = \frac{\text{True Positives}}{\text{All Positives}} \times 100$$

$$= \frac{a}{(a+b)} \times 100 \qquad (15.3)$$

The *negative predictive value* (NPV) is the *percentage of all people who test negative who really do not have the condition* (99% in the example). To calculate it, simply divide the number of true negative results (d) by the total number of negative results ($c + d$):

$$\text{Negative Predictive Value } (\%) = \frac{\text{True Negative}}{\text{All Negative}} \times 100$$

$$= \frac{d}{(c+d)} \times 100 \qquad (15.4)$$

These measures of test performance are best thought of as operational measures of the overall programme. They reflect both the *accuracy of the test* (sensitivity and specificity) and the *prevalence* of the condition in the population tested. Even a superb test (very high sensitivity and specificity) will yield a low PPV if the condition is rare.

An example – testing blood donors for HIV infection

It is routine practice in most countries to screen all blood donors for HIV, but what is the probability that someone who tests positive really is infected with HIV?

What measure do we need to calculate to answer this question?

To answer this, we must calculate the positive predictive value of the test. Assume that we are using the test to screen a high-risk population of

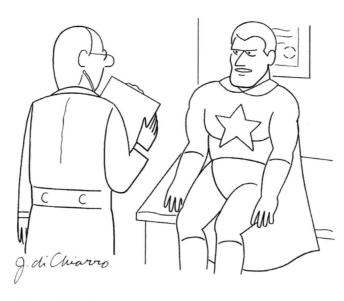

"Normal! What do you mean my test results are 'normal'?"

intravenous drug users in New York City who have an HIV prevalence of 5500 per 10,000. Using this information and your answers to the following questions, construct a table similar to Table 15.1 to show these data.[1]

How many in a group of 10,000 intravenous drug users would you expect to have HIV infection?

Of these, how many would test positive if the test had a sensitivity of 99.5%, and how many would falsely test negative?

How many of the drug users will not be HIV-positive and, of them, how many would test negative if the test had a specificity of 99.5%? How many would falsely test positive?

What proportion of the people who test HIV-positive would truly have HIV infection?

Given the known prevalence of HIV infection in this group, we would expect 5500 of the 10,000 intravenous drug users to be HIV-positive and the remaining 4500 would be HIV-negative, giving the 'total' row at the bottom of the table. Of the HIV-positive group, 99.5% or 5473 would correctly test

---

[1] If you are faced with questions about the performance of a screening of diagnostic test, the easiest way to look at the data is in the form of a 2×2 table (so-called because it has 2 main columns and 2 rows of data) like this.

positive and the remaining 27 would falsely test negative (giving the numbers for cells *a* and *c* in the table) and among the HIV-negative group 99.5% or 4478 would correctly test negative (*d*) and the remaining 22 would falsely test positive (*b*). Your table should then show a total of 5495 positive test results, of which 5473 or 99.6% are true positives (the PPV). Similarly, of the 4505 negative test results, 4478 or 99.4% are true negatives (the NPV). The test therefore performs very well in this high-risk population.

Now repeat the calculations for a low-risk population of new blood donors where the prevalence of HIV is only 4 per 10,000.

Among the blood donors we would expect only about 4 out of 10,000 people to be truly HIV-positive and the remaining 9996 would be HIV-negative. All four of the HIV-positive people should correctly test positive (Table 15.2). Among the HIV-negative group 99.5% or 9946 would correctly test negative and the remaining 50 would falsely test positive. This means that we now have a total of 54 positive test results but, of these, only 4 or 7.4% are true positives (PPV). This means that 93% or more than 9 of every 10 positive test results would be false positives.

Thus, even with a very high sensitivity and specificity, the same test performs badly in this low-risk population. The profound influence of changes in disease prevalence and test accuracy on the positive predictive value of a test is shown in Table 15.3. In practice, the lower values for sensitivity and specificity included in the table are often encountered, and for most diseases of consequence the prevalence in the general population is also quite low; for example, recent Australian data suggest the prevalence of breast cancer

Table 15.2 Positive and negative predictive values of an HIV test in high- and low-risk populations.

Test	True HIV status Positive	Negative	Total	
Intravenous drug users				
Positive	5,473	22	5,495	PPV = 5,473 ÷ 5,495 = 99.6%
Negative	27	4,478	4,505	NPV = 4,478 ÷ 4,505 = 99.4%
Total	5,500	4,500	10,000	
New blood donors				
Positive	4	50	54	PPV = 4 ÷ 54 = 7.4%
Negative	0	9,946	9,946	NPV = 9,946 ÷ 9,946 = 100%
Total	4	9,996	10,000	

Table 15.3 Variation in the positive predictive value of a test with prevalence of disease and accuracy of test.

Prevalence (%)	Sensitivity and specificity[a]			
	99%	95%	90%	80%
20	96.1%	82.1%	69.2%	50.0%
10	91.7%	67.9%	50.0%	30.8%
5	83.9%	50.0%	32.1%	17.4%
1	50.0%	16.1%	8.3%	3.9%
0.1	9.0%	1.9%	0.9%	0.4%

[a] Assuming, for convenience, that sensitivity and specificity have the same value.

among women aged 50–69 who attend for mammographic screening (the target age group) is around 0.3% (AIHW and NBOCC, 2009).

The prevalence of prostate cancer in 60-year-old men is approximately 1%. Using Table 15.3, how accurate would you want an ultrasound screening test to be before you would consider starting a screening programme to detect early prostate cancer?

With such a low prevalence, even a test with 99% sensitivity and specificity would give a positive predictive value of only 50%; i.e. half of all positive test results would be false positives. While this is less than ideal, in practice this is not necessarily the sole consideration in initiating a screening programme. For example, most studies of screening mammography have demonstrated that it achieves a positive predictive value in the range of only 10%–20% for women aged between 50 and 69 years. However, the reduction in breast cancer mortality associated with screening women over the age of 50 is deemed by most (but not all, see Box 15.5 at the end of the chapter) to outweigh the consequences of the large number of false positives that inevitably result.

Parallels with clinical diagnostic tests

Although tests used for screening and diagnosis may look similar, it is important to remember that these are two fundamentally different processes as shown in Table 15.4, which compares the attributes of a screening test and a test used for clinical diagnosis. However, the aspects of accuracy and predictive values that we have just discussed in relation to screening also apply to all **diagnostic tests**, although this is another situation where clinical epidemiologists use different terms for the same things. Box 15.3 shows an example.

Table 15.4 A comparison of screening and diagnostic tests.

	Screening tests	Diagnostic tests
Use	To identify people likely to have pre-clinical disease	To establish presence/absence of disease
Timing	Performed before development of clinical disease	Performed after onset of symptoms or when disease is suspected
Target population	Large numbers of asymptomatic but potentially at-risk individuals	People with symptoms to establish diagnosis, or asymptomatic individuals with a positive screening test
Characteristics	Relatively cheap, very safe, and acceptable to someone who has no symptoms	May be expensive, possibly invasive but justifiable if necessary to establish diagnosis
Performance	High sensitivity desirable so potential cases are not missed	High specificity important (to minimise false positives) as well as high sensitivity
Positive result	Identifies people who may have the disease and in whom further investigations are required	Result provides a definite diagnosis

Box 15.3 Accuracy and predictive values of diagnostic tests

A red tympanic membrane is generally considered a good predictor of acute otitis media (AOM) or middle-ear infection in children. However, in a study conducted to determine the accuracy of this sign compared with the results of the 'gold standard' test, myringotomy (incising the tympanic membrane), the sensitivity and specificity were found to be only 18% and 84%, respectively (Karma *et al.*, 1989). If we assume a **pre-test probability*** or prevalence of AOM of 50%, this means that only 53% of children with a red tympanic membrane will actually have AOM (the PPV or **post-test probability**), the other positive test results will be false positives. Similarly, 49% of those who do not have a red tympanic membrane will have AOM (false negatives). On its own, then, this is not a very accurate marker of AOM, but if seen together with other signs such as bulging and reduced mobility of the tympanic membrane the accuracy of diagnosis improves. Clinical decision rules based on the presence or absence of several known clinical features of a condition are useful tools to enhance diagnostic accuracy.

*This is another situation in which clinical epidemiologists use different terms to describe the same things. In clinical epidemiology the term '*pre-test probability*' is often used synonymously with *prevalence*. It represents the probability that the patient had the condition on the basis of information available before the test was undertaken, i.e. the prevalence of the condition and the patient's clinical picture. Similarly, the predictive values, which represent the probability that the patient has (or does not have) disease on the basis of test results, are often called '*post-test probabilities*'.

The trade-off between sensitivity and specificity

Let us assume that we have developed a new blood test that will screen people for a debilitating but treatable disease. The test involves measuring blood levels of a marker M and is far less invasive than the 'gold standard' test. To evaluate the new test, levels of M were measured in 225 people believed to be at moderately high risk for the disease and the results were compared with the 'gold standard' test. For the blood test, anyone with an M level of 20 mg/l or higher was said to have the disease. Figure 15.3 shows the distribution of M levels in people with and without the disease as diagnosed by the 'gold standard' test. The light bars on the left represent the 99 people who truly do not have the disease and the dark bars on the right represent the 126 people who truly do. When compared with the 'gold standard' results, 115 of 126 with disease tested positive (M levels ≥ 20 mg/l) as did 10 of 99 without disease; the remaining 11 with disease and 89 without had negative test results. We can summarise the data as shown in Table 15.5.

How accurate is the M test? (i.e. what are the sensitivity and specificity?)

How well has the test performed in this population? (i.e. what are the predictive values of the test?)

Figure 15.3 Distribution of M levels by disease status according to the 'gold standard' test.

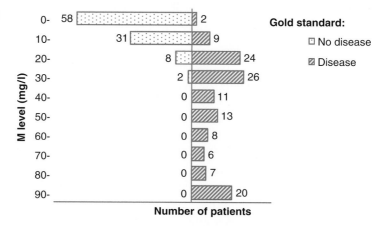

Table 15.5 A summary 2 × 2 table for the M test with a cut-off point of 20 mg/l.

	True disease status		
M test	Positive	Negative	Total
≥20 mg/l (positive)	115	10	125
<20 mg/l (negative)	11	89	100
Total	126	99	225

Using a cut-off of ≥ 20 mg/l to classify people as positive or negative we can calculate the following:

$$\text{Sensitivity} = \frac{115}{126} \times 100 = 91.3\%$$

$$\text{Specificity} = \frac{89}{99} \times 100 = 89.9\%$$

$$\text{PPV} = \frac{115}{125} \times 100 = 92.0\%$$

$$\text{NPV} = \frac{89}{100} \times 100 = 89.0\%$$

These look pretty good, but ideally we would like to have all of these values as close to 100% as possible. The M test has, for instance, missed the 11 people with the disease whose M values were less than 20 mg/l. So what if we were to lower the cut-off point to 10 mg/l? Looking again at Figure 15.3, this would mean that 9 of the 11 false negative people would now be correctly diagnosed as having the disease, but it would also mean that an extra 31 people without the disease would be included in the diseased group.

Calculate the sensitivity, specificity and PPV for this new cut-off point. (*Hint: use Table 15.5 as a guide to lay out a 2 × 2 table for the new cut-off point.*)

How do the values compare with those obtained using the higher cut-off point (20 mg/l)?

If we change the cut-off point to 10 mg/l the results are now as shown in Table 15.6. We can calculate the new sensitivity, specificity, PPV and NPV as we did above:

$$\text{Sensitivity} = \frac{124}{126} \times 100 = 98.4\%$$

$$\text{Specificity} = \frac{58}{99} \times 100 = 58.6\%$$

Table 15.6 Results of the M test using a cut-off point of 10 mg/l.

	True disease status		
M test	Positive	Negative	Total
≥ 10 mg/l (positive)	124	41	165
< 10 mg/l (negative)	2	58	60
Total	126	99	225

$$\text{PPV} = \frac{124}{165} \times 100 = 75.2\%$$

$$\text{NPV} = \frac{58}{60} \times 100 = 96.7\%$$

By changing the cut-point to ≥ 10 mg/l the sensitivity is now excellent and there are very few false negatives, but the specificity has markedly decreased. With the drop in specificity, the PPV of the test has fallen from 92% to 75% because there are now far more false positives (41 instead of 10).

Looking at the distribution of M levels in the two groups of people (Figure 15.3), we can see that, although they are clearly different, there is some overlap between the two. Where we decide to make the cut-off to try to differentiate between 'disease' and 'no disease' determines how many false positive and false negative test results we find. *There is, therefore, a trade-off to be made between sensitivity and specificity.* For any disease, the optimum point has to be selected depending on the consequences of missing a few positives if the cut-off point is set higher or falsely classifying more negatives as positive if the cut-off point is set lower. If early detection greatly reduced mortality from the disease, and if false positives could be identified fairly quickly and cheaply, and without adverse consequences by further testing, then clearly we would set the cut-point lower than if the reverse were the case. (See Box 15.4 for more about how we can assess the performance of a screening test.)

Box 15.4 ROC curves and likelihood ratio tests

One way to visualise the relation between sensitivity and specificity is with a 'receiver operating characteristic' or *ROC curve*. These were developed by the British during World War II to measure how well their radar receivers (hence the name) could discriminate between incoming German planes and flocks of birds. To generate a ROC curve we plot the *sensitivity* of a test against 1 (or 100%) minus the specificity of the test. Figure 15.4 shows the ROC curve for the M test (dark blue line). The closer the curve goes to the top left-hand corner of the graph where the sensitivity = 100% and specificity = 100% (i.e. 1 – specificity = 0%) the better the test, so the light blue curve shows a test that performs less well than the M test. One way to assess how well a test discriminates between people with and without disease is by calculating the *area under the curve* (often referred to as the AUC or C-statistic) where a value of 1.0 indicates a perfect test

(*continued*)

Box 15.4 (continued)

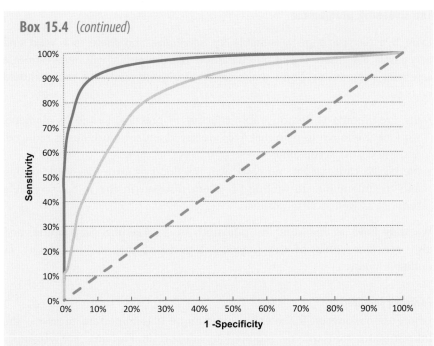

Figure 15.4 ROC curve for use of M levels (dark blue) to diagnose disease compared to an inferior test (light blue).

and a value of 0.5 indicates the test is performing no better than chance (shown by the dashed line in the figure).

You will also hear clinicians talking about the *likelihood ratio* (LR) for a test. This is the probability of getting a particular test result in someone who truly has the condition of interest divided by the probability of getting the same result in someone who does not have the condition. For a positive result this is equal to the sensitivity ÷ (1 – specificity). So for the M test with a cut-off of ≥ 20 mg/l the LR for a positive test is 91.3 ÷ 10.1 = 9.0. For a negative test the likelihood ratio is equal to (1 – sensitivity) ÷ specificity or 8.7 ÷ 89.9 = 0.1.

The large LR positive and small LR negative indicate that someone who is positive on this test is much more likely to actually have the disease than not, while someone who tests negative is very unlikely to have it. Their new 'post-test' probability of having/not having the disease depends on their 'pre-test' probability (before the test) and the LR and can be estimated using *Bayes' nomogram* (Attia, 2003).

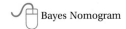 Bayes Nomogram

The screening programme

Even if a disease appears suitable for screening and there is a valid and acceptable test, there is still no guarantee that the public will benefit from a screening programme. Some major concerns beyond predictive values should be that:

- the programme is demonstrably effective in practice, i.e. all its elements work near enough to plan that lives are saved and/or morbidity is reduced, and the cost is acceptable;
- the health care system can cope with the flood of extra diagnostic testing and treatment due to finding prevalent disease (in the initial screening rounds) as well as false positives.

We thus have to measure the outcomes of a screening programme, and also consider some of the practical aspects of maintaining quality as outlined below.

Facilities required

Before embarking on a screening programme it is important to assess the infrastructure that will be required to support it. Facilities are obviously needed for the screening process but, equally importantly, they are also needed for the subsequent confirmatory testing and diagnosis, treatment and follow-up of those who test positive. Estimates are needed as to the likely uptake of screening, the total number of positive test results (including false positives) expected based on the prevalence of the disease and the sensitivity and specificity of the test, and the likely effect that this will have on the demand for medical services. *It is of no use, and is indeed unethical, to initiate a screening programme if the resources required in order to act upon the results are not available.*

Treatment

The proposed treatment must be effective and early initiation of treatment must improve the disease outcome. If it does not, then by diagnosing the disease earlier we will simply lengthen the time a person is aware of, and worrying about, the disease.

Cost

When a screening programme is introduced we must consider not only the financial cost, but also the emotional cost of both the screening and subsequent treatment for those who test positive and then weigh this against the costs of treating those who develop disease later. A positive balance is required between the costs of screening and the consequences of not screening.

Evaluation of a screening programme

The fact that a screening programme ought to work does not mean that it will in practice (see Box 15.1 at the start of the chapter). No mass screening should be introduced without convincing evidence of its likely effectiveness and it is imperative that the programme be evaluated as a whole. We will now look at the initial research that should precede the introduction of any full-scale population screening, and provide some comment on the necessary in-service monitoring that should follow its introduction.

It can be difficult to assess whether a programme will work. There are some relatively simple early *process measures* that can give an idea of how things are going, but ultimately we also have to show that the programme delivers improved *outcomes*. To see whether we have succeeded in detecting disease earlier than usual, we can compare the *stage of disease* in patients whose disease was detected at screening with the stage of disease in those in whom it was detected in the normal way. If cases identified at screening are less advanced, then at least the potential for benefit has been demonstrated. Another simple check on the process is the positive predictive value of the screening test being used. A high PPV reflects a good combination of an accurate test and an appropriate population (reasonably high prevalence).

A low PPV implies that the programme may be in trouble. Why?

As you saw above, a low PPV indicates that, of all the positive test results, only a few reflect true instances of disease, and the large number of false positives will lead to unnecessary concern and expense for those individuals. Because virtually all diseases considered serious enough for screening in the general population will have a fairly low prevalence, the PPV of any test will be less than optimal however high its sensitivity and specificity (refer back to Table 15.3). Health authorities and the general public need to agree explicitly on what level of false positives is acceptable, in the light of what these people will suffer. The community should also be given the chance to declare that they believe that a large benefit for a minority (only *some* of the 'true positives') outweighs the smaller losses (and the costs) suffered by a much larger group (the 'false positives').

Turning to outcome evaluation, the ultimate judge of the potential value of a screening programme, there are four areas we need to address:

- the health outcomes to be considered,
- potential sources of bias in the evaluation of a screening programme,
- the design of an evaluation study, and
- the negative consequences of screening.

Health outcomes to be considered

Quality of life is a particularly important issue for a disease like prostate cancer, where standard treatments can convey substantial morbidity.

It is important to identify the most important health outcomes that it is hoped the screening programme will deliver. For fatal conditions such as many cancers, a reduction in mortality is the most important outcome to be gained from a screening programme. However, mere prolongation of life might not adequately justify screening if the quality of the additional life is poor. Thus we should also consider absence or reduction of serious morbidity and improvement in quality of life as essential target outcomes for a screening programme. The quality-adjusted life years or QALYs that you met in Chapter 2 can help with this. Other sensible endpoints need to be set for non-fatal conditions: for example, we would want to know that detecting impaired hearing in school children led to some measurable benefits of consequence – perhaps improved performance at school.

Potential sources of bias in the evaluation of a screening programme

At first glance, it might seem that all we need to do is follow-up people who have and have not been screened to see what effects the screening has on their morbidity and mortality. However, such simple cohort comparisons are unreliable as bias is a major problem and, as you will see, what we really need is evidence from randomised trials. There are three major sources of bias to be dealt with in any evaluation of the effects of screening: *volunteer bias*, *lead-time bias* and *length bias*. All are special forms of selection bias and will lead to inappropriate comparisons unless dealt with properly.

Volunteer bias

People who attend for screening are likely to differ from those who do not. They tend to be of higher socioeconomic status, to be more health-conscious and more likely to comply with prescribed advice. Thus, better results for a screening programme of volunteers compared with disease outcomes in non-volunteers may relate to factors associated with the 'volunteerism', rather than benefits of treatment following earlier diagnosis. (This is the same volunteer bias that you saw when we discussed selection bias in Chapter 7.)

In the HIP trial of mammographic screening (described in Box 15.5), only about two-thirds of the 31,000 women randomly allocated to the mammography group actually took up the initial offer to be screened and less than half attended all four annual examinations. After 5 years of follow-up of all women in the intervention arm, i.e. all those who were offered screening, those women who had refused breast screening had much higher mortality from all causes and from cardiovascular disease than those who were screened (Table 15.7).

Table 15.7 Volunteerism among women randomly allocated to the mammography group in the HIP study, showing that mortality was lower among women who took up the offer of mammography than among those who did not.

Women randomly allocated to mammography	Deaths per 10,000 women per year	
	All causes	Cardiovascular
Women who underwent mammography	42	17
Women who refused the offer of mammography	77	38
Total	54	24

(Sackett *et al.*, 1991)

Because the screening was directed only at breast cancer, why might women who came for screening have lower mortality rates for causes other than breast cancer?

The most likely reason is 'volunteer bias' – the women who took up the offer of screening were different in important ways from those who did not. (And note that Table 15.8 shows that the overall rates of total and cardiovascular mortality were essentially the same in both arms of the trial, reinforcing the fact that the mammographic screening itself did not affect these outcomes.)

The only reliable way to avoid this type of bias is to recruit a pool of volunteers and then *assign them randomly* to receive screening or no screening, just as they did in the HIP trial (Box 15.5). It is also important to ensure that as many as possible of those assigned to screening are actually screened. The correct analysis is then by **intention to treat**, i.e. comparing the groups as they were originally randomised, regardless of whether women were actually screened. If only those who actually received the screening are compared with the rest, we lose all the benefits of the randomisation in terms of controlling for confounding and avoidance of selection bias. (As you saw in Table 15.7, those who do take up screening are likely to have inherently better health outcomes than those who do not, regardless of the screening.) This analysis is not only theoretically correct, but also reflects the reality of public health practice because not all of us will eagerly take up each preventive opportunity. Details of this analysis are described below, and shown in Table 15.8.

Lead-time bias

Lead-time is the period between when disease is detected by screening and when it would have become symptomatic and been diagnosed in the usual way. Consider a situation in which breast cancer starts to develop (disease onset)

Table 15.8 Detection of new breast cancers and mortality from breast cancer, all causes other than breast cancer and cardiovascular disease in the HIP study.

Study group	Breast cancer cases in the first 10 years (per 1000 person-years[a])	Deaths (per 10,000 women per year[a])				
		Breast cancer			All other causes	Cardiovascular disease
		Age 40–49	Age 50–59	Age 60–69		
Control	2.1	2.4	5.0	5.0	54	25
Mammography	2.1	2.5	2.3	3.4	54	24
Change	–	+4%	–54%	–32%	–	–4%

[a] Units as reported.
(Shapiro, 1989; Sackett *et al.*, 1991)

Box 15.5 Mammographic screening for breast cancer – still generating controversy

Mammographic (X-ray) screening for breast cancer has been evaluated in a number of different countries. One of the first randomised trials conducted to determine its efficacy was the Health Insurance Plan (HIP) study in New York – an inspired initiative that linked the introduction of breast screening to a health insurance scheme. In this large-scale trial, 62,000 women aged 50–64 years who were members of this insurance plan were invited to participate in the early 1960s. About 31,000 women were randomly allocated to the intervention group and offered an initial mammographic (and physical) screening examination followed by three additional screening examinations at yearly intervals. Another 31,000 women were randomly allocated to the control group and were not offered the screening programme. After 18 years of follow-up, breast cancer mortality was 23% lower in the group offered screening (Shapiro *et al.*, 1985). These promising first results were the basis for many countries to consider mammography as a valuable public health tool, particularly in 50–64-year-old women.

However, there are still controversial issues to be resolved.

- The results of most studies have not shown a marked benefit of screening women aged under 50 years.
- There have been criticisms of this and other core mammographic screening trials and, although these have generally been rebutted, they indicate that there are complex issues involved, both in conducting the studies and in interpreting the results. This has been highlighted by two

(continued)

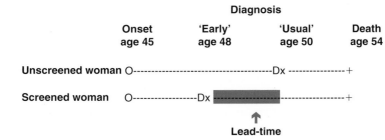

Figure 15.5 The lead time associated with screening in two individuals. The shaded area represents the lead time.

in two women at age 45. One attends for mammography and the tumour is detected at age 48, while the other is diagnosed at the age of 50 when she notices a lump in her breast. Both women die of their cancer at age 54 (Figure 15.5). The first woman has survived for 6 years following the discovery of the tumour while the second has lived for only 4 years following diagnosis.

Without knowledge of the time of onset of disease, the screening process appears to have increased the survival time by 2 years for the woman who was screened when in fact their disease courses were identical. Both women have lived for 9 years following the initial development of the tumour. The first woman has just known and worried about her disease, and perhaps been without one breast, for 2 years longer than the second woman. This is known as 'lead-time bias' and, if ignored, it would distort a direct comparison of survival rates in screened and unscreened groups. Conventionally, survival is often calculated for a 5-year period after diagnosis of cancer: in this example, the woman diagnosed clinically (unscreened) who died 4 years after diagnosis would not be in the numerator of the survival rate, i.e. she would be defined as a 'non-survivor'. However, her exact counterpart in the screened group who died 6 years after diagnosis would be included as a survivor, incorrectly suggesting a benefit from screening. If lead-time bias is ignored, the survival among women who were screened would appear to be higher than that among women diagnosed clinically, even if their disease courses were identical. A related phenomenon is the apparent transient increase in incidence seen when a screening programme is first introduced as the screening detects prevalent cases in the population earlier than they would normally have been detected (e.g. see Törnberg *et al.*, 2006).

So unless we have some idea of the actual lead time, perhaps from previous studies, we should not use survival time from diagnosis to evaluate a screening programme. Instead, we should consider the effects on longer-term age-specific morbidity or mortality rates of the disease. These rates are less likely to be affected by early diagnosis than time-limited survival rates, and should therefore better reflect the true benefits of early treatment. Table 15.8 shows such results from the HIP study evaluating the effectiveness of mammography, based on a 10-year follow-up.

Describe the data reported in Table 15.8 above. Would you implement a breast-screening programme on the basis of these results?

Table 15.8 compares breast cancer detection rates and breast cancer mortality rates (separately for three age groups) among the group randomly allocated to mammography (regardless of whether they actually underwent the procedure) and the control group. It also shows the mortality rates for cardiovascular disease and for all causes other than breast cancer. Cardiovascular and 'all-other-cause' mortality rates were similar for the two groups (implying that the randomisation process had created two equivalent, i.e. 'exchangeable', groups of women), but breast cancer mortality rates in women aged 50–59 and 60–69 years were substantially lower in the group randomly allocated to screening. On the basis of these data alone it would appear that a breast cancer screening programme for women between the ages of 50 and 64 (the maximum age of women when they entered the study) should certainly be considered. In practice, it would also be important to consider other aspects of this study, to ensure that the results were valid; and given that we are making our judgement many years after these data were published, we must also examine the results of other studies in this area, ideally through a formal systematic review and meta-analysis (see Chapter 11).[2]

Over the 10 years of follow-up in the HIP Study, **breast cancer detection rates** in the two groups were very similar. Screening does not alter the underlying incidence of disease (although introduction of screening may be associated with an apparent transient increase in incidence due to detection of prevalent cases, and/or a small ongoing increase due to detection of clinically insignificant tumours), but simply improves the outcome after diagnosis.

---

[2] As noted in Box 15.5 this has been done, and there has been sufficient variation in the results of subsequent RCTs to leave the policy implications less certain than they appear from the HIP data.

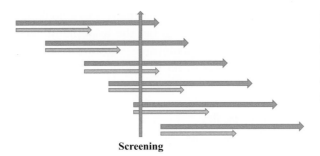

Figure 15.6 Length bias. Dark bars represent slowly developing and light bars rapidly developing disease. The length of the bar indicates the duration of the detectable pre-clinical state.

Screening

Length bias

When we screen for disease we are also more likely to detect cases where the disease is progressing slowly. This is because, as we discussed earlier (look back to 'The disease'), rapidly developing disease will become clinically apparent sooner and so be more likely to be diagnosed outside a screening programme. These cases that are diagnosed between regular screening visits are sometimes called 'interval' cases. The 'slower' cases that are more likely to be detected by screening (remember, prevalence is a function of incidence and duration) are likely to have an inherently more favourable outcome, and the effect of this will again tend to make screening appear more favourable than it really is. **Length bias** refers to this over-representation of slowly progressing disease among cases detected by screening (see Figure 15.6 which shows that at any point in time there will be more slowly developing cases in the population than rapidly developing cases). Randomisation should give an even balance of each type of case in screened and unscreened groups, again eliminating this as a problem for comparisons of age-specific mortality.

Design of a study to evaluate a screening programme

The preceding discussion should make it clear that the initial evaluation of a novel screening programme requires a randomised trial to allay concerns about these varied threats to validity; no other design can be wholly convincing in this regard. However, it is important to note that there are situations where this is not possible, for example for ethical reasons, as in the case of cervical cancer screening (see below), and in this case we need to rely on other sources of evidence. Moreover, once a screening programme has been rolled out as part of a health service's disease control activities it needs further monitoring and evaluation in that setting. As randomisation to the intervention will no longer be an option, this will generally include careful assessment of the process measures we discussed above and monitoring of population-wide descriptive data including trends in incidence and mortality rates. Making sound judgements from such data is challenging, but the example of cervical cancer below gives a sense of what is achievable. However, before we look at these non-randomised designs, let us return to consider some examples of random-ised studies.

Randomised studies

Secure long-term benefits of a screening programme must be documented before it can be adopted for widescale use. Ideally, this demands a number of randomised trials with persons assigned to be offered screening or not, and then followed for some time (usually many years) to assess their health. Inevitably, in the short term more disease will be found among those screened, so the real issue is whether their survival or quality of life is enhanced in the long term. The HIP study mentioned above was a landmark in this respect, with the investigators showing great foresight in realising the need for a very large long-term trial. It included over 60,000 women and the length of follow-up was 18 years, but even so, from the point of view of obtaining reliable results, the numbers of deaths from breast cancer were not very great in the earlier years of the study. A smaller study, or one that was conducted for only a short period of time, would not have been sufficient to show with any certainty (i.e. precision) whether breast cancer screening was of benefit. Additional data from subsequent RCTs, combined in the form of a meta-analysis, have allowed more reliable assessment of the value of mammographic screening (National Cancer Institute, 2015). However, as noted above, this is still not definitive; nonetheless, both the National Cancer Institute and the US Preventive Services Taskforce continue to recom-mend biennial mammography for women 50–75 (US Preventive Services Taskforce, 2015).

Large bowel cancer is the only other cancer for which strong evidence from randomised studies shows a consistent mortality benefit from screening using a simple test for blood in a person's stools (Ee and Olynyk, 2009). The widely accepted benefits of screening for cervical cancer by a smear test to detect abnormal cells are based on much weaker evidence (see non-randomised studies below), as it had become an accepted part of medical practice before the benefits of RCTs for assessing screening programmes were realised. And while prostate cancer screening by testing PSA levels in blood is widely practised in the USA, and to a lesser degree in some other countries (essen-tially large-scale case-finding, as there are no organised public programmes), supportive trial data are lacking. A number of large RCTs have now reported interim results, although these have not resolved the questions of the magni-tude (if any) of any absolute benefit from screening, nor the trade-offs

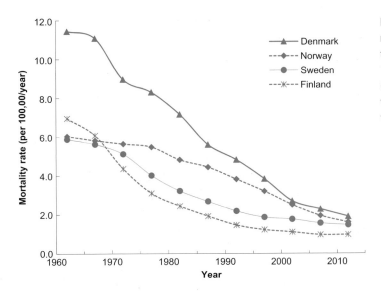

Figure 15.7 Cervical cancer mortality rates (5-year averages, standardised to the world population) from 1960–2012 in the Nordic countries. (*Data source*: NORDCAN, http://www-dep.iarc.fr/NORDCAN/english/frame.asp, accessed 14 March 2015.)

(expected to be substantial, see below) in terms of extra morbidity and costs of screening (Ilic *et al.*, 2013).

Non-randomised studies

As you saw in Chapters 7 and 8, non-randomised studies are much more prone to selection bias and confounding than are randomised studies. However, they are sometimes the only source of evidence available. Ecological studies have been used as the primary evidence to evaluate the impact of cervical screening on rates of cervical cancer and, as an example, Figure 15.7 shows changes in cervical cancer mortality rates over time in Scandinavia.

What are the most striking elements of this figure?

Perhaps the most conspicuous feature of the graph is the fact that, until about 1975, cervical cancer mortality rates in Denmark were double those elsewhere in Scandinavia. Leaving Denmark aside for the moment, we can see that between 1965 and 1980, mortality fell more rapidly in Finland and Sweden, where nationwide screening programmes had been introduced in the early 1960s, than it did in Norway, where, at that time, only 5% of the population was covered by screening (nationwide screening was not introduced until 1995). This visual impression is reinforced by a more formal analysis that indicated that, between 1965 and 1982, cumulative cervical cancer mortality rates fell by 50% in Finland and 34% in Sweden compared with a drop of only 10% in Norway (Laara *et al.*, 1987). Since 1980 the rates have continued to fall in all three countries.

So what about Denmark? Mortality has also fallen there, but, although the *absolute* drop is quite dramatic, the *relative* fall between 1965 and 1982 was only 25%, i.e. somewhere between that in Sweden and that in Norway, and this fits with the intermediate level of screening in Denmark – about 40% coverage of the population by 1980. Thus the data appear to support the hypothesis that screening does reduce mortality from cervical cancer, but, as you saw in Chapter 3, the results of an ecological study can be hard to interpret. For example, it has been pointed out that the fall in cervical cancer rates in some of these countries actually began before the introduction of screening, emphasising the problems of separating out other temporal effects, such as social change. It is difficult from these data to say how much of an impact the screening really had, although other evidence now supports the claim that cervical cancer screening confers a real benefit in terms of saving life.

Case–control studies have also been used to compare those with and without disease with respect to their history of screening. For example, case–control studies of bowel cancer have shown that screening sigmoidoscopy is associated with 50%–70% lower mortality from cancers in the parts of the bowel that are within reach of the sigmoidoscope, but with no difference in mortality from tumours in parts of the bowel that cannot be reached (Selby *et al.*, 1992). This design has a number of practical advantages over prospective studies, including the fact that case–control studies can often be conducted more quickly and at relatively low cost; however, considerable care must go into the design stage and interpreting the data can pose a number of additional challenges (Walter, 2003).

Non-randomised studies are most important once a screening programme has been established as a standard public health intervention, as ongoing monitoring and evaluation is required to check that the benefits shown in the research trials are actually achieved in practice. In the early stages, process measures of the sort noted above (e.g. a shift towards diagnosis of cancer at an earlier stage, high predictive values) will be prominent. In the longer term the focus needs to change to disease-specific outcomes, for example ecological-type assessments of the contributions of a screening programme to any changes in disease patterns seen, as for the cervical cancer example you saw above (see National Cancer Institute, 2015 for more examples). This need for ongoing monitoring using routine data holds for all large-scale population interventions, not just for screening programmes, and emphasises the importance of high-quality administrative data for in-service programme evaluation.

The negative consequences of a screening programme

Our prime focus in the previous discussion was how to validly assess whether screening provides a health benefit. However, this is only part of the story; the potential harms that may follow screening also have to be considered and must be found to be substantially less than the benefits before screening can proceed. We therefore summarise below the sorts of problems that can follow from offering screening to healthy individuals as a counterbalance to any unbridled enthusiasm you may have developed for screening as a strategy for disease control.

The negative effects or harm that can result from screening are different for those people with positive test results and those with negative test results. Potential harm for those with a positive test result includes the possibilities of:

- complications arising from investigation,
- adverse effects of treatment,
- unnecessary treatment of persons with true positive test results who have inconsequential disease (this is central to doubts over prostate cancer screening, and almost certainly important for breast cancer as well (National Cancer Institute, 2015; Independent UK Panel on Breast Screening, 2012),
- adverse effects of labelling someone as having disease or early diagnosis,
- anxiety generated by the investigations and treatment, and
- costs and inconvenience incurred during investigations and treatment.

For example, it has been estimated that, of 1000 women aged less than 50 years screened every two years by mammography for 10 years, 251 women will have an abnormal mammogram (Barratt *et al.*, 2005). This group will then undergo more than 300 additional procedures, with 60 women having at least one biopsy, but only 12 women will finally be diagnosed as having cancer and three of these cancers will be ductal carcinoma in situ, a pre-cancerous lesion for which the benefit of surgical and medical intervention remains uncertain. This represents a PPV for mammography of about 5% for all cancers and 4% for invasive cancer among women aged under 50 years. The other 239 women whose mammograms were abnormal will have undergone the stress of follow-up testing for no clear benefit. Another nine of the women whose mammogram is negative for breast cancer will be diagnosed with *interval cancers* when they present with symptoms between their regular screening visits. The corresponding PPVs for women over the age of 50 are 10%–19% and 7%–16%, i.e. two to four times higher, thus the benefits of screening will also be higher. (Improvements in technology may improve the situation somewhat, but the fundamental problem of very low prevalence remains.) We also noted above the uncertainties that still surround screening for prostate cancer; as at 2009, the trial data show an approximate doubling of major interventions (surgery, radiotherapy, both of which have serious side effects) in the men offered screening, for at best a modest lowering of mortality (Barry, 2009).

Potential harm for those with a negative test result includes the possibilities of:

- false reassurance if the result turns out to be a false negative and there is delayed presentation of symptomatic disease later,
- anxiety generated by the screening test and waiting for the result, and
- costs and inconvenience incurred during the screening test.

Harm from screening programmes can therefore include the following.

(1) *Physical harm* from complications, invasive tests and/or treatments, especially if falsely positive, or from delayed presentation if falsely negative.
(2) *Psychological harm* from anxiety, anger or depression from waiting, distress from invasive tests or procedures, knowing a serious diagnosis earlier without improved prognosis, and from falsely negative or positive test results.
(3) *Financial harm* from the costs of tests, medical appointments, possible hospitalisation and treatments.

We detail these negatives to emphasise the need to take a balanced view of what we are really offering the public when we introduce a screening programme. If we overemphasise the potential benefits, and neglect serious consideration of how a community might view and be impacted by the harms, we do everyone a disservice.

Summary

A recent systematic review concluded that reductions in disease-specific mortality are uncommon and reductions in all-cause mortality are rare or non-existent for most currently available screening tests (Saquib *et al.*, 2015).

Screening is an inherently attractive public health strategy for controlling some diseases, particularly when no or few feasible avenues for primary prevention exist, as early diagnosis of disease among apparently well people can certainly lead to better outcomes. Nonetheless, its popularity among some segments of the public and the health professions may over-represent its capabilities, especially if people expect the results of a screening test to be 100% accurate all of the time. A cool-headed approach is required, and some simple questions make a good starting point when considering screening.

- Is this disease appropriate for screening?
- Do we have a truly valid test?
- How well could a screening programme work in our community?

Points to look for when evaluating the potential benefits of screening include the stage of disease in cases detected by screening, a high positive predictive value for the screening test and, most importantly, demonstrated and worthwhile improvement in outcomes in randomised trials.

These are the scientific aims. We then have to think practically and ethically. Other questions we should ask include the following.

- Do we have the resources to implement the programme, and to deal with the extra clinical and psychological load that will ensue?
- If we are taking resources from other public health programmes, are we sure that we are improving the overall cost–benefit ratio for the community?
- Does our community truly understand and accept the inherent trade-off – namely, that there will be a large benefit for only a few and some costs (mostly smaller) for many others, and that some disease will be missed?

These are not light challenges to be faced.

Questions

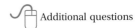 Additional questions

1. Papanicolau (Pap) smear screening is currently the accepted method for early detection of cervical cancer and women with an abnormal Pap smear result are referred to a gynaecologist for colposcopy for definitive diagnosis. To see whether repeat Pap screening would reduce the number of unnecessary referrals, 110 women with an abnormal Pap smear were given both a second Pap smear and colposcopy. The colposcopy showed that 13 women had high-grade lesions and 97 did not. The result of the repeat Pap test was abnormal for 12 of the women with and 72 without high-grade lesions.
   (a) Construct a 2 × 2 table comparing repeat Pap test with colposcopy.
   (b) Calculate the sensitivity and specificity of the repeat Pap test.
   (c) What is the positive predictive value of the repeat Pap test?
   (d) What is the probability that a woman whose repeat Pap test gives a negative result actually has a high-grade lesion?
   (e) Could a second Pap smear be used to identify women who should be referred for colposcopy?

2. An experimental screening test for hepatitis B has a sensitivity of 82% and a specificity of 93%. The prevalence of hepatitis B in the population to be screened is estimated to be 3%.
   (a) What is the probability that an individual with a positive test result does not have hepatitis B?
   (b) Using this test, what proportion of a population free of hepatitis B would falsely test positive?

3. You are considering introducing a prostate cancer screening programme using the PSA (prostate-specific antigen) test. You know that the test has a sensitivity of 85% and a specificity of 80% for detecting prostate cancer and that the prevalence of prostate cancer in men over 60 years of age is 4%.
   (a) Among a group of 10,000 men aged over 60, how many would be expected to have prostate cancer and how many of these would be expected to have a positive PSA test?

(b) How many men would not have prostate cancer and, of these, how many would have a positive PSA test?

(c) Summarise these data in a table and calculate the positive predictive value of a positive PSA test.

(d) How useful is the PSA test in this population? Consider both the negative and positive outcomes for men who are screened.

(e) If the prevalence of prostate cancer among men older than 70 years is 15% would it be better to restrict screening to this age group?

(f) What characteristics of a disease make it one for which we would consider introducing a screening programme?

For further questions relating to screening, see an excellent case study, '*Screening for antibody to the human immunodeficiency virus*' from the Epidemic Intelligence Service of the US Centers for Disease Control and Prevention (CDC-EIS, 2003, Student Guide #871–703), which is freely available from their website: http://www.cdc.gov/eis/casestudies.html.

REFERENCES

 References

AIHW (Australian Institute of Health and Welfare) and NBOCC (National Breast and Ovarian Cancer Centre). (2009). *Breast Cancer in Australia: An Overview, 2009*. Cancer series no. 50. Cat. no. CAN 46. Canberra: AIHW.

Attia, J. (2003). Moving beyond sensitivity and specificity: using likelihood ratios to help interpret diagnostic tests. *Australian Prescriber*, 26(5): 111–113.

Barratt, A., Howard, K., Irwig, L., Salkeld, G. and Houssami, N. (2005). Model of outcomes of screening mammography: information to support informed choices. *British Medical Journal*, 330: 1–5.

Barry, M. J. (2009) Screening for prostate cancer – the controversy that refuses to die. *New England Journal of Medicine*, 360: 1351–1354.

Ee, H. C. and Olynyk, J. K. (2009). Making sense of differing bowel cancer screening guidelines. *Medical Journal of Australia*, 190: 348–349.

Gøtzsche, P. C. and Jørgensen, K. J. (2013). Screening for breast cancer with mammography (Review). *Cochrane Database of Systematic Reviews*, Issue 6. Art. No.: CD001877. DOI: 10.1002/14651858.CD001877.pub5.

Ilic, D., Neuberger, M. M., Djulbegovic, M. and Dahm, P. (2013). Screening for prostate cancer. *Cochrane Database of Systematic Reviews*, Issue 1. Art. No.: CD004720. DOI: 10.1002/14651858.CD004720.pub3.

Independent UK Panel on Breast Cancer Screening. (2012). The benefits and harms of breast cancer screening: an independent review. *The Lancet*, 380: 1778–1786.

Karma, P. H., Penttila, M. A., Sipila, M. M. and Katajs, M. J. (1989). Otoscopic diagnosis of middle ear effusion in acute and non-acute otitis media. I. The value of otoscopic findings. *International Journal of Pediatric Otorhinolaryngology*, 17: 37–49.

Laara, E., Day, N. E. and Hakama, M. (1987). Trends in mortality from cervical cancer in the Nordic countries: association with organised screening programmes. *Lancet*, 1: 1247–1249.

Martin, R. M. (2007). Commentary: Prostate cancer is omnipresent, but should we screen for it? *International Journal of Epidemiology*, 36: 278–281.

National Cancer Institute. (2015). PDQ® Cancer Information Summaries: Screening/Detection (Testing for Cancer). http://www.cancer.gov/cancerto pics/pdq/screening, accessed 19 February 2015.

Sackett, D. L., Haynes, R. B., Guyatt, G. H. and Tugwell, P. (1991). *Clinical Epidemiology. A Basic Science for Clinical Medicine*, 2nd edn. Boston, MA: Little Brown and Co.

Saquib, N., Saquib, J. and Ioannidis, J. P. A. (2015). Does screening for disease save lives in asymptomatic adults? Systematic review of meta-analyses and randomized trials. *International Journal of Epidemiology*, 44: 264–277.

Selby, J. V., Friedman, G. D., Quesenberry Jr, C. P. and Weiss, N. S. (1992). A case–control study of screening sigmoidoscopy and mortality from colorectal cancer. *New England Journal of Medicine*, 326: 653–657.

Shapiro S. (1989) Determining the efficacy of breast cancer screening. *Cancer*, 63: 1873–1880.

Shapiro, S., Venet, W., Strax, P., Venet, L. and Roeser, R. (1985). Selection, follow-up, and analysis in the Health Insurance Plan Study: a randomized trial with breast cancer screening. *National Cancer Institute Monograph*, 67: 65–74.

The South-East London Screening Group. (1977). A controlled trial of multiphasic screening in middle-age: results of the South-East London Screening Study. *International Journal of Epidemiology*, 6: 357–363; reprinted in 2001; *International Journal of Epidemiology*, 30: 935–940.

Törnberg, S., Kemetli, L., Lynge, E., *et al.* (2006). Breast cancer incidence and mortality in the Nordic capitals, 1970–1998. Trends related to mammography screening programmes. *Acta Oncologica*, 45: 528–535.

US Preventive Services Taskforce. (2015). *Breast Cancer Screening Draft Recommendations*. http://www.uspreventiveservicestaskforce.org/Page/Topic/rec ommendation-summary/breast-cancer-screening, accessed 7 June 2015.

Various. (2001). Commentaries on the South-East London Screening Study. *International Journal of Epidemiology*, 30: 940–947.

Walter, S. D. (2003) Mammographic screening: case–control studies. *Annals of Oncology*, 14: 1190–1192.

Wilcken, B., Wiley, V., Hammond, J. and Carpenter, K. (2003). Screening newborns for inborn errors of metabolism by tandem mass spectrometry. *New England Journal of Medicine*, 348: 2304–2312.

RECOMMENDED FOR FURTHER READING

- The original paper from screening study discussed in Box 15.1 plus a series of commentaries on this:

  The South-East London Screening Group. (1977). A controlled trial of multi-phasic screening in middle-age: results of the South-East London Screening Study. *International Journal of Epidemiology*, 6: 357–363; reprinted in 2001; *International Journal of Epidemiology*, 30: 935–940.

  Various. (2001). Commentaries on the South-East London Screening Study. *International Journal of Epidemiology*, 30: 940–947.

- A discussion of the history and current relevance of screening for prostate cancer:

  Martin, R. M. (2007). Commentary: Prostate cancer is omnipresent, but should we screen for it? *International Journal of Epidemiology*, 36: 278–281.

- A systematic review looking at whether screening for disease really saves lives:

  Saquib, N., Saquib, J. and Ioannidis, J. P. A. (2015). Does screening for disease save lives in asymptomatic adults? Systematic review of meta-analyses and randomized trials. *International Journal of Epidemiology*, 44: 264–277.

Epidemiology and the public's health

Box 16.1 The role of epidemiology in translational research

Translational research can be divided into five separate phases (T0–T4) and epidemiology has a key role to play in all of these (from Khoury *et al.*, 2010):

T0: *Description and discovery*: describing patterns of health and disease by person, place and time; observational studies to identify potential 'causes' of health outcomes.

T1: *From discovery to application (e.g. tests, interventions)*: clinical and population studies to further characterise discoveries from T0 and identify potential interventions to improve health.

T2: *From application to evidence-based guidelines*: observational and experimental studies to assess the efficacy of an intervention to inform guidelines and recommendations.

T3: *From guidelines to practice*: studies to assess the implementation and uptake of guidelines (e.g. identifying barriers to uptake).

T4: *From practice to health outcomes*: evaluation studies to assess the effectiveness of interventions (e.g. a screening programme) in practice.

In the preceding chapters we have covered the core principles and methods of epidemiology and have shown you some of the main areas where epidemiological evidence is crucial for policy and planning. You will also have gained a sense of the breadth and depth of the subject from the examples throughout the book. To finish off we will take a broader look at the role of epidemiological practice and logic in improving health. This process where research evidence is used to change practice or policy is known as *translation* (see Box 16.1).

Translating epidemiological research into practice

When epidemiological evidence is both sufficient and sound it has the potential for direct translation into public health (and clinical) practice and policy. In addition to providing primary research evidence to identify and test potential interventions to improve health, you saw in Chapter 11 the fundamental role of epidemiology in *knowledge synthesis* through systematic reviews and meta-analyses to better inform all stages of the research and translation continuum. You have also encountered many examples of the application of simple descriptive tools to evaluate disease control programmes once they have been implemented. However, policy makers must have confidence in the quality of our data and the soundness and impartiality of our interpretations of those data. As you have seen, the evidence will often not include any data from experiments. How then can we give assurances as to the soundness of our data and their meaning?

Sometimes the data almost 'speak for themselves', but this is uncommon. The role of cigarette smoke in the lung cancer epidemics perhaps comes closest. Here the accumulated mass of causal evidence – very strong associations from observational studies, powerful dose–response effects, consistency across multiple studies, the proven carcinogenicity of many ingredients of tobacco smoke, and clear evidence that smoking preceded the onset of cancer (temporality) – made a compelling case. The fact that the associations became stronger when 'dose' of smoking was measured more accurately through detailed questioning, together with validation of self-reported smoking status using serum or saliva cotinine levels, a biomarker for nicotine intake, made measurement error an unlikely explanation. But perhaps most influential were the huge relative risks, generally of the order of 10–20 for smokers compared to non-smokers, which made it virtually impossible for confounding to explain away the link. In many countries these observational data were rapidly translated into anti-smoking programmes, the beneficial results of which you have seen in previous chapters. However, over 60 years after the original case–control studies, and 50 years since the influential policy document from the US Surgeon General (U.S. Department of Health, Education, and Welfare, 1964) on the harmful effects of smoking, smoking in Western societies has not been eliminated, despite a raft of legislative and behavioural science-driven interventions. Even with strong evidence, full translation is tricky, and goes well beyond science.

Box 16.2 Beta-carotene: an epidemiological tale

The history of nutritional epidemiology is based on the identification and correction of specific deficits in what came to be called vitamins, as well as the need to provide adequate energy for growth. In the second half of the twentieth century, observations from descriptive studies comparing populations with adequate energy intake led to hypotheses that much of the uneven distribution of non-infectious diseases, especially cancers and heart diseases, could be due to dietary differences between populations. This led to a flood of analytic epidemiology and parallel laboratory work as scientists tried to identify specific cancer-causing agents (carcinogens) and possible cancer preventives.

Observational studies suggested that a number of cancers occurred less commonly among individuals and groups who ate more fruit and vegetables, and laboratory studies showed (amongst many other factors) that vitamin A and related compounds (retinoids) were promising anti-carcinogens. The strands were woven together and beta-carotene, the principal dietary precursor of vitamin A, was identified in the laboratory and in case–control and cohort studies as a substance that might underlie the beneficial effects of fruits and vegetables. Beta-carotene's appeal as a preventive agent was substantial: it combined a number of theoretical anti-cancer properties and appeared to be entirely safe (vitamin A itself being far more toxic at effective anti-cancer doses).

This message was captured most cogently in a paper published in Nature (Peto *et al.*, 1981), and several research groups were stimulated to conduct randomised trials using beta-carotene. These experiments were required to quantify the 'beta-carotene effect' separately from effects of other inter-related dietary elements. When put to the test in this way, the hypothesis failed to stand up; in fact beta-carotene may actually have been harmful to some smokers: in one trial the incidence of lung cancer was 18% (95% CI 3–36%) higher among smokers randomised to receive beta-carotene than among those randomised to the placebo group. (ATBC, 1994). The overall trial evidence led the US Food and Drug Administration to disallow health claims for beta-carotene related to cancer prevention (FDA, 1998).

Unfortunately, the evidence is rarely as convincing as that seen for smoking. Box 16.2 summarises the research that led to the conclusion that beta-carotene was not the cancer preventive that scientists had initially hoped it might be. The unexpected trial results, which firmly contradicted the preventive promise of the non-experimental research, were seen by some as a strong indictment of observational epidemiology. So what went wrong? Why did the observational studies get the 'wrong' answer?

Clearly we need more information to answer this question fully. If we first consider the complex make-up of our diets, a first thought might be that there is likely to be real potential for confounding when studying effects of one nutrient among many and, given the general imprecision of dietary measures (as discussed in Chapter 7), control for confounding by other dietary factors will not be wholly successful. Additionally, people who eat diets high in fruit and vegetables (the main contributors of beta-carotene) are likely to differ from those with low fruit and vegetable intake with respect to other personal and lifestyle factors such as smoking, alcohol consumption and physical activity, which also affect cancer risk. Some of these other factors will also be very hard to measure and so hard to control for in the analyses. Furthermore, the associations found in the observational research were generally small to modest (50%–100% increases in risk or RRs of 1.5–2.0) thus, despite great consistency of effects across studies and strong biological support for the hypothesis, a cautious interpretation was required. These challenges to interpreting the results of the observational studies were the reason that scientists promoted the need for randomised experiments as the only way to make a strong test of the hypothesis (Peto *et al.*, 1981). (A more detailed overview is provided by Hercberg, 2005.)

Despite the outcome, the full research sequence from the beta-carotene case study is actually a good example of how science should operate: a sound hypothesis that may have strong public health value emerged from a variety of sources (Peto *et al.*, 1981); it was then tested via a series of large and rigorous experiments in different populations; it failed the test, leading to quite rapid formal direction from the US Government that beta-carotene (and vitamin A) supplements were not approved as cancer prevention agents (FDA, 1998).

Challenges

So what have we learned from this? The totality of evidence indicates that beta-carotene is a good marker of (and part of) a beneficial diet, but is insufficient on its own to provide any protection. We have also learned that dietary epidemiology is more challenging than was initially appreciated, and that due attention needs to be given to the challenges of measurement and confounding in observational studies; we want to

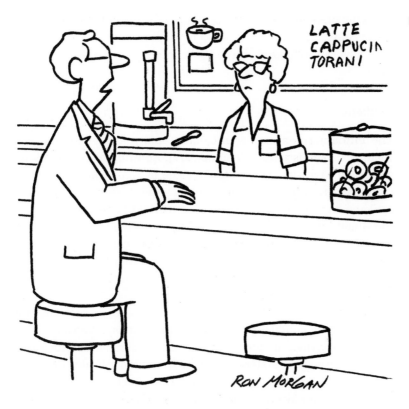

LATTE
CAPPUCIN
TORANI

RON MORGAN

"I haven't read the health columns this morning.
Is coffee *out* or *in* today?"

minimise dilemmas such as those depicted in the cartoon for the public
and for policy makers.

Compelling observational data such as those seen for smoking are, unfortunately, the exception. The multivariable and often hard-to-identify and remote causes of many chronic diseases are generally much weaker, leaving many studies under-powered with more room for results to vary by chance, quite apart from the real potential for weak effects to be due to residual confounding or bias. The resulting papers report weak or moderate effects (RRs less than two) which may well differ among studies investigating the same relationship. One result is a flow of sometimes contradictory newspaper headlines and journal articles depicting new panaceas or lifestyle risks. This highlights the importance of a sound systematic review to provide a balanced explanation and presentation of *all* relevant data (Chapter 11) and the need for authors, editors and medical journalists to show restraint and avoid the premature trumpeting of 'interesting' findings from the report of a single study.

So how can we address these challenges?

Synthesis and integration

> The research outputs from epidemiology fit well with the growing desire for public health and medical research to be 'translational', i.e. directly applicable to a population or patient. Hiatt (2010) puts epidemiology at 'the epicenter of translational science'.

The increasing focus on translational epidemiology (Khoury *et al.*, 2010; Hiatt, 2010) offers a useful counter to those who have questioned the value of epidemiology, by promoting the value of *data synthesis* and *collaborative engagements* across research groups, as well as increased *integration* of epidemiology with other disciplines relevant to public health, especially social and laboratory sciences. The first two endeavours help minimise the play of chance and allow direct assessment of consistency of findings, while the third broadens causal perspectives and, through advances at the molecular and genetic level, permits sharper measures of both diseases and exposures.

The Cochrane Collaboration has set a superb example by encouraging investigators to conduct practically directed data syntheses in a standardised manner and, since its inception in 1993, Cochrane contributors have produced thousands of systematic reviews evaluating health care interventions (Ferrie, 2015). Collaboration among researchers is also becoming more common and an increasing number of groups of epidemiologists are sharing their data to permit direct pooling of their results with results from other studies. One of the first of these was established at Oxford University to help pin down the long-contentious relationship between use of the oral contraceptive pill and a woman's risk of breast cancer (Collaborative Group on Hormonal Factors in Breast Cancer, 1996). Finally, recognising the need for integration across disciplines, funding bodies are increasingly demanding that research be 'multidisciplinary', bringing together scientists from a range of relevant fields. In addition to epidemiologists, these groups may include demographers, geographers, social scientists and health policy experts who provide perspective on the upstream 'macro' level drivers of health as well as geneticists and molecular biologists who add insights at the 'micro' level regarding individual susceptibility to disease and more sophisticated ways to classify disease (see, for example, serotyping of infectious agents in Chapter 13). The rapidly increasing integration with bench (laboratory) science, where new, sophisticated tools and the mapping of the human genome provide a welter of molecular, genetic and epigenetic data, complements the standard personal and health information of traditional epidemiology. However, although it is easy to focus on individual-level risk factors when searching for the causes of disease, we should not ignore the fact that that these exist

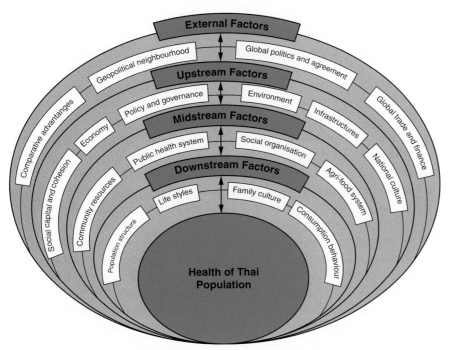

Figure 16.1 Multilevel model adopted for the Thai Health-Risk Transition Study. (*From*: Sleigh *et al.*, Cohort Profile: The Thai Cohort of 87,134 Open University students. *Int J Epidemiol*, 2008; 37: 266–272, by permission of the International Epidemiological Association.)

within a much broader and more complex web of social and environmental factors (McMichael, 1999).

A qualitative sense of some of these multifactorial approaches is given in Figure 16.1, which shows the eco-social model which guided the design and research questions of the Thai Health-Risk Transition Study, a large-scale cohort study established in 2005 to evaluate forces behind changing disease patterns in Thailand (Sleigh *et al.*, 2008).

At another level, we have also briefly discussed *lifecourse epidemiology* (Kuh and Ben-Shlomo, 2004) which brings temporal integration. It aims to identify and integrate exposures and other influences across a person's life (as far back as conception, and possibly beyond) and relate them to their health at different ages. Capturing details of habits, diets and other aspects of early life is mostly too much to expect from retrospective questioning in adulthood, but historical records from early surveys, schools and hospitals have proved invaluable. For example, a group of Bristol epidemiologists identified good dietary records from the 1930s for over 4000 children, more than 85% of whom have been followed up to the present for mortality, and a proportion resurveyed six decades later (the Boyd Orr study; Frankel *et al.*, 1998). A number of pregnancy and birth cohorts have also been established to collect detailed early-life data prospectively, with the intention of life-long follow-up of the study participants (for example the ALSPAC Study, see Box 4.3). Improvements in data linkage will help these studies ensure high follow-up rates, something that will be critical to avoid selection bias in the long term.

Limiting error

We have given a lot of attention to the challenges of error and confounding throughout the book so will not revisit these in detail here, but dealing with these biases effectively is crucial for epidemiology to be a consistently useful translational discipline. New analytic methods for identifying, quantifying and (to a degree) dealing with bias and confounding provide some tools to help us achieve this. By making the relationships between the variables we are studying explicit, directed acyclic graphs (DAGs) can sharpen our causal thinking and improve our ability to identify and control for confounders appropriately. Some of the newer methods we have alluded to like instrumental variables and Mendelian randomisation, itself a spinoff of our new genetic knowledge, offer the potential to remove, or at least reduce, the bias in our analyses. And perhaps most importantly, keeping an eye on the exchangeability of the groups we are comparing can help us design better studies as well as in assessing whether selection bias or confounding might affect our results. In addition to this we must continually strive to sharpen our measurement – not just of exposures and the outcome we are interested in, but also of confounders so that we can adjust for these more fully. In particular, anything we can do to decrease random misclassification will increase the precision of our estimates and so help clarify weaker associations that lie close to the null.

Improving measurement

As epidemiology is, at its core, a measurement science we will expand a little further on this here. New technologies now allow more sophisticated measurement both of exposure (e.g. serum biomarkers, DNA damage in cells) and of outcome (e.g. early cellular changes, molecular subtypes of disease based on genetic profiles). Increasing the precision and accuracy of our measurement is paramount, but we also need to be highly specific about what we mean by exposure and outcome. A single infectious agent may have different strains, cigarettes have varying levels of tar, menopausal hormone therapy comes in different formulations and doses, and so on. Duration, intensity, pattern and timing of exposure may be critical. Is someone who drinks a glass or two of wine each night getting the same 'causal dose' of alcohol as their neighbour who drinks only on Friday nights but then drinks a bottle or two? For liver cirrhosis the answer might be 'yes', but for risk of injury it would clearly be 'no'. Similarly, we need maximum precision in defining outcomes.

Uterine cancer was recorded as one disease until the mid-twentieth century when cancers of the body of the uterus were separated from those of the cervix (neck of the uterus), as they are histologically quite distinct. They were then found to have completely different risk factors: obesity and oestrogen exposure for endometrial cancer and human papillomavirus (HPV) infection for cervical cancer, requiring very different preventive strategies. We now know that risk factors also differ for different histological types of cancer at the *same* site – for example, cigarette smoking is associated only with the rare mucinous type of ovarian cancer (Collaborative Group on Epidemiological Studies of Ovarian Cancer, 2012) while a history of endometriosis is associated only with two other histological types (endometrioid and clear cell) (Pearce *et al.*, 2012). With our increasing genetic and molecular capability we can now subdivide the histological types of cancer further based on their molecular characteristics. In many cases these 'molecular subtypes' have a very different prognosis and, in the case of breast cancer, they are now used to determine treatment as different drugs target different molecular characteristics of the cancers.

Box 16.3 The evolving epidemiology of cancer of the cervix

1713: Cancer of the whole uterus (including what we now know as the cervix) noted to be uncommon in nuns (Ramazzini, 1713) leading to the hypothesis that it was related to sexual activity.

1928: Papanikolaou reported that 'uterine' cancer could be diagnosed by vaginal smear.

1950s: Cancer of the cervix identified as a separate entity.

1960s: Introduction of cervical cancer screening using the 'Pap' smear in the USA.

1974: The evidence shows a strong relation between sexual activity and cervical cancer mortality suggesting an infectious cause (Beral, 1974).

1960s–1970s: Herpes simplex virus initially suspected as the cause.

1976: Harald zur Hausen identifed human papillomavirus (HPV) DNA in cervical cancer and genital warts and was later awarded the Nobel Prize for Medicine for this work; subsequently multiple HPV strains were identified and refined testing showed specific strains including HPV16, 18, 31 and 45 were very strongly associated with the cancer.

1999: HPV proposed as a necessary cause of cancer of the cervix (Walboomers *et al.*, 1999).

2006: First HPV vaccine approved by the US FDA.

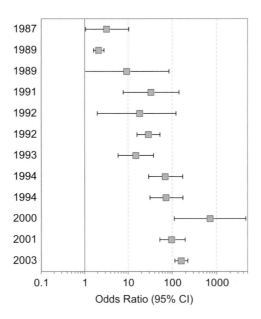

Figure 16.2 Odds ratios and 95% confidence intervals (CI) for the association between human papillomavirus (HPV) infection (via HPV DNA detection) and invasive cervical cancer risk in successive molecular epidemiologic studies. (*Adapted from*: Franco and Tota, Invited commentary: Human papillomavirus infection and risk of cervical precancer – using the right methods to answer the right questions, *Am J Epidemiol.*, 2010; 171, p. 166, by permission of the Society for Epidemiological Research.)

For example, Herecptin® is given only to women with breast cancer if their cancer tests positive for human epidermal growth factor receptor 2 (HER2). This sophisticated molecular information also allows us to refine our case definitions and thus has the potential to increase our ability to identify causal relationships by allowing us to study more homogeneous groups that are more likely to share a common aetiology.

A dramatic example of the effects of clearly defining both exposure and outcome comes from studies of the relation between HPV infection and cervical cancer (see also Box 16.3). In early studies HPV was detected in 30%–60% of cases and the observed associations suggested a 2- to 5–fold increase in risk. Improved detection methods mean that HPV is now identified in 99% of cases and, as a result, we now see odds ratios of 100–900 for the association between the presence of HPV DNA and risk of invasive cervical cancer (Franco and Tota, 2010). The massive effects of this improvement in measurement on the magnitude of the observed association are shown in Figure 16.2. This increasing precision has in turn helped identify the best targets for the recently introduced vaccines against HPV intended to prevent cancer of the cervix. Good translation thanks to improved measurement.

Good measurement is also essential for descriptive epidemiology. As you saw in Chapters 2 and 3, international organisations such as the United Nations and World Health Organization are trying to tackle health at a global level. Similarly, as you saw in Chapter 12, good surveillance data are essential to detect and effectively control outbreaks of infectious diseases. These efforts require accurate information to quantify the problem (by person, place and time) and to track changes over time. High-income countries usually have the luxury of well-developed civil registration and surveillance systems, often covering the entire country; however, the same cannot be said for lower- and middle-income countries. While many are making great improvements in this area, comprehensive data collection requires resources and reliable systems and so is difficult in areas of conflict or with limited resources or in countries with a very large and geographically dispersed population such as India. This makes tracking of progress towards the Millennium Development Goals (see Box 2.10) and other health targets a challenge. Initiatives like the INDEPTH Network which encourages low- and middle-income countries to establish health and demographic surveillance systems to collect routine data are helping to improve data in some areas, but there is still a long way to go.

A final word

We hope that by now you have a good sense of what epidemiology has offered and continues to offer the study of public health and indeed health in general. As we alluded to right at the start, perhaps epidemiology's most important role is the rigour it brings to the collection, analysis and interpretation of all aspects of health data, because without reliable data we cannot move forward. As you have seen, this is often not straightforward – the study of free-living people, their environment and society is necessarily highly complex and the various elements are often closely inter-related making it hard to study the effects of individual components. However, by applying sound epidemiological principles with a pragmatic approach that is alert to the pitfalls but also practical about assessing the likely effects of any error on the data we see, there is much we can learn and contribute to improving health.

REFERENCES

ATBC (The Alpha-Tocopheral Beta Carotene Prevention Study Group). (1994). References
The effect of vitamin E and beta carotene on the incidence of lung cancer and other cancers in male smokers. *New England Journal of Medicine*, 330: 1029–1035.

Beral, V. (1974). Cancer of the cervix: a sexually transmitted infection? *The Lancet*, 1(7865): 1037–1040.

Collaborative Group on Epidemiological Studies of Ovarian Cancer. (2012). Ovarian cancer and smoking: individual participant meta-analysis including 28,114 women with ovarian cancer from 51 epidemiological studies. *Lancet Oncology*, 13: 946–956.

Collaborative Group on Hormonal Factors in Breast Cancer. (1996). Breast cancer and oral contraceptives: collaborative reanalysis of individual data on 53 297 women with breast cancer and 100 239 women without breast cancer from 54 epidemiological studies. *Lancet*, 347: 1713–1727.

FDA (Food and Drug Administration). (1998). Food labeling: health claims: antioxidant vitamin A and β-carotene and the risk in adults of atherosclerosis, coronary heart disease, and cancers: interim final rule. *Federal Register*, 63: 34092–34097.

Ferrie, J. E. (2015). Evidence and policy: mind the gap. *International Journal of Epidemiology*, 44: 1–7.

Franco, E. L. and Tota, J. (2010). Invited commentary: Human papillomavirus infection and risk of cervical precancer – using the right methods to answer the right questions. *American Journal of Epidemiology*, 171: 164–168.

Frankel, S., Gunnell, D. J., Peters, T. J., Maynard, M. and Davey Smith, G. (1998) Childhood energy intake and adult mortality from cancer: the Boyd Orr cohort study. *British Medical Journal*, 316: 499–504.

Hercberg, S. (2005). The history of B-carotene and cancers: from observational to intervention studies. What lessons can be drawn for future research on polyphenols? *American Journal of Clinical Nutrition*, 81(suppl): 218S–222S.

Hiatt, R. A. (2010). Invited commentary: The epicentre of translational science. *American Journal of Epidemiology*, 172: 525–527.

Khoury, M. J., Gwinn, M. and Ioannidis, P. A. (2010). The emergence of translational epidemiology: from scientific discovery to population health impact. *American Journal of Epidemiology*, 172: 517–524.

Kuh, D. and Ben-Shlomo, Y. (eds). (2004). *A Life Course Approach to Chronic Disease Epidemiology*, 2nd edn. Oxford: Oxford University Press.

McMichael, A. J. (1999). Prisoners of the proximate: loosening the constraints on epidemiology in an age of change. *American Journal of Epidemiology*, 149: 887–897.

Pearce, C. L., Templeman, C., Rossing, M. A., *et al.* (2012). Association between endometriosis and risk of histological subtypes of ovarian cancer: a pooled analysis of data from 13 case–control studies. *Lancet Oncology*, 13: 385–394.

Peto, R., Doll, R., Buckley, J. D. and Sporn, M. B. (1981). Can dietary beta-carotene materially reduce human cancer rates? *Nature*, 290: 201–208.

Ramazzini, B. (1713). *Diseases of Workers. Translation of Latin text of 1713*. Chicago, IL: University of Chicago Press, 1940.

Sleigh, A. C., Seubsman, S., Bain C. and the Thai Cohort Study Team. (2008). Cohort profile: the Thai cohort of 87,134 Open University students. *International Journal of Epidemiology*, 37: 266–272.

US Department of Health, Education, and Welfare. (1964). *Smoking and Health: Report of the Advisory Committee to the Surgeon General of the Public Health Service*. Public Health Service Publication No. 1103. Washington, DC: US Department of Health, Education, and Welfare.

Walboomers, J. M. M., Jacobs, M. V., Manos, M. M., *et al.* (1999). Human papillomavirus is a necessary cause of invasive cervical cancer worldwide. *Journal of Pathology*, 189: 12–19.

RECOMMENDED FOR FURTHER READING

- A thoughtful piece about the role of epidemiology:
  McMichael, A. J. (1999). Prisoners of the proximate: loosening the constraints on epidemiology in an age of change. *American Journal of Epidemiology*, 149: 887–897.

Answers to questions

Chapter 2

1. (a) Incidence proportion = 15 cases ÷ 1000 women = 1.5% in 8 years.
   (b) Incidence rate = 75 strokes ÷ 5000 person-years
       $$= 1.5/100 \text{ person-years } or$$
       $$15/1000 \text{ person-years } or$$
       $$1500/10^5 \text{ person-years}$$
   (c) Incidence rate = 27 cases ÷ 50,000 = 54 per 100,000 per year
2. (a) Prevalence at age 55 = 100 ÷ 2000 = 0.05 or 5%
       Prevalence at age 65 = 400 ÷ 2000 = 0.20 or 20%
   (b) Number of women 'at risk' = 2000 – 100 (who already had high blood pressure) = 1900
   (c) Incidence proportion = 300 ÷ 1900 = 0.16 or 16% in 10 years
       It is an incidence proportion (or cumulative incidence) because the same women have been followed for the 10-year period.
   (d) We could estimate the total number of person-years at risk by assuming that all 1900 initially healthy women were followed for the whole 10 years, giving
       $$1900 \times 10 = 19,000 \text{ py}$$
       but 300 of the women developed high blood pressure and so were not at risk for the whole period. If we assume that, *on average*, they developed it half way through the follow-up period, we can improve our estimate of the number of person-years to
       300 women who developed high blood pressure × 5 years = 1500
       + 1600 women with no high blood pressure × 10 years = 16,000
       giving a total of 17,500 py.
   (e) Incidence rate = 300 ÷ 17,500 = 17.1/1000 person-years or $1710/10^5$ person-years (actually 1714 but we have rounded this off to 1710).
3. Answer = (a) community A has a younger population than community B.
   If a disease is more common in older people (true for most diseases, including IHD), then if the age-standardised rate is *higher* than the crude rate this tells us that the average age in the standard population is higher than that in the community. Conversely, if the age-standardised rate is *lower* than the crude rate, then the average age in the standard population

is lower than in the community. The age-standardised rate was higher in community A but lower in community B so community A must have a younger population.

4. Table 2.10 shows that chronic obstructive pulmonary disease (COPD) and lower respiratory infections are the third and fourth most common causes of mortality with each causing approximately 3.1 million deaths worldwide each year. However, if we consider the burden of each disease measured in DALYs, lower respiratory infections accounted for greater loss of healthy life (146.9 million DALYs) than COPD (92.4 million DALYs). This is because COPD is primarily a disease of older age while deaths from lower respiratory infections are relatively more common in children; as a result, more years of life are lost following the death of a child from a lower respiratory infection than following the death of an adult from COPD.

Chapter 3

1. While this graph is rather different from any you have seen so far, if you consider the title and the labels of the x and y axes a clear picture emerges: over one decade there has been a very large shift in mortality. Over 600 of every 10,000 deaths have been deferred from early life (most from before 1 year of age) until after age 60, with the majority of them now occurring after the age of 70. The proportions of deaths occurring at intermediate ages are largely unchanged. Clearly some major changes to the environment and/or care of infants (resulting in reduced infant mortality) and young children occurred during this time. It is difficult to identify these changes precisely in retrospect, but they coincided with campaigns to improve the quality of primary care and maternal care, as well as the initiation of programmes to improve the quality of water supply and sanitation across much of Thailand.

2. A sample of people surveyed at a shopping mall on a weekday morning is very unlikely to be representative of the general population because it will not include the vast majority of those who work during the week. These people are more likely to be captured by a survey conducted in the evening or at a weekend, but this may miss those who do not work and so might be more likely to shop during the day.

3. The shape of the curve for the USA in Figure 3.6 looks very different from that in Figure 3.7 because while Figure 3.7 shows rates from 1950 to 2010, Figure 3.6 only shows data from 1970 and so misses the upsurge in incidence that occurred prior to 1970.

Chapter 4

1. This is not a straightforward task and there are no absolute right or wrong answers – it will always be partly a matter of judgement depending on the specific circumstances. A completed version of Table 4.1 below shows the main issues and some specific exceptions are noted below.

Comments and exceptions:

Ecological study: it may be possible to study rare diseases and exposures if the populations are large enough. If it uses routinely available data it may also be quick and cheap to run; however, if new data collection is required the converse may be true. The major drawbacks are that populations often differ in many ways other than the characteristic of interest and the results seen at the population level may not apply to the individual.

Cross-sectional study: relatively simple, cheap and quick to conduct. Not good for studying rare conditions and hard to establish temporality. The ethical issues are likely to be minor although for any study, collection of blood samples for genetic testing adds ethical complexity.

Case–control study: good for studying multiple causes of rare diseases. Ensuring that exposure occurred before the disease can be a challenge but is less of an issue for things that do not change over time (e.g. blood type, genetic markers, early life exposures). Not good for studying rare

Table 4.1 Comparing the strengths and weaknesses of different study designs.

	Ecological	Cross-sectional	Case-control	Cohort	Randomised controlled trial	Nested case-control
Investigation of rare disease or outcome	4	2	5	2	1	2
Investigation of a rare exposure	1	1	1	2–5	5	2
Testing multiple effects of an exposure	2–4	3	1	5	3	1
Study of multiple exposures	2–4	5	5	3	1	3
Establishing temporality[a]	N/A	1	1–3[a]	4	5	4
Give a direct measure of incidence	N/A	1	1	5	5	3
Explore exposures which change over time	1	1	2	5	1	5
Time required[b]	4	4	3	1	1	4
Costs[b]	1–3	4	3	1	1	4
Ethical Problems[b]	N/A	4	4	4	1	4

[a] That is, that the exposure came before the outcome. N.B., even in a case–control study, some exposures will clearly pre-date the development of disease – for example, gender, genetic characteristics, blood group.
[b] For these attributes, a score of 1 = poor indicates a lot of time required, high costs or major ethical problems; a score of 5 = excellent indicates least time required, lowest costs or no ethical problems.

exposures. In a true population-based study it is possible to estimate disease incidence.

Cohort study: population-based cohort studies are not very good for studying rare exposures, but rare exposures can be studied if participants are selected to over-represent those who are 'exposed' to the factor of interest, for example an occupational cohort exposed to a specific chemical. Very large cohort studies (such as EPIC and the Million Women Study), with sufficient follow-up, can investigate rare outcomes. If information is collected at regular intervals it is possible to study effects of exposures that change over time. Establishing temporality can still be a problem for cases diagnosed very early in the follow-up period.

Randomised controlled trial: this shares many of the attributes of a cohort study except it is an excellent design to study rare exposures (because a large proportion of the population can be intentionally exposed) but is usually less good for studying multiple outcomes of one exposure as an RCT will usually be designed to focus on a small number of 'end-points'. However, the ethical implications and, because of the increased regulatory issues, sometimes the cost are much greater.

Nested case–control study: this combines many of the benefits of the cohort and case–control designs but can only be conducted in the context of an existing cohort study. The incremental costs are likely to be low.

2. The aim of the control group is to tell us what the rate of polio would have been in the vaccinated group if the children had not been vaccinated. The vaccine and control groups must therefore be as similar as possible in every way except vaccination status. A major advantage of using other groups of second-grade children as controls is that they would be the same age as the vaccinated children. However, it is very likely that exposure to the polio virus would vary geographically and over time. This means that control children selected from a different area or from a different calendar year might have a much higher or lower chance of being exposed to the virus than the children in the study group making comparisons very problematic. Although first- and third-grade children would be slightly younger and older, respectively, than second-grade children, by comparing rates in these groups to the rate in the vaccinated second-graders in the same area in the same year, the investigators were able to ensure that, as far as possible, the children in both groups had a similar chance of being exposed to the virus.

3.

Nuremberg Code Statement	Relevant moral principle
1. Requirement for voluntary consent	Respect for autonomy
2. The experiment should yield fruitful results	Beneficence
3. The experiment should be designed based on prior knowledge so the results justify performing the experiment	Beneficence and non-maleficence
4. Avoid unnecessary suffering	Non-maleficence
5. Experiments should not be conducted if death or disabling injury is a possibility	Non-maleficence
6. The degree of risk should not exceed the importance	Beneficence and non-maleficence
7. Proper precautions should be taken to avoid adverse events	Non-maleficence
8. Scientists should be properly qualified	Beneficence and non-maleficence
9. The subject should be able to withdraw at any time	Respect for autonomy
10. The scientist should discontinue the study if continuation is likely to risk in injury/death	Non-maleficence

Note that the principle of *Justice* is not explicitly covered by any of the statements, although it could be seen as implicit in some. This is because the primary focus is on protecting the individual, reflecting the circumstances from which the Nuremberg Code arose.

Chapter 5

1. (a) $Incidence\ proportion = \dfrac{Number\ of\ people\ who\ get\ disease}{Number\ of\ people\ at\ risk\ at\ the\ start\ of\ the\ period}$

   So the incidence proportion in
   (i) exposed workers = $40 \div 2500 = 1.6\%$ in 10 years
   (ii) unexposed workers = $60 \div 7500 = 0.8\%$ in 10 years
   (iii) all workers = $100 \div 10{,}000 = 1.0\%$ in 10 years

   (b) The relative risk $= \dfrac{Incidence\ in\ exposed\ group}{Incidence\ in\ unexposed\ group}$

   $$= IP_e \div IP_o$$
   $$= 1.6 \div 0.8 = 2.0$$

   Workers exposed to pesticides were twice as likely to develop the disease as those not exposed.

   (c) The attributable risk
   = Incidence in exposed group − Incidence in unexposed group

$= IP_e - IP_o$

$= 1.6 - 0.8 = 0.8\%$ in 10 years

An additional 0.8 cases of disease will occur in every 100 men (or 8 in 1000 men) exposed to pesticides for 10 years (over and above the background rate of disease in the unexposed group). This is the amount of disease that can be said to be *attributable to the pesticides* assuming that we believe that pesticide exposure is actually causing the disease.

Note: the attributable fraction would be $0.8 \div 1.6 = 50\%$

(d) The population attributable fraction $= (IP_T - IP_o) \div IP_T$

$$= (1.0 - 0.8) \div 1.0$$
$$= 0.2 \text{ or } 20\%$$

This tells us that *if pesticide exposure is a cause of the disease* then 20% of all cases occurring among the workers (regardless of whether they were exposed to pesticides) could be attributed to pesticide exposure.

Note: the population attributable risk would be $1.0 - 0.8 = 0.2\%$ in 10 years.

The difference between the *population attributable fraction* (PAF) and the *attributable fraction* (AF) depends on the prevalence of the exposure. An exposure with a high AF may have a low PAF if the exposure is very rare (very few of the cases in the whole population could be attributed to the exposure). Conversely, an exposure with a lower AF may have almost as high a PAF if the exposure is very common.

2. (a) Relative risk $= IR_e \div IR_o = 53 \div 6 = 8.8$

(b) (i) RR for low dose versus never used $= 39 \div 6 = 6.5$

(ii) RR for high dose versus never used $= 62 \div 6 = 10.3$

Results such as these are often presented as follows:

OC use	Incidence rate	Relative risk (versus never/past user)
Never/past user	6	1.0
Low-dose user	39	6.5
High-dose user	62	10.3

(Note: the relative risk in never/past users is set as 1.0 because this is the reference to which we are comparing the other groups; $IR_o \div IR_o = 1.0$.)

(c) The results suggests that, compared with women who have never used OCs, users of low-dose oestrogen OCs have a 6.5-fold risk of thromboembolism and users of high-dose oestrogen OCs have a 10.3-fold risk of thromboembolism. The risk of thromboembolism therefore increases with increasing level of oestrogen. This pattern is called a 'dose–response' relationship.

3. (a) A case–control study of smoking and lung cancer

	Cases	Controls	Total
Ever smokers	647	622	1269
Never smokers	2	27	29
Total	649	649	1298

(b) To answer this question you need to calculate the *odds ratio*:

$$\text{Odds Ratio} = \frac{a \times d}{b \times c} = \frac{647 \times 27}{622 \times 2} = 14.0$$

(c) and (d) You need to calculate first the *attributable fraction* and then the *population attributable fraction*:

$$\text{Attributable Fraction} = \frac{(\text{OR} - 1)}{\text{OR}} \quad \frac{(14 - 1)}{14} \times 100 = 92.9\%$$

If smoking is a cause of lung cancer then 93% of lung cancers *among smokers* can be attributed to their smoking and, theoretically, would not have occurred if the men had never smoked.

Population Attributable Fraction

$$= \frac{P_e(\text{OR} - 1)}{P_e(\text{OR} - 1) + 1} = \frac{(0.958 \times 13)}{(0.958 \times 13) + 1} \times 100 = 92.6\%$$

where P_e = prevalence of exposure among controls = 622 ÷ 649 = 0.958. While the AF told us the proportion of lung cancers *among smokers* that could be attributed to smoking, the PAF tells us the proportion of *all* lung cancers attributable to smoking. In this particular example the prevalence of exposure is so high that the AF and PAF are almost identical.

4. (a) The incidence rates can be calculated as follows:

	Cases	Person-years (py)	Incidence rate (per 100,000 py)	Rate ratio
7–8 hours sleep	541	451,393	120	1.0
6 hours sleep	267	175,629	152	1.27
≤5 hours sleep	67	30,115	222	1.85
All women	875	657,137	133	

(b) The rate of CHD increases as the length of time a woman sleeps decreases. A woman who sleeps for 6 hours is 27% more likely, and a woman who sleeps for 5 hours or less is 85% more likely, to develop CHD than a woman who sleeps for 7–8 hours.

(c) To answer this you need to calculate the *population attributable fraction*:

$$PAF = (CI_T - CI_o) \div CI_T$$
$$= (133 - 120) \div 133$$
$$= 0.098 \text{ or } 9.8\%$$

The PAF is quite low because most women, or at least most of the person-time, is for women who sleep for 7–8 hours.

Chapter 6

1. The results from the first study suggest that alcohol is associated with an 80% increase in risk of the cancer. The confidence interval is quite narrow, suggesting that the study was fairly large and the estimate of the RR is quite precise. The results of the second study suggest that caffeine may also be associated with an 80% increase in risk of the cancer, but in this case the confidence interval is very wide, implying that it was a small study and hence that the estimate of the OR is very imprecise. It is possible that the association seen in the second study could simply represent the play of chance because the confidence interval includes the no-effect value of 1. Overall, the data suggest that there is a moderately strong association between alcohol and the cancer (although we would still like to see additional data to support this), but they tell us little about the risks of caffeine other than to flag a possible association that needs evaluating in a larger study.

2. The answer is (b). There will always be some random sampling error in a study even when study participants are selected at random and a 95% confidence interval will just give an indication of how much random sampling error is present. Exposure measurement is a completely different issue.

3. The answer is (c). The 'no-effect' value for a relative risk is 1.0 – this means that the risk is the same in the two groups being compared. Because the confidence interval does not include the value 1.0 (both the lower and upper bounds are below 1.0), this means that the result is statistically significant. Without having more information about the size of the relative risk we cannot say whether this is clinically significant.

4. If a result is statistically significant it means that it is unlikely to have arisen by chance while clinical significance describes whether or not a result is

clinically or practically meaningful. In a large study even quite small differences can be statistically significant, but if the difference is so small that it has no practical effect, e.g. a drug that reduces the duration of flu symptoms by only a couple of hours, then it may not be clinically significant. Conversely, a study may see a large difference that would be clinically meaningful but, if the study was quite small, this may not be statistically significant and it would be hard to be sure the difference had not arisen just by chance.

Chapter 7

1. Women who read health magazines obviously have an interest in health and so are probably more likely to be vegetarian than are women who do not read such magazines. On top of this, the vegetarian readers may also be more likely to respond to the questionnaire. Both of these biases would mean that the percentage of vegetarians in the community would be overestimated. Note also that the study would provide information just about women and men might be very different.

2. (a) People with high alcohol intake are probably less likely to agree to take part.

   (b) Alcohol consumption in the control group is, therefore, likely to be lower than in the whole community.

   (c) Assuming that patients with liver disease tend to have a higher than average alcohol consumption, the difference between the cases and controls would be exaggerated because of the falsely low level of consumption among the controls. This would make the association between alcohol consumption and liver disease look stronger than it really was.

3. (a) The misclassification is *systematic* (because the measurement instrument *systematically* overestimated people's exposure) and *non-differential* (because it has occurred among both cases and controls).

   (b) In the presence of non-differential misclassification, the observed odds ratio is likely to underestimate the true odds ratio.

   (c) In this situation, (i) 15% or 15 of the 100 unexposed cases and (ii) 15% or 23 of the 150 unexposed controls would have been misclassified as exposed.

   (d) The best way to answer this is to draw up a 2 × 2 table showing the results that would have been obtained:

	Cases	Controls	Total
Exposed	300 + 15 = 315	250 + 23 = 273	588
Unexposed	100 − 15 = 85	150 − 23 = 127	212
Total	400	400	800

Therefore, in this situation, (i) 315 of the cases would be classified as exposed and 85 as unexposed, and (ii) 273 of the controls were exposed and 127 were unexposed.

(e) $OR = \dfrac{315 \times 127}{85 \times 273} = 1.7$

This compares to the 'true' value of 1.8. *Non-differential* misclassification will usually bias the results towards the null value regardless of whether it is random (as you saw in Table 7.5) or systematic, as in this example.

4. (a) The misclassification is *systematic*, because cases systematically underestimated their exposure, and is *differential*, because it occurred only among cases, and not controls.

   (b) There are 300 exposed cases so if misclassification affects 20% this means that 60 cases will be misclassified as unexposed. We can draw up a 2 × 2 table to show the results that would be obtained:

	Cases	Controls	Total
Exposed	300 – 60 = 240	250	490
Unexposed	100 + 60 = 160	150	310
Total	400	400	800

$OR = \dfrac{240 \times 150}{160 \times 250} = 0.9$

The observed OR is therefore much lower than the true OR of 1.8, in fact the bias is so great that the observed OR is less than 1.0 when the true OR is greater than 1.0.

   (c) This contrasts with the situation in Table 7.7, where cases systematically *overestimated* their exposure to the same extent and the OR was biased *upwards* to 2.40.

5. (a) The misclassification is *systematic* because non-exposed people are misclassified as exposed but the reverse is not occurring. It is *non-differential*, as would be expected in a cohort study, because it affects *all* exposed people regardless of whether or not they go on to develop disease.

   (b) If exposed people, who have a higher incidence of disease, are misclassified as unexposed then the incidence of disease in the unexposed group will increase. The incidence in the exposed group should not be affected.

   (c) The effect of the misclassification will therefore be to make the two groups look more similar than they really are and the observed RR will be closer to 1.0 than the true RR.

Misclassification is just as much a problem in cohort studies as it is in case–control studies.

6. (a) In the situation where 20% of the controls are misclassified with regard to their exposure status, 50 of 250 exposed controls will be misclassified as unexposed and 30 of 150 unexposed controls will be misclassified as exposed:

	Cases	Controls	Total	
Exposed	300	250 – 50 + 30 = 230	530	$OR = \dfrac{300 \times 170}{100 \times 230}$
Unexposed	100	150 – 30 + 50 = 170	270	
Total	400	400	800	$= 2.22$

(b) This misclassification is *differential*; exposure measurement among the cases was perfect, and the misclassification only occurred among controls.

(c) Differential random misclassification can make an association look stronger or weaker than it really is. In this situation, we would observe a higher odds ratio (2.2 compared to the 'true' odds ratio of 2.0), making the association seem stronger than it really is.

(d) If we had misclassified cases instead of controls the bias would have gone the other way and we would have underestimated the 'true' odds ratio (an observed OR of 1.11), making the association seem weaker than it really is.

Chapter 8

1. Odds Ratio $= \dfrac{a \times d}{b \times c} = \dfrac{20921 \times 94183}{64422 \times 7827} = 3.9$

2. (i) Moped drivers: Odds Ratio $= \dfrac{17869 \times 86212}{51900 \times 7342} = 4.0$

   (ii) Moped passengers: Odds Ratio $= \dfrac{3052 \times 7971}{12522 \times 485} = 4.0$

3. The crude and stratum-specific odds ratios are almost identical suggesting that position on the moped does not confound the association between not wearing a helmet and head injury.

4. The crude association between rider position (drivers versus passengers) and head injury:

$$\text{Crude Odds Ratio} = \frac{25211 \times 20493}{138112 \times 3537} = 1.1$$

(i) No helmet: Odds Ratio $= \dfrac{17869 \times 12522}{51900 \times 3052} = 1.4$

(ii) Helmet: Odds Ratio $= \dfrac{7342 \times 7971}{86212 \times 485} = 1.4$

The crude odds ratio suggests that rider position does not affect the risk of head injury (OR = 1.1) but when we stratify by helmet use we see that moped drivers have a 40% higher risk of head injury (OR = 1.4) than moped passengers regardless of whether or not they wear a helmet. The crude association was therefore confounded by helmet wearing.

5. For something to be a confounder it must be (i) a risk factor for disease among those who are not exposed to the factor of interest; (ii) be associated with the exposure of interest; and (iii) not lie on the causal pathway between exposure and outcome. Therefore, in the situation of drinking coffee and heart disease:

(a) Heart disease occurs more frequently in older people, and among males. It is possible that older people might drink less coffee than younger people, or that men might drink more (or less) coffee than women. If either of these conditions is true then the potential confounding effects of age and/or sex should be considered (certainly age and sex do not lie on the causal pathway between coffee drinking and heart disease).

(b) The confounding effects of *smoking* should definitely be considered. As you have seen in previous chapters, heart disease occurs more frequently in smokers, and those who drink coffee may be more likely to smoke. Also, while coffee drinking and smoking often go together, coffee drinking does not 'cause' someone to smoke.

(c) Heart disease occurs more frequently among those who do not exercise, and people who drink coffee may exercise less (for example, people who work in an office may drink more coffee and have less opportunity to exercise). Therefore, the confounding effects of *physical activity* should also be considered.

(d) While consumption of fruit and vegetables may be protective against heart disease; it is also possible that people who drink a lot of coffee eat less of these foods so *fruit and vegetable intake* might confound the effects of coffee drinking on heart disease.

6. (a) The overall incidence rate of heart disease among those with a high energy intake is 720 ÷ 60,000 = 12.0/1000 person-years (py) and the

incidence rate among those with a low energy intake is 700 ÷ 55,000 = 12.7/1000 py, giving a *crude* rate ratio of 0.9 (12.0 ÷ 12.7).

(b) When we stratify by level of physical activity we see a different picture: in the active group, the incidence rate of heart disease among those with a high energy intake is 500 ÷ 50,000 = 10.0/1000 py, whereas that among those with a low energy intake is 100 ÷ 15,000 = 6.7/1000 py, giving a rate ratio of 1.5; in the inactive group, the incidence rate of heart disease among those with a high energy intake is 220 ÷ 10,000 = 22.0/1000 py, whereas that among those with a low energy intake is 600 ÷ 40,000 = 15.0/1000 py, again giving a rate ratio of 1.5.

(c) As in the case–control example in Table 8.4, when we remove the effects of physical activity the true association between a high energy intake and heart disease is stronger (RR = 1.5) than when we did not allow for the effects of physical activity. Confounding is just as much a problem in cohort studies (or any other non-randomised follow-up studies, including non-randomised trials) as it is in case–control studies.

7. If either (i) half as many people participated in the study, or (ii) twice as many people participated in the study, the odds ratios will not change. Increasing or decreasing the size of a study will not make any difference to the amount of confounding (except in the context of a randomised controlled trial, when the bigger the study is, the less likely it is that there will be any confounding).

Results of the study shown in Table 8.7 assuming that the study had half as many people (the minor differences are due to rounding).

Energy intake	Total		High physical activity		Low physical activity	
	Heart disease	Controls	Heart disease	Controls	Heart disease	Controls
High	236	116	26	26	210	90
Low	605	398	5	8	600	390
OR	1.3		1.6		1.5	

Results of the study shown in Table 8.7 assuming that the study had twice as many people.

Energy intake	Total		High physical activity		Low physical activity	
	Heart disease	Controls	Heart disease	Controls	Heart disease	Controls
High	944	462	104	102	840	360
Low	2420	1590	20	30	2400	1560
OR	1.3		1.5		1.5	

Chapter 10

1. (a) and (d)

(a) We should always consider chance as a possible explanation and we know nothing of the sample size or the width of the confidence interval around the risk estimate. (d) If cases could not remember how much cauliflower they ate this is likely to lead to misclassification in this group. If this is random then the true association would probably be even stronger than that observed but if cases (but not controls) had systematically under-estimated how much cauliflower they ate, this might falsely make it look as if they ate less cauliflower than controls and thus that eating cauliflower protected against stroke.

Although it is likely that there is random misclassification of the expos-ure, this would probably have biased the results to the null so the true association would be even stronger than that observed. Misclassification of the outcome is less likely, but if some cases are incorrectly classified as controls and vice versa then the true association is again likely to be stronger than that observed.

2. The other issues that we should consider are:

Confounding: a single food (cauliflower here) will be highly correlated with other elements of a diet, and probably other lifestyle factors too; if any of these are causes of stroke then at least part of the apparent cauliflower 'effect' will be due to them, i.e. it could be confounded. Appropriate control for these factors in the analysis may at least partially solve the problem, provided all variables are measured reasonably accurately.

Selection bias: this is always a concern in case–control studies. We have no information here on which to make a judgement, but when interpreting the result you would need to argue for the appropriateness of your choice of control group on theoretical (if one of them suffered a stroke they would be very likely to be enrolled as a case) and practical (a high response rate) grounds.

3. Other factors to consider when assessing whether an association is likely to be causal are:

   - The strength of the association: the point estimate (OR in this case, otherwise RR) is ~0.5 so moderately strong but still more likely to be due to chance or bias than a much stronger effect would be.
   - A dose-response - i.e. a clear trend of increasing effect at higher levels of exposure - is reassuring; however, a variety of dose–response patterns are possible, including thresholds (below which no effect is observed) and plateaus (a maximum possible effect, beyond which further dose increases are irrelevant to outcomes). Thus, absence of a clear trend does not exclude causality.

- Consistency of the effect across a number of studies: if your finding is aberrant (e.g. most others show little or no effect of cauliflower on stroke) any causal claim you make will be very weak and likely to be dismissed, unless you can argue convincingly that your research is of far higher quality than what has gone before. This might be so if you were reporting results from a large, well-conducted randomised trial which refuted prior observational data supporting a causal relation, especially if uncontrolled confounding was a concern in the earlier research. An example from observational dietary research is shown in the beta-carotene example on p 419.
- Temporality: it should be clear that the exposure or dose in question preceded the outcome by sufficient time that it could plausibly have induced (or prevented) the relevant pathological change underlying disease occurrence (for cauliflower and stroke this might be the slowing down of the development of atheromatous plaque in the cerebral blood vessels). While the precise timing and dose of a causal exposure is rarely known with certainty, your questions must have been clearly formulated to avoid (or at least minimise) the potential that cases who ate a lot of cauliflower then gave it up, perhaps because of altered taste sensation, and thus the stroke caused them to avoid the vegetable and not the reverse.
- Plausibility: it is reassuring if there is a known or plausible biological mechanism through which exposure could produce or prevent disease.
- Another factor that could be considered is the 'specificity' of the association but, as described on page 284, this can be a more tricky. For discussion of this and some other possible aids to causal arguments it can be helpful to read Bradford-Hill's excellent speech on the subject (Hill, 1965).

Hill, A. B. (1965). The environment and disease: association or causation? *Proceedings of the Royal Society for Medicine*, 58: 295–300.

Chapter 11

1. The primary ways to identify relevant literature for a systematic review include:
   - a Pubmed search of mainstream literature,
   - searching reference lists of papers identified,
   - looking for papers that have cited the papers identified,
   - a search of the Cochrane CENTRAL database (or other clinical trials registers) if it is an area where trials have been conducted,
   - talking to investigators in the field.

2. The grey literature is that outside the mainstream journals and it includes documents such as reports, theses, conference abstracts, etc. When feasible, it is a good idea to look beyond the mainstream literature when conducting a systematic review because:
   - there is the possibility of publication bias – mainstream journals may be more likely to publish reports that find an association than studies that do not find an association;
   - authors may be less likely to write up null results for publication although they may present them at a conference, in which case they will probably be available in abstract format;
   - results from studies conducted by a student or by a health department may be available in a student thesis or government report but may never be published in the mainstream literature;
   - if a review is restricted to published papers it may miss studies that did not find an association, so the conclusions may be biased in favour of concluding there is an association. Studies that don't find a significant result may be more likely to be reported in abstracts, student theses, etc. Searching this literature can, however, be challenging.
3. It would be inappropriate to include the data from both reports in a meta-analysis because the two sets of results would not be independent and including both reports would give too much weight to the results from this one study. Unless the focus of the meta-analysis was specifically on short-term follow-up, it would be usual to include the more recent paper with longer follow-up.

Chapter 12

1. Answer = (a). If the number of cases detected by surveillance increases, this suggests the incidence of disease may be increasing.
2. Answer = (c). Undercount represents the cases that are not reported to a surveillance system. It may be presented as the proportion of cases that are not reported, or as the ratio of the total number of cases to the number reported, e.g. for hepatitis C in the USA it is estimated there may be ~10 times as many cases in the community as are counted by a surveillance system.
3. An event-based surveillance system establishes an organised framework for rapidly capturing information about events that are a potential risk to public health and it relies on a wide variety of information sources. Data collected are on specific 'events', such as multiple reports of similar illnesses, an outbreak, or potential high-risk exposures in a population. The information can be rumours or ad-hoc unstructured reports and may be

sourced from recorders or automated information extracted from Internet sources. The advantages of an event-based system are that it may provide for early detection of outbreaks, detection of rare but potentially high impact outbreaks and/or emerging or unknown diseases. A disadvantage of event-based surveillance is that there is a need to verify reports or information therefore resources are required to follow up reports. In addition, there is a lot of 'noise' in the system and it may be very sensitive to potential events but not very specific, i.e. many reports will not be potential events of interest.

4. Indicator-based surveillance is conducted for a number of notifiable infectious diseases and for cancer to:
   – count cases to quantify the burden of disease
   – establish trends in occurrence and/or to monitor elimination
   – identify epidemics, outbreaks and clusters
   – evaluate the effect of interventions to control the diseases.

Chapter 13

1. In a hypothesis-generating interview it is important to have a wide range of inquiry about illness and possible sources. The types of information that could be collected include: (1) demographic details including place of residence, occupation, etc., (2) signs and symptoms of illness to characterise disease and develop a case definition, (3) contact with other people who were ill with similar symptoms, (4) recent travel, (5) exposure to potential sources of infection, such as contact with animals, swimming in recreational water, eating foods, visiting shopping centres, etc.

2. Answer (d): OR = 3.6 (95% CI = 1.00 – 6.45) because, although this is not the largest relative risk, it is statistically significant and so least likely to be due to chance.

3. Hepatitis B is a vaccine-preventable disease. The main control measures in this prison setting are to: (1) offer screening to inmates to identify those who are susceptible, (2) immunise susceptible prisoners, (3) interview inmates about high-risk activities and possible illness, (4) educate inmates about the spread of hepatitis B, including unprotected sex, sharing needles and injecting equipment, tattooing and sharing razors, hair clippers and toothbrushes, (5) provide condoms and equipment for safe injection, and (6) offer post-exposure prophylaxis to high-risk contacts of cases. The key measures to preventing the spread of hepatitis B through the prison population are to break the chains of transmission through immunisation and education.

Chapter 14

1. Relative measures (e.g. relative risk, RR; odds ratio, OR) evaluate the relative *strength of an association* between exposure and disease, and they are most useful for identifying the causes of a disease. Absolute or difference measures (e.g. attributable risk, AR; population attributable risk, PAR) are a better measure of the *burden of disease attributable to an exposure* and, therefore, potentially preventable by removal of that exposure. The attributable risk and attributable fraction tell us how much disease in an exposed group can be attributed to the exposure and the population attributable risk and population attributable fraction tell us how much disease in the whole population can be attributed to the exposure. Of all these measures, the PAR is most directly useful to assess the likely benefits of a prevention programme for the whole community.

2. We can see that lowering smoking rates will reduce mortality from both lung cancer and coronary heart disease (CHD), given that we accept both associations are causal. The maximum benefits achievable if in the future no-one smoked depend on the prevalence of smoking, which was very high amongst these doctors (83% in 1951). The crucial marker, the PAR, would therefore be approximately 80% of the ARs shown. A very large number of CHD deaths could therefore be averted, as could a lesser, but still considerable, number of lung cancer deaths. (Of course, mortality from other diseases would also be lessened, increasing the attraction of anti-smoking campaigns.) The AFs and high prevalence indicate that a non-smoking population would experience very low mortality from lung cancer, but there are many other contributors to CHD mortality so this would continue as a public health challenge, despite more lives being saved by avoiding CHD deaths than from lowering lung cancer deaths.

   In applying these data to other populations, it seems reasonable to accept the RRs as being widely applicable (and other data support this), but other crucial factors will be the base mortality rates among non-smokers, especially for CHD, and, more importantly, the prevalence of smoking (and average amounts smoked, which we have ignored for simplicity) in the population. If the prevalence of smoking was lower, the benefits would be more limited. The actual benefits realised by such campaigns also depend on the success of efforts to induce current smokers to quit, as well as from those discouraging non-smokers from starting, and this is hard to predict.

   A later paper from the original investigators looking at mortality in this cohort gives a good description of the long-term fate of this cohort and a good sense of the complexities of studying influences of exposures over long periods (Doll *et al.*, 2004).

Doll, R., Peto, R., Boreham, J. and Sutherland, I. (2004). Mortality in relation to smoking: 50 years' observations on male British doctors. *British Medical Journal*, 328: 1519–1528.

Chapter 15

1. (a) The 2 × 2 table for repeat Pap smear:

	Colposcopy		
Pap smear	Positive	Negative	Total
Positive	12	72	84
Negative	1	25	26
Total	13	97	110

   (b) Sensitivity and specificity for Pap smear:
       Sensitivity = 12 ÷ 13 = 0.923 or 92%
       Specificity = 25 ÷ 97 = 0.258 or 26%
   (c) Positive predictive value = 12 ÷ 84 = 14%
   (d) Probability of high-grade disease in women testing negative by Pap smear = 1 ÷ 26 = 0.038 or 4%
   (e) The repeat Pap smear had low specificity. In this population with a prevalence of 11.8% (pre-test probability), the positive predictive value is low, and all women testing positive would still have to go on to colposcopy. So, although only 8% of higher-grade lesions would have been missed, this is not a very helpful extra step to add to the diagnostic process.
2. The first thing to do is complete a 2 × 2 table based on an artificial population of, say, 1000 people. We know that about 30 (3% × 1000) will be hepatitis B-positive and that the test will detect 82% or about 25 of them (82% × 30), leaving 5 false negatives. With a specificity of 93%, 902 of the 970 who are truly hepatitis B negative will correctly test negative, leaving 68 false positives:

	True status		
Hepatitis B test	Positive	Negative	Total
Positive	25	68	93
Negative	5	902	907
Total	30	970	1000

(a) The probability that an individual with a positive test result does not have hepatitis B is thus 68 ÷ 93 = 73%.

(b) In a population free of hepatitis B, 7% (68 ÷ 970) of people would falsely test positive.

3. (a) The prevalence of prostate cancer in men over 60 years is 4% so 400 of a group of 10,000 men would be expected to have prostate cancer (4% × 10,000). The test has a sensitivity of 85% so 340 of the men with prostate cancer (85% × 400) would be expected to have a positive PSA test.

(b) The remaining 9600 men would not have prostate cancer and, as the test has a specificity of 80%, 7680 of them (80% × 9600) would be expected to have a negative PSA test and the remaining 1920 would test positive.

(c) The table below summarises the results.

Properties of the PSA screening test

PSA test	Prostate cancer		
	Yes	No	Total
+	340	1920	2260
–	60	7680	7740
Total	400	9600	10,000

The PPV is the proportion of all positive test results that are true positives = 340 ÷ 2260 = 15.0%.

(d) The positive predictive value of 15% tells us that for every prostate cancer the PSA test identifies in this population ('true positives'), another 6 or 7 more men without cancer will also test positive and thus have to be investigated ('false positives'). The PPV is low because of the combination of relatively poor specificity and quite a low prevalence of disease (although 4% is higher than for many other cancers). Whether this means the programme should be abandoned depends on the amount of harm suffered by the false positives and the benefits of detecting the disease earlier in the minority who do have cancer. Widespread screening, for example for breast and large bowel cancer, is conducted with PPVs of this order; however, the public should be made more aware of the likelihood of false positive results when involving them in a decision of whether to screen or not.

On a more positive note, someone who has a negative test result is not too badly off. The negative predictive value of the test is very high (7680 ÷ 7740 = 99%), although you can see that the test would will still miss 60 cancers in every 10,000 men screened.

(e) If the prevalence of disease is higher, then the positive predictive value will also increase – in this case to 43% (1275 ÷ 2975). Now only about one in two PSA-positive men will be incorrectly labelled as having prostate cancer, a far more acceptable situation. However, as can be seen from the table below, we now miss more cases (225 instead of 60), and have a slightly reduced NPV of 97% (6800 ÷ 7025). And of course we have missed the opportunity for any early detection of prostate cancers in men in their 60s. Neither choice will please everyone!

Properties of the PSA screening test among men aged over 70 years.

| PSA test | Prostate cancer | | Total |
	Yes	No	
+	1275	1700	2975
–	225	6800	7025
Total	1500	8500	10,000

(f) For a disease to be considered for a screening programme it should be a serious threat to health (and be perceived as such by the population); be reasonably common (but this can still mean very low prevalence in practical terms); and have a fairly well-understood natural history/ clinical course. There must also be a good screening test for it and it should have been demonstrated, ideally in randomised trials, that outcomes are improved if treatment is initiated sooner.

Direct standardisation

To use direct standardisation you need to know:

(1) the age-specific disease rates in your study population and
(2) the age distribution of the standard population

An example: standardising the IHD mortality rate for males in Germany to the world standard population

See Table 1. You first multiply each age-specific rate (Column D) by the number of people in that age group in the standard population (Column E) to calculate the number of events that you would expect to see in the standard population if it had the same rates as your study population (Column F).

You then divide the total number of events expected (the total of column F) by the total number of people in the standard population (the total of Column E) to calculate the standardised rate.

Crude mortality rate = Total deaths ÷ total population
= 211 per 100,000 per year

Standardised mortality rate = Expected deaths ÷ standard population
= 121 per 100,000 per year

Table 1 Standardising the IHD mortality rate for males in Germany to the world standard population.

A Age group (years)	B Number of IHD deaths (males) in Germany	C Number of males in Germany	D Mortality rate in Germany (per 100,000) (B ÷ C)	E World standard population	F Cases expected in standard population (D × E)
0–4	0	2,032,000	0.00	12,000	0.00
5–9	0	2,296,000	0.00	10,000	0.00
10–14	0	2,362,000	0.00	9,000	0.00
15–19	11	2,353,000	0.47	9,000	0.04
20–24	15	2,283,000	0.66	8,000	0.05
25–29	42	2,990,000	1.40	8,000	0.11
30–34	142	3,722,000	3.82	6,000	0.23
35–39	407	3,548,000	11.47	6,000	0.69
40–44	839	3,061,000	27.41	6,000	1.64
45–49	1,484	2,801,000	52.98	6,000	3.18
50–54	2,396	2,295,000	104.40	5,000	5.22
55–59	5,352	2,903,000	184.36	4,000	7.37
60–64	8,080	2,505,000	322.55	4,000	12.90
65–69	11,562	1,844,000	627.01	3,000	18.81
70–74	12,605	1,350,000	933.70	2,000	18.67
75–79	12,700	869,000	1461.45	1,000	14.61
80–84	12,727	403,000	3158.06	500	15.79
85+	16,213	376,000	4311.97	500	21.56
TOTAL	**84,575**	**39,993,000**	**211.47**	**100,000**	**120.89**

(*Source for raw data:* Global Cardiovascular Infobase, www.cvdinfobase.ca, accessed 23 September 2003.)

Standard populations

Table 2 Examples of some commonly used standard populations

Age (years)	Segi World Standard (1960)[a]	African Standard[b]	European Standard[a]	Proposed New European Standard[c]	New WHO World Standard 2000–2025[a]	INDEPTH Standard for LMIC 2013[d]
0–4	12,000	10,000	8,000	5,000	8,860	14,630
5–9	10,000	10,000	7,000	5,500	8,690	13,660
10–14	9,000	10,000	7,000	5,500	8,600	12,640
15–19	9,000	10,000	7,000	5,500	8,470	10,800
20–24	8,000	10,000	7,000	6,000	8,220	8,540
25–29	8,000	10,000	7,000	6,000	7,930	7,050
30–34	6,000	10,000	7,000	6,500	7,610	6,040
35–39	6,000	10,000	7,000	7,000	7,150	5,230
40–44	6,000	5,000	7,000	7,000	6,590	4,540
45–49	6,000	5,000	7,000	7,000	6,040	3,890
50–54	5,000	3,000	7,000	7,000	5,370	3,230
55–59	4,000	2,000	6,000	6,500	4,550	2,740
60–64	4,000	2,000	5,000	6,000	3,720	2,290
65–69	3,000	1,000	4,000	5,500	2,960	1,820
70–74	2,000	1,000	3,000	5,000	2,210	1,320
75–79	1,000	500	2,000	4,000	1,520	840
80–84	500	300	1,000	2,500	910	440
85+	500	200	1,000	2,500[e]	630	320
TOTAL	100,000	100,000	100,000	100,000	100,000[f]	100,000[f]

LMIC: Low- and middle-income countries.

[a] From Ahmad *et al.* (2001); [b] from Waterhouse *et al.* (1976); [c] from Eurostat (2013); [d] from Sankoh *et al.* (2014); [e] includes 1500 age 85–89, 800 age 90–94 and 200 age 95+; [f] the numbers do not sum to exactly 100,000 because of rounding.

REFERENCES

Ahmad, O., Boschi-Pinto, C., Lopez, A., *et al.* (2001). *Age Standardization of Rates: a New WHO Standard*. EIP/GPE/EBD World Health Organization. Report No.: GPE Discussion Paper Series: No. 31. Geneva: World Health Organization.

Eurostat Task Force. (2013). Revision of the European Standard Population: Report of Eurostat's task force. Luxembourg, European Union. Available from http://ec.europa.eu/eurostat/.

Sankoh, O., Sharrow, D., Herbst, K., *et al.* (2014). The INDEPTH standard population for low- and middle-income countries, 2013. *Global Health Action*, 7: 23286. Available at: www.globalhealthaction.net/index.php/gha/article/view/23286, accessed 2 May 2015.

Waterhouse, J., Muir, C., Correa, P. and Powell, J. (eds). (1976). *Cancer Incidence in Five Continents*, Volume III. IARC Scientific Publication No. 15. Lyon: International Agency for Research on Cancer.

Calculating risk and lifetime risk from routine data

The 'quick and dirty' method

If a disease is rare, it is possible to make a rough estimate of the risk (or incidence proportion or cumulative incidence) by adding up the incidence rates for *each year* of life from 0 to 74. Because incidence rates are usually presented for 5-year age groups, e.g. 0–4 years, 5–9 years, etc., the rate at age 0 is the same as that at ages 1, 2, 3 and 4 years; similarly, the rate at age 5 is the same as that at ages 6, 7, 8 and 9 years; and so on for each 5-year age group. This means that, if the incidence in a 5-year band is 3/100,000, the chance a person develops disease during one of the 5 years is 3/100,000 and it is 15/100,000 for the whole 5-year period. One way to add up all the incidence rates to age 74 is therefore to multiply each of the age-specific rates by 5 (assuming that they are for 5-year age groups) and then to add them up. Or, to save time, you can do it the other way around and add up the 5-year rates and then multiply by 5 to obtain the same answer. This is then usually presented as a percentage:

$$\text{Lifetime risk} \approx 5 \times (\text{sum of rates from } 0-74) \times 100 \qquad \text{(A3.1)}$$

As an example, consider the age-specific IHD mortality rates in Germany shown in Appendix 1. If we add up the rates from ages 0–4 up to 70–74, we find a total of 2,270/100,000 = 0.0227, so

$$\text{Lifetime risk} \approx 5 \times 0.0227 \times 100 = 11.4\%$$

The proper method

Technically, the measure above is called the 'cumulative rate' because it is just the incidence rates summed or 'accumulated' for all ages from 0 to 74 years. To calculate a more accurate estimate of the lifetime risk you have to use a slightly more complicated formula:

$$\text{Lifetime risk} = 1 - \exp(-\text{ cumulative rate}) \qquad \text{(A3.2)}$$

Where $\exp(x)$ means e^x, where e = 2.7183, the base for *natural* logarithms (as opposed to 10 which is the base for standard logarithms).

So, if the cumulative rate of IHD mortality is 11.4% (=0.114) then the lifetime risk is

Lifetime risk $= 1 - e^{-0.114} = 1 - 0.892 = 0.108$ or 10.8%

Note that this figure of 10.8% is slightly lower than the 'quick and dirty' value of 11.4% we calculated above. This difference arises because IHD is quite common. The rarer the disease and, therefore, the lower the lifetime risk, the closer the answers from the two methods will be.

Another way to express the lifetime risk is in the form of '1 in X' where X is calculated by dividing 1 (or 100% if the lifetime risk is expressed as a percentage) by the lifetime risk:

$$= 1 \text{ in } (1 \div \text{lifetime risk}) \tag{A3.3}$$

So the lifetime risk of IHD mortality in Germany could be expressed as:

$$1 \text{ in } (1 \div 0.108) = 1 \text{ in } 9$$

It is important to note that, in this context, the lifetime risk is an artificial measure. It assumes that people do not die of any other causes along the way and it is also based on the current rates of disease without taking into account the fact that these may change over time. However, despite these limitations it can be a useful measure for comparing the burdens of various diseases within a population or for comparing the same disease across different populations.

Indirect standardisation

To use indirect standardisation you need to know:

(1) the age distribution of your study population and
(2) the age-specific disease rates in the standard population

An example: calculating the SMR for IHD in males in Brazil compared with Germany

See Table 3. You first multiply each age-specific rate in the standard population (Column C) by the number of people in that age group in the study

Table 3 Calculating the SMR for IHD in males in Brazil compared with Germany.

A Age group (years)	B Male population in Brazil ($\times$1000)	C Mortality rate (males) in Germany (per 100,000)	D Expected deaths in Brazil ($C \times B$)
0–4	9,025	0.00	0.00
5–9	8,703	0.00	0.00
10–14	8,604	0.00	0.00
15–19	8,109	0.47	37.91
20–24	7,360	0.66	48.36
25–29	6,841	1.40	96.09
30–34	6,642	3.82	253.40
35–39	5,622	11.47	644.91
40–44	4,707	27.41	1290.16
45–49	3,745	52.98	1984.14
50–54	2,912	104.40	3040.15
55–59	2,454	184.36	4524.22
60–64	1,957	322.55	6312.40
65–69	1,583	627.01	9925.51
70–74	1,138	933.70	10625.55
75–79	721	1461.45	10537.05
80+	583	3715.02	21658.57
TOTAL	**80,706**	**211.47**	**70978.43**

(*Source for raw data:* Global Cardiovascular Infobase, www.cvdinfobase.ca, accessed 23 September 2003.)

population (Column B) to calculate the number of events you would expect to see in the study population *if* it had the same rates as the standard population (Column D). You then divide the total number of events actually *observed* in the study population by the number of events *expected* (the total of column D) if the study population had had the same rates as the standard population. This gives you the *standardised mortality ratio* (SMR) (or *standardised incidence ratio* (SIR) if you are using incidence rates).

Observed number of deaths in Brazil = 39,437

Expected number if Brazil had same mortality rates as Germany = 70,978

∴ Standardised Mortality Ratio (SMR) = O ÷ E = 39,437 ÷ 70,978 = 0.56

The *crude* mortality rate from IHD in Brazilian men was less than one-quarter of that in Germany (47 versus 211/100,000 per year) but the average age of the population is much lower in Brazil than in Germany. When we standardise for age, the SMR=0.56 suggests that IHD mortality in Brazil is about half that in Germany.

Calculating life expectancy from a life table

Life expectancy is calculated based on what we expect to happen to a hypothetical cohort of 100,000 newborn infants if they experience the same mortality rates that currently operate within the population. (The cohort size is often denoted I_x, where x is the age of interest, thus at the start age = 0 and I_0 = 100,000.) Table 4 shows the first and last few rows of a standard life table for Australian males based on mortality rates from 2005 to 2007.

If the probability of a male dying before his first birthday (q_o) is 0.00527 then we would expect 527 deaths in our cohort in the first year of life ($d_0 = I_o \times q_0$) leaving 99,473 survivors at age = 1 (i.e. I_1 = 99,473). We can also estimate the numbers of years of life lived between the ages of 0 and 1. Because most infant deaths occur shortly after birth, this is estimated as 99,535 years, but for older ages we assume that those who died did so, on average, halfway through the year and thus contribute 0.5 years of life. Thus, for example, at age = 3 the total

Table 4 Life table for Australian males, 2005–2007.

Age	Life table Cohort I_x	Probability of dying q_x	Number of deaths $d_x = I_x \times q_x$	Years of live lived $L_x = I_x - (d_x \div 2)$	Cumulative years of life $T_x = T_{x+1} + L_x$	Life expectancy $e_x = T_x \div I_x$
0	100,000	0.00527	527	99,535	7,902,203	79.0
1	99,473	0.00040	40	99,452	7,802,668	78.4
2	99,434	0.00025	25	99,420	7,703,216	77.5
3	99,409	0.00019	19	99,399	7,603,796	76.5
...	...	...	...	...	...	...
97	3,879	0.27159	1,054	3,330	10,862	2.8
98	2,825	0.28593	808	2,403	7,532	2.7
99	2,018	0.30026	606	1,700	5,129	2.5
100	1,412	0.31460	445	3,429	3,429	2.4

Where: I_x = the proportion of persons surviving to that age
q_x = the proportion of persons dying between exact age x (I_x) and exact age x+1 (I_{x+1})
d_x = the number of deaths occurring between exact age x and exact age x+1
L_x = the years of life lived by the cohort between exact age x and exact age x+1
(*Source for raw data:* Australian Bureau of Statistics. (2007). Life Tables Australia: 2005–2007. ABS Publication 3302.0.55.001. http://www.abs.gov.au, accessed 12 September 2009.)

years of life $L_3 = 99{,}409 - (19 \div 2) = 99{,}399$. If we repeat these calculations for each year of age up to 100 we end up with 1412 men from our original cohort of 100,000 who survive to age 100, 445 of whom will die before their 101st birthday.

We then go on to calculate the total number of years lived by our cohort. Most life tables do not go beyond 100 years, although there are still some survivors at this point. We therefore have to estimate the total amount of life they have left; in this case 3429 years. We can then add on the total years of life lived at every other year of life giving a total of 7,902,203 years for the entire cohort. By dividing the years of life remaining at any given age by the number of survivors at that age ($T_x \div I_x$), we can then calculate life expectancy at that age. For example, at age 3 the 99,409 survivors have a total of 7,603,796 years life remaining giving a life expectancy at age 3 of 76.5 years.

Why the odds ratio approximates the relative risk for a rare disease

Table 5 shows the results of a hypothetical cohort study.

$$Relative\ risk = \frac{IP_e}{IP_o} = \frac{a}{(a+b)} \div \frac{c}{(c+d)} = 0.75\% \div 0.25\% = 3.0$$

However, if the disease is rare then

$a\ (= 75)$ is very small in comparison to $b\ (= 9{,}925)$, so $a + b \approx b$
and
$c\ (= 25)$ is very small in comparison to $d\ (= 9{,}975)$ so $c + d \approx d$
This means that the

$$Relative\ risk = \frac{a}{(a+b)} \div \frac{c}{(c+d)} \approx \frac{a}{b} \div \frac{c}{d} = \frac{a \times d}{b \times c} = Odds\ Ratio$$

To show that this is true, imagine we conducted a case–control study in this population with all 100 cases and the same number of controls. Half of the population is exposed and half is unexposed, so we would expect about 50 controls to be exposed and 50 to be unexposed and the

$$Odds\ ratio = \frac{75 \times 50}{25 \times 50} = 3.0$$

Table 5 Results of a hypothetical cohort study.

	Cases	Non-cases	Total	Incidence proportion (%)
Exposed	75 (a)	9,925 (b)	10,000 ($a + b$)	0.75
Unexposed	25 (c)	9,975 (d)	10,000 ($c + d$)	0.25
Total	100	19,900	20,000	

Formulae for calculating confidence intervals for common epidemiological measures

Although statistical packages routinely calculate confidence intervals for you, it is helpful to understand where they come from and sometimes useful to be able to calculate them by hand. We show below the formulae for estimating confidence intervals for some of the most common measures. The general rule for a 95% confidence interval is that the lower bound is equal to the point estimate minus $1.96 \times$ the standard error and the upper bound is equal to the estimate plus $1.96 \times$ the standard error. For 90% intervals you simply substitute 1.645 for 1.96 (giving a narrower interval but less certainty that it contains the correct value) and for 99% intervals you use 2.575 (giving a wider interval and more certainty that it contains the correct value).[1]

i.e. 95% confidence limits = estimate $\pm 1.96 \times$ standard error

It is important to remember, though, that some intervals have to be calculated on a log scale and then back transformed to the original scale (see, for example, the formula for the odds ratio below).

So, assuming that your data are set out in a standard way as follows:

	Cases/ affected	Controls/ unaffected	Total people	Total person-years
Exposed	a	b	N_1	PY_1
Unexposed	c	d	N_0	PY_0

Then Table 6 shows you how to calculate the standard error for some common epidemiological measures.

---

[1] These intervals are calculated on the assumption that the estimate comes from a 'normal' distribution or bell-shaped curve and this distribution can therefore be used to identify the multiplier for any width of CI although 90%, 95% and 99% are those most commonly used.

Table 6 Formulae for calculating the standard error for some common epidemiological measures.

Measure	Estimate	Standard deviation
Risk (in exposed)*	$\dfrac{a}{N_1}$	$\sqrt{\dfrac{a(N_1 - a)}{N_1{}^3}}$
Incidence rate (in exposed)	$\dfrac{a}{PY_1}$	$\sqrt{\dfrac{a}{PY_1{}^2}}$
Log odds ratio	$\ln\left(\dfrac{a \times d}{b \times c}\right)$	$\sqrt{\dfrac{1}{a} + \dfrac{1}{b} + \dfrac{1}{c} + \dfrac{1}{d}}$
Log risk ratio	$\ln\left(\dfrac{a}{N_1} \div \dfrac{c}{N_0}\right)$	$\sqrt{\dfrac{1}{a} - \dfrac{1}{N_1} + \dfrac{1}{c} - \dfrac{1}{N_0}}$
Log rate ratio	$\ln\left(\dfrac{a}{PY_1} \div \dfrac{c}{PY_0}\right)$	$\sqrt{\dfrac{1}{a} + \dfrac{1}{b}}$

* Can be used for any proportion, e.g. incidence proportion or prevalence.

So if a case-control study gives the following results:

Table 7 Hypothetical results from a case–control study.

	Cases	Controls	Total
Exposed	130	45	175
Unexposed	87	198	285

$$\text{Odds ratio} = \frac{130 \times 198}{87 \times 45} = 6.57$$

Log odds ratio = ln(6.57) = 1.883

$$\text{Standard error of log odds ratio} = \sqrt{\tfrac{1}{130} + \tfrac{1}{45} + \tfrac{1}{87} + \tfrac{1}{198}} = 0.216$$

So to calculate the 95% confidence interval for the log odds ratio:

Lower bound = 1.883 – (1.96 × 0.216) = 1.460

Upper bound = 1.883 + (1.96 × 0.216) = 2.306

and the 95% confidence interval for the odds ratio itself is then obtained by exponentiating to move back from the (natural) log scale to the more familiar arithmetic scale:

Lower bound = $exp^{1.460}$ = 4.3

Upper bound = $exp^{2.306}$ = 10.0

The final result might thus be presented as OR = 6.6 (95% CI = 4.3 – 10.0).

The Mantel–Haenszel method for calculating pooled odds ratios

When you do a stratified analysis to control for confounding you end up with a number of different odds ratios – one for each stratum. If these are all fairly similar, the next stage is to combine them into a single **adjusted odds ratio** that summarises the effect of the exposure *adjusted* for the confounder. Note that it is practical to do this only when you have a fairly small number of strata; once you need to adjust for more than one or two confounders it is better to use multivariable modelling techniques.

An adjusted odds ratio is essentially a *weighted average* of the stratum-specific odds ratios. We calculate a weighted average rather than a straight average so that strata with more people (and therefore greater precision) have a bigger influence on the final result than small strata. To calculate a weighted average, each individual value is multiplied by its weight and these new values are then added up and divided by the sum of the weights. Various sets of weights can be used for pooling odds ratios, but those proposed by Mantel and Haenszel (1959) are commonly used.

Imagine a case–control study with a total of T people in each stratum (T may be different for each stratum) as follows:

	Cases	Controls	
Exposed	a	b	
Unexposed	c	d	$T = a + b + c + d$

The odds ratio in each stratum is $\text{OR} = \dfrac{a \times d}{b \times c}$

The weight for each stratum is $w = \dfrac{b \times c}{T}$ ⟶ (A8.1)

So for each stratum we calculate:

$$\text{OR} \times w = \frac{a \times d}{b \times c} \times \frac{b \times c}{T} \qquad (A8.2)$$

We then add these values up for each stratum (= $\Sigma[(a \times d) \div T]$, where Σ (sigma) means summed over all strata), and divide by the sum of the weights = $\Sigma[(b \times c) \div T]$, so:

Mantel-Haenszel pooled OR $= \dfrac{\sum \left[(a \times d) \div T \right]}{\sum \left[(b \times c) \div T \right]}$

As an example, imagine a case–control study in which we are concerned about possible confounding by socioeconomic status (SES) because high SES is associated with a lower risk of disease but an increased risk of exposure:

Table 8 A hypothetical case–control study, stratified by SES.

	High SES		Low SES		Total	
	Cases	Controls	Cases	Controls	Cases	Controls
Exposed	460	490	90	45	550	535
Unexposed	60	150	70	95	130	245
Total	520	640	160	140	680	245
Odds Ratio	2.35		2.71		1.94	

To calculate the Mantel–Haenszel adjusted odds ratio:

1. first calculate *for each stratum separately:* $(a \times d) \div T$ and add these up for all of the strata,
2. then calculate *for each stratum separately:* $(b \times c) \div T$ and add these up for all of the strata, and
3. then divide (1) by the result from (2).

Table 9 Calculation of the Mantel–Haenszel adjusted odds ratio.

	High SES	Low SES	Total
(1) (a × d) ÷ T	(460 × 150) ÷ 1160 = 59.48	(90 × 95) ÷ 300 = 28.50	59.48 + 28.50 = 87.98
(2) (b × c) ÷ T	(60 × 490) ÷ 1160 = 25.34	(70 × 45) ÷ 300 = 10.50	25.34 + 10.50 = 35.84
(3) $\dfrac{\sum[(a \times d) \div T]}{\sum[(b \times c) \div T]}$			87.98 ÷ 35.84 = 2.45

In this example the pooled or adjusted OR of 2.45 is higher than the crude OR of 1.94, confirming that there was some confounding by SES. The adjusted OR is much closer to the OR in the high SES group (2.35) than it is to the OR in the low SES group (2.71) because the high SES group is much larger.

Meta-analysis

Exactly the same method can also be used to pool odds ratios from different studies in a meta-analysis.

REFERENCE

Mantel, N. and Haenszel, W. (1959) Statistical aspects of the analysis of data from retrospective studies of disease. *Journal of the National Cancer Institute*; 22: 719–748.

Glossary

Note: We have used italics to indicate other terms that are defined in this glossary.

Absolute risk reduction (ARR), Absolute risk increase (ARI) – clinical epidemiology terms for the *attributable risk*, used when then the risk in the exposed group is lower (ARR = $I_o - I_e$) or higher (ARI = $I_e - I_o$) than the risk in the control group.

Accuracy – this is achieved when the observed result is close to the true value. See also *precision*.

Adjustment – the process of correcting an estimate (e.g. odds ratio or relative risk) to reduce the *confounding* effects of some other factor; analogous to the process of *standardisation*.

Age-specific rate – incidence or mortality rate calculated for a specific age-group (usually a one, five or 10 year age band) to remove the *confounding* effects of age. See also *crude rate, age-standardised rate*.

Age-standardised rate – incidence or mortality rate that has been standardised for age by the process of *direct standardisation*. In practice an age-standardised rate is a weighted average of the *age-specific rates* where the weights are obtained from the age-distribution of a pre-defined standard population. See also *crude rate, standardised incidence (mortality) rate*.

Airborne transmission – transmission of an infectious agent via infectious droplet nuclei that can be inhaled. See also *direct transmission* and *indirect transmission*.

Ascertainment bias – see *selection bias*.

Attack rate – a measure of risk or the *incidence proportion* often used for an outbreak that occurs over a relatively short time period. See also *secondary attack rate*.

Attributable fraction – the proportion of all disease occurring in an exposed group that can be attributed to their exposure; equal to the *attributable risk* $(I_e - I_o)$ divided by the incidence of disease in the exposed group (I_e).

Attributable risk – a measure of the excess amount of disease occurring in one group over and above that in a comparison or reference group $(I_e - I_o)$. It can be calculated using *incidence rates* in which case it is also known as a *rate difference*, or *incidence proportions* in which case it is a *risk difference*.

Background rate or risk – the rate or risk of disease in an unexposed population; i.e. the amount of disease that will occur in the absence of the exposure or risk factor of interest.

Case–cohort study – a study conducted within the context of a *cohort study*, where cases are all those diagnosed with a particular disease and the comparison group is a random sample (subcohort) of the whole cohort population. The main difference from a *nested case–control study* is that the subcohort may include some people with the disease of interest; also, because it is selected to represent the whole cohort, the same subcohort can be used for studies of different outcomes.

Case–control study – a study where a group of people with disease (cases) are compared to a group without the disease (controls), selected to represent the population from which the cases came.

Case–crossover study – a study where each case acts as their own control thereby controlling for many known and unknown confounders. Exposure in a defined period prior to disease onset is compared with exposure in a defined 'control' period. Only suitable for studying transient exposures – for example studies of sexual activity and myocardial infarction.

Case–fatality ratio (CFR) – the proportion of people with a given disease or condition who die from it in a given period. It is a common measure of the short-term severity of an acute disease and allows a direct assessment of the effectiveness of an intervention.

Case-finding – opportunistic attempts at early detection of disease when someone comes into contact with the health system for another reason.

Cause – something (an event, condition, characteristic or combination of these) that plays an essential role in producing an effect (e.g. the occurrence of disease). See also *component cause, necessary cause, sufficient cause*.

Clinical significance – see *significance, clinical*.

Cluster – a group of cases of a rare (usually non-infectious) disease that occur in the same area or time period at a level greater than would be expected by chance.

Cohort study – a study where a sample of people (the cohort) are followed up over time to see who develops the disease of interest. The cohort may be a single population group who are then stratified on the basis of their exposure level, or it may be a group who have experienced a specific exposure (for example, an occupational or military group) who are then compared with e.g. the general population.

Common-source outbreak or epidemic – see *point-source outbreak or epidemic*.

Community trial – a trial in which the intervention is implemented at the community level, usually because it would be impossible to offer (or evaluate) the intervention at the individual level, for example studies of water fluoridation and dental health.

Competing cause – a cause of death other than the disease of interest. For example, in a long-term cohort study some people will die from other causes before they develop the condition of interest and in this case the investigator will never know if they might have developed the condition if they had lived longer.

Component cause – something (an event, condition, characteristic or combination of these) that, in conjunction with other factors, plays a role in producing an effect (e.g. the occurrence of disease). However it is neither necessary to cause disease, nor sufficient to cause disease on its own. See also *necessary cause, sufficient cause.*

Confidence interval (CI) – the range placed around a *point estimate* in which the true result is likely to lie and a way of quantifying the amount of *random sampling error* in a study or, conversely, the *precision* of an estimate. Most common are 95% confidence intervals and these are often interpreted as the range that will include the true value 95% of the time. However what they really mean is that if we were to repeat a study many times with different samples of people, then 95% of the 95% confidence intervals we calculated would include the true value. Other percentages can also be used, for example 99% intervals are wider but more likely to include the true value whereas 90% intervals are narrower but less likely to include the true value.

Confounding – a mixing or muddling of effects that can occur when the relationship we are interested in is confused by the effect of something else – the 'confounder'.

Confounding by indication – a type of confounding common in non-randomised studies looking at the effects of treatment. It occurs because, even among a group of people who all have the same medical condition, those who choose to take or who are prescribed a particular medication may well differ from those who do not take it or who are not prescribed it. For example, most drugs have one or more contraindications and people with these conditions would not be prescribed that drug and so would all be in the non-exposed group.

Control event rate (CER) – a term sometimes used in clinical trials to describe the risk or *incidence proportion* of the outcome of interest in the control or placebo group. See also *experimental event rate.*

Correlation study – see *ecological study.*

Counterfactual – a situation or condition that did not occur but could, would, or might have occurred under differing conditions.

Critical point – the theoretical (and usually unknown) point during the development of disease after which the disease process is irreversible and treatment will confer little or no benefit. Depending on the disease, this may occur very early in the disease process or may not occur at all.

Cross-level bias – bias that is due to the aggregation at the population level of causes or effects that are unlike those at the individual level. This form of bias is also referred to as the *ecological fallacy* when aggregate-level associations in ecological studies are interpreted as individual-level associations.

Crossover trial – a clinical trial where the same group of participants forms both the experimental and the control group. Participants are randomised such that they either receive the active treatment for the first time period and placebo for the second, or receive placebo for the first study period and the active treatment for the second. This design can only be used for exposures that have a fairly transient effect such that the effect of treatment does not carryover from one time period to the next.

Cross-sectional study – a survey of a random sample or cross-section of the population where information about potential *exposures* and outcomes is collected at the same time. Distinct from *cohort studies* and most *case–control studies* because it does not just consider *incident* (new) *cases* but all those in the population at the time of the survey (*prevalent cases*).

Crude estimate – an unadjusted measure of disease occurrence or association that has been calculated without consideration of the potential *confounding* effects of other variables.

Crude rates – overall incidence or mortality rates calculated for a whole population (IR = number of events in one year $\div$ total population or IR = number of events $\div$ person-time at risk) with no *adjustment* for the potential *confounding* effects of other variables e.g. age. See also *age-specific rate, age-standardised rate, standardised incidence (mortality) rate.*

Cumulative incidence – see *incidence proportion.*

DAG – see *directed acyclic graph.*

Data linkage – see *record linkage.*

Density sampling – a scheme for selecting controls for a *case–control study* (or *nested case–control study*) where controls are selected from all those in the population who are disease-free but at risk of developing the disease at the time when a case is diagnosed. In practice this means that someone can be recruited as a control for a study and then recruited again as a case if they go on to develop the disease of interest.

Diagnostic test – a definitive test used to diagnose disease in those suspected of being affected. See also *screening test.*

Differential error or misclassification – *measurement error* or *misclassification* that occurs to a greater extent in one study group than another, for example it is more likely to occur in cases than controls (or vice versa) in a *case–control study.*

Direct standardisation – the process where the rate of disease (or mortality) in a population is calculated on the assumption that the population had a standard age-sex distribution. If this is done for several different study populations then the resulting *standardised incidence (mortality) rates* can be directly compared because any differences in age/sex between the populations have been removed. Direct standardisation is most commonly performed for age and sex but can be performed for other characteristics such as race or socioeconomic status. See also *indirect standardisation*.

Direct transmission – transmission of an infectious agent through close personal contact with an infected individual, for example by touching infectious secretions or excreta. See also *indirect transmission* and *airborne transmission*.

Directed acyclic graph (DAG) – a pictorial representation of the causal relationships between variables. It is 'directed' because arrows indicate the direction from causes to outcomes, and 'acyclic' because no variable can affect itself (i.e. the arrows cannot form a loop).

Disability-adjusted life year (DALY) – a measure of the burden of a disease or risk factor on a population that counts not only years of life lost completely due to premature death, but also years of health lost through disability where the extent of disability is weighted from zero (perfect health) to one (death). See also *quality-adjusted life year*.

Disability-free life expectancy – the number of years of life an individual of a given age is expected to live free of disability, based on current morbidity and mortality rates. See also *life expectancy* and *health adjusted life expectancy*.

Ecological fallacy – an error made when information about groups of people is used to make inferences about individuals. For example, if suicide rates are lower in areas with high unemployment it would be tempting to assume this means that the unemployed are less likely to commit suicide than the employed. However, we do not know who is actually committing suicide. It is possible that it is unemployed people committing suicide, but that they are more likely to do so if they live in an area where the overall unemployment rate is low.

Ecological study – a study comparing the levels of exposure and or disease across populations rather than individuals. For example a study relating average income to child mortality rates in different countries. Susceptible to *ecological fallacy*.

Effect modification – when the association between an *exposure* and outcome (the 'effect') differs across levels of a third variable – the 'effect modifier'.

Eligibility criteria – criteria used to define the target population and establish whether an individual is eligible to participate in a study. See also *exclusion criteria*.

Endemic disease – a disease that is constantly present in a given population.

Epidemic – the occurrence of disease at a level greater than would normally be expected.

Event-based surveillance – see *surveillance*.

Excess rate – see *rate difference*.

Excess risk – see *risk difference*.

Exchangeability – two groups are exchangeable when individuals in the 'exposed' group of a study do not differ in any respect from individuals in the 'unexposed' group (with the exception of their exposure status). Ensuring the exposed and unexposed groups are exchangeable reduces the likelihood of confounding.

Exclusion criteria – criteria on which potential participants who are eligible for a study are excluded, usually for practical reasons such as their level of health, ability to give informed consent, ability to complete the study requirements. See also *eligibility criteria*.

Expected years of life lost (EYLL) – see *years of life lost*.

Experimental event rate (EER) – a term sometimes used in clinical trials to describe the risk or *incidence proportion* of the outcome of interest in the treatment or intervention group.

Exposure – a generic term used to describe the genetic, phenotypic, behavioural, lifestyle, environmental factors (or potential *causes*) being studied in relation to an outcome of interest.

External validity – see *generalisability*.

False negative – a negative test result in a person who actually has the condition being tested for and thus should have tested positive.

False positive – a positive test result in a person who does not actually have the condition being tested for and thus should have tested negative.

Force of morbidity – a synonym for the *incidence rate*.

Generalisability – the degree to which the results of a study can be reliably applied to a broader population than that included in the study. This depends on how representative the *study population* is of the target population (i.e. the response rate) and also how representative the *target population* is of other populations of interest. When applied to a causal association it is usually a decision based on judgement – for example, can the results of a study of American men be applied to men (or women) in Russia?

Health-adjusted life expectancy (HALE) – the equivalent number of years an individual can expect to live in full health based on current morbidity and mortality rates. Unlike *disability-free life expectancy* where years of life lived with disability are ignored, HALE includes this extra time but includes a weighting to allow for the fact that it is not lived in full health. See also *life expectancy*.

Health expectancy measures – measures that focus on what is being achieved such as *life-expectancy*. See also *health gap measures*.

Health gap measures – measures that focus on what is not being achieved such as *potential years of life lost*. They have the useful property that they can be calculated separately for different diseases or for different causes of disease. See also *health expectancy measures*.

Healthy worker effect – a problem that arises in occupational studies because workers are inherently healthier than the general population which includes all those too sick to work. As a result, employed groups will naturally tend to have lower morbidity/mortality rates than the overall population and it can be difficult to know whether this might mask an increase in risk due to a specific occupational *exposure*. Similar issues arise in comparisons of other healthy groups, such as the armed forces, to the general population.

Heterogeneity – when something varies across different groups it is heterogeneous. See also *homogeneity*.

Historical (or retrospective) cohort study – a *cohort study* where participants are identified in the present and historical records are used to measure their *exposure* in the past. This past measure of exposure can then be linked to the incidence of disease over the intervening years. This preserves the major benefit of a cohort study in that exposure is documented prior to the outcomes occurring, but avoids the lengthy time delay in that the outcomes have already occurred.

Homogeneity – when something is constant across different groups it is homogeneous. See also *heterogeneity*.

Host – the human or animal to which an infectious agent acquires entry and in which it multiplies.

Hypothesis test – a statistical test to assess the probability that the observed result would have arisen if the true result was something different. Usually calculated to assess the probability that a result as great as or greater than that observed would have arisen if there is really no association (the *null hypothesis*).

Incidence – new cases of disease; somewhat confusingly the term is commonly used to describe the actual number of new cases and also as a synonym for both the *incidence rate* and *incidence proportion* (or cumulative incidence).

Incidence density – see *incidence rate*.

Incidence proportion – the proportion of a defined population that develop the outcome of interest in a specified time period (IP = number of cases in a given time period $\div$ number of people at risk during the same period). Synonyms are risk or cumulative incidence.

Incidence rate – the rate at which new cases of disease occur in a population. Can be calculated from population data as IR = number of new cases in a one-year period $\div$ the number of people at risk during the same period. If it is not reasonable to assume that everyone has been at risk for the whole period, for example in a *cohort study* where people have been recruited to the study over a period of time, then it can be calculated as IR = number of new cases in a one-year period $\div$ total *person time* at risk.

Incident case – a new case of disease that is diagnosed during a specified time period.

Incubation period – the time between initial infection (entry of an infectious agent into a susceptible host) and the onset of clinical disease (symptoms).

Indicator-based surveillance – see *surveillance*.

Indirect standardisation – the process where the observed number of events in a study population is compared to the number of events that would have been expected to occur if the study population had the same characteristics as a standard population. Indirect standardisation is most commonly performed for age and sex but can be performed for other characteristics such as race or socioeconomic status. The results are usually presented as a *standardised incidence (mortality) ratio*. See also *direct standardisation*.

Indirect transmission – transmission of an infectious agent that involves a *vehicle* which may be inanimate, such as bedding, clothes or utensils (collectively called 'fomites'), food or water, or the soil; or alive in which case it is called a *vector*. See also *direct transmission* and *airborne transmission*.

Infection – the entry of a microbial agent into a higher-order host and its multiplication within the host.

Infectivity –the ability of an organism to invade and multiply in a host. It is the proportion of exposures that result in infection.

Infestation – when a lower organism lives on an external surface of another (usually higher) organism, for example, lice and scabies.

Information bias – see *measurement bias*.

Intensity (of infection) – a measure of the number of organisms infecting an individual.

Intention to treat analysis – analysis of data from a randomised trial that compares the groups as they were originally randomised, regardless of whether people actually received the intervention or not. Usually the most appropriate way to analyse data from a randomised study because if only those who actually received the intervention are compared with the rest, the benefits of the randomisation in terms of controlling for confounding and avoidance of selection bias are lost.

Internal validity – the degree to which the results of a particular study are free from bias and confounding.

Interval case – a case of disease that is diagnosed clinically between routine visits for screening.

Interviewer (observer) bias – a bias that can arise in exposure (disease) measurement when an interviewer (or observer) is aware of the disease (exposure) status of an individual. For example: an interviewer may ask questions somewhat differently, and thus potentially get different answers, when they know they are talking to someone they know has disease; a clinician may be more likely to diagnose disease in someone they know has been exposed to a particular factor.

Latent period (of an infectious agent) – the time from entry of an infectious agent into a host until the onset of infectiousness; may be longer or shorter than the *incubation period*. If it is shorter then infected persons may pass on the infection before they become ill (as with influenza) and if it is longer they will be ill before they are very infectious (like with SARS).

Lead time – the period between the first detectable signs of disease (i.e. detection by screening is possible) and the overt symptoms that normally lead to diagnosis.

Lead time bias – bias introduced into screening studies when groups of screened and unscreened individuals are compared without consideration of *lead time* such that screened individuals appear to do better simply because their disease was detected earlier than among those who are not screened.

Length bias – the over-representation of slowly progressing disease, which is more likely to have a favourable outcome, among cases detected by *screening*.

Life expectancy – the average number of years that an individual of a given age is expected to live if current mortality rates continue; see also *health adjusted life expectancy*.

Life table – a table that shows, amongst other things, the probability that an individual of any given age will die before reaching their next birthday (or the next age-group if the table is not calculated for individual years of age), and their future life-expectancy. Also known as a mortality table or actuarial table.

Measurement (or information) bias – any error in the measurement of either *exposure* or disease that differs between study groups. Can lead to *differential misclassification* of exposure or disease status.

Measurement error – any error in the measurement of either *exposure* or disease. Can lead to *misclassification* of exposure or disease status.

Meta-analysis – a technique for combining the results of multiple different studies into a single estimate, essentially a weighted average of the study-specific results where more reliance is placed on bigger studies with more precise estimates.

Migrant study – a comparison of disease incidence/mortality between groups who have migrated to a new country and those who stayed in their home country, for example Japanese people in Hawaii and Japanese in Japan. As both groups are likely to be genetically similar, differences between the groups suggest the condition under study is at least partly determined by environmental causes.

Misclassification – occurs when errors in measurement of exposure or outcome mean that people are classified into the wrong groups. For example someone with disease is wrongly classified as disease-free or vice versa, or someone who has been exposed to the factor of interest is wrongly classified as unexposed, or exposed at a lower level. See also *non-differential misclassification, differential misclassification.*

N-of-1 trial – a *crossover trial* where each participant serves as their own control such that they are randomised to periods of active treatment and placebo and their outcomes during the different time periods are compared. This design can only be used for exposures that have a fairly transient effect such that the effect of treatment does not carryover from one time period to the next.

Necessary cause – a *component cause* that is necessary for an outcome to occur; for example infection with influenza virus is a necessary cause of influenza.

Negative predictive value (NPV) – a measure of the performance of a screening programme in a specific population; the NPV of the test is the probability that someone who tests negative truly does not have the condition of interest. See also: *sensitivity, specificity, positive predictive value.*

Nested case–control study – a study conducted within the context of a *cohort study*, where cases are all those diagnosed with a particular disease and the comparison group is selected from those without disease at the time the cases were diagnosed. For this reason, the comparison group is specific to the particular case-group and cannot be used to study other outcomes as is possible in a *case–cohort study.*

Non-differential error or misclassification – *measurement error* or *misclassification* that occurs to the same extent in all study groups, for example in both cases and controls in a *case–control study.*

Null hypothesis – the hypothesis that there is no difference between the groups being studied or no association between an exposure and outcome.

Null value – the value that indicates no effect or association between two factors; equal to 0 for a difference measure (*absolute risk*) and 1.0 for a relative measure (*relative risk*).

Number needed to treat – the estimated number of people who would have to be given a new treatment in order to save one life (or prevent one adverse event if death is not the relevant outcome) in a specified time period, often one year. Calculated as $1 \div$ *absolute risk reduction.*

Observer bias – see *interviewer bias.*

Odds – the ratio of the number of people within a particular group who meet a specified condition divided by the number of people in the group who do not meet that condition. Identical to the odds commonly used in betting.

Odds ratio – the *odds* of disease in a group of people exposed to a potential risk factor divided by the odds of the same disease in a second or reference group who are unexposed. In practice this is equal to the odds that someone with disease (case) is exposed to a potential risk factor divided by the odds that someone without the disease is exposed to the same factor. In some circumstances (the outcome is rare or controls in a case–control study are selected via *density sampling*) the odds ratio is equal to the *relative risk*.

Outbreak – the occurrence of cases of disease in a community or region where it would not normally be expected, or at a much greater level than expected. See also *epidemic*.

Pathogenicity – the power of an organism to produce overt illness among those infected. It is measured as the proportion of those exposed to infection that goes on to develop clinical or overt illness.

Period prevalence – the proportion of a population affected by the condition of interest at any point during a specified time interval; period prevalence = the *prevalence* at the start of the time interval + the *incidence* of new cases during the time interval. See also *point prevalence*.

Person-time or person-years – the total amount of time lived by a defined group of people. For example, if 100 people are followed for an average of 5.7 years this is a total 570 person-years (100×5.7) of follow-up.

Point estimate or effect estimate – the main measure of association calculated in a study, for example an *odds ratio* or *relative risk*.

Point prevalence – the proportion of a population affected by the condition of interest at a specific point in time.

Point-source outbreak or epidemic – an epidemic that occurs when many people are suddenly exposed to the same source of infection, leading to a clear increase in incidence of disease. May also be called a common-source or extended-source outbreak, the latter implying that the exposure may be spread over a period.

Population attributable fraction – the proportion of disease occurring in a population that can be attributed to the exposure of interest. Equal to the *population attributable risk* ($I_T - I_o$) divided by the incidence of disease in the whole population (I_T). See also *population attributable risk, attributable fraction*.

Population attributable risk – the amount of disease (usually measured as *incidence* rate or *incidence proportion*) occurring in a population that can be attributed to the exposure of interest ($I_T - I_o$). See also *population attributable fraction, attributable risk*.

Positive predictive value (PPV) – a measure of the performance of a screening programme in a specific population; the PPV of the test is the probability that someone who tests positive actually has the condition of interest. See also: *sensitivity, specificity, negative predictive value*.

Post-test probability – a clinical epidemiology term for the probability that someone has disease based on the results of a specific test; a synonym for the *positive predictive value*.

Potential years of life lost (PYLL) – also known as years of potential life lost; the number of years of life lost because of deaths that occur prior to some pre-defined age.

Power – probability that the study will detect an association of a particular size if it truly exists in the general population.

Precision – little variation between the results; the converse of random error. A precise estimate will have a narrow *confidence interval*, conversely a wide confidence interval indicates a lack of precision.

Pre-test probability – a clinical epidemiology term for the probability that someone has disease based on the evidence available before a test is performed; often used synonymously with *prevalence*.

Prevalence – the proportion of a population affected by the condition of interest. See also *point prevalence, period prevalence*.

Prevalence ratio – the *prevalence* of disease in one group divided by the prevalence in a second or reference group.

Prevalent case – a case of disease that is already present in the population at a given point in time.

Primary prevention – all interventions that attempt to prevent disease from occurring, i.e. to reduce the incidence of disease.

Propagative epidemic – an epidemic that arises from the introduction of an infection into a susceptible population with subsequent transmission from person to person and a progressive increase in incidence. Also known as a contagious epidemic.

Proportional mortality ratio (PMR) – the proportion of deaths due to a specific cause in a group of interest divided by the proportion of deaths due to the same cause in a comparison group.

Publication bias – a form of selection bias that can occur in a systematic review or *meta-analysis* where studies with unexpected or null findings are less likely to be published than studies with new or positive findings or that confirm expectations.

***p*-value (probability value)** – the probability that we would have seen a difference as big as (or bigger than) we did if there were really no difference between the groups.

Quality-adjusted life year (QALY) – a measure of *life expectancy* that weights each year of life based on the quality of that life from one (perfect health) to zero (death). See also *disability-adjusted life year*.

Random error – or poor precision is the divergence, by chance alone, of a measurement from the true value. See also *systematic error*.

Randomisation – the process of allocating study participants to different exposure groups (e.g. intervention and control) at random such that each person has an equal chance of being allocated to the intervention group. Not to be confused with *random selection*.

Randomised controlled trial – a study where people are allocated to the exposure and control groups at random; the best design to avoid *confounding*.

Random sampling error – the introduction of error into the results of a study because only a sample of the population was studied instead of the whole population, for example in a population-based case–control study where a sample of people without disease are recruited to represent the broader population. Random sampling error is unavoidable in most situations but can be minimised by taking as large a sample as possible. It can also be quantified by the use of *confidence intervals*.

Random selection – the selection of participants for a study on the basis of chance such that each person in the source population has the same chance of being included in the study. Note, this does not mean that exposure is assigned at random, see *randomisation*.

Rare disease assumption – when a disease (or any health condition) is relatively rare (e.g. <10%) then the *odds ratio, risk ratio* and incidence *rate ratio* will all be approximately equal and the odds ratio can be used as an estimate of the *relative risk* (the risk of disease in one group relative to a reference group).

Rate difference – the *incidence rate* of disease in one group minus the *incidence rate* in a second or reference group ($IR_e - IR_o$); also described as *attributable risk*.

Rate ratio – the *incidence rate* of disease in one group divided by the *incidence rate* in a second or reference group ($IR_e \div IR_o$); also described as *relative risk*.

Recall bias – a type of bias that occurs when one group in a study tends to recall or report information differently from the comparison group. Most likely in a *case–control study* (or *cross-sectional study*) when cases, who may have thought extensively about what caused their disease, may recall their past exposures differently from controls, who do not have disease.

Record linkage – a process where records from different sources, for example prescribing records and death records, are combined at the individual level. In some countries this is facilitated by the use of a unique identification number to match records for a single person.

Relative risk – the term *relative risk* is synonymous with *risk ratio* but in practice it is also commonly used to describe a *rate ratio* and, in some circumstances, an *odds ratio* since all three measures compare the amount of disease in one group *relative* to that in another.

Relative risk reduction (RRR), Relative risk increase (RRI) – clinical epidemiology terms used to describe the reduction (or increase) in *relative risk* in a study group compared to the reference level of 1.0. For example, a RRI of 0.3 would mean that the relative risk in the study group was 1.3; a RRR of 0.3 would mean that the relative risk was 0.7.

Relative survival rate – the *survival rate* adjusted to allow for the fact that some people would have died anyway from other causes. A relative survival rate of 100% thus does not indicate that no one has died, but that mortality did not differ from that experienced by the general population.

Reservoir – the natural habitat of an infectious agent; may be human, animal or environmental.

Residual confounding – in practice adjusting for a confounding variable is unlikely to remove its confounding effect completely. Any remaining confounding is known as residual confounding. The more a variable confounds an association (i.e., the bigger the change in an effect estimate when you adjust for the confounder), the more likely there is to be some remaining uncontrolled confounding.

Retrospective cohort study – see *historical cohort study*.

Reverse causality – occurs when the outcome precedes and causes the exposure, instead of the exposure preceding and causing the outcome.

Risk difference – the *incidence proportion* or risk of disease in one group minus the *incidence proportion* or risk in a second or reference group ($IP_e - IP_o$); also described as *attributable risk*.

Risk factor – a factor (genetic, behavioural, environmental, societal) that is thought to increase risk of developing a particular health state. For example, smoking is a strong risk factor for lung cancer. The term was coined by investigators on the Framingham Heart Study.

Risk ratio – the *incidence proportion* or risk of disease in one group divided by the *incidence proportion* or risk in a second or reference group ($IP_e \div IP_o$); also described as *relative risk*.

Screening – the widespread use of a simple test for disease in an apparently healthy (asymptomatic) population.

Screening programme – an organised system using a *screening test* among asymptomatic people in the population to identify early cases of disease in order to improve outcomes.

Screening test – a test, usually relatively cheap and simple, used to test large numbers of apparently healthy people to identify individuals suspected of having early disease who will then go on to have further *diagnostic tests* to confirm the diagnosis. A screening test differs from a diagnostic test in that there is greater emphasis on cost and safety (as large numbers may be tested and most will not have disease) and less on definitive diagnosis.

Secondary attack rate – the number of cases of infection that develop among the susceptible contacts of an infected case as a proportion of the total number of exposed contacts; a measure of *infectivity*.

Secondary prevention – efforts to reduce the burden of disease by detecting it sooner (e.g. by *screening*) and thereby making treatment more effective and improving outcomes. Secondary prevention does not affect the incidence of disease, in fact it may actually lead to a transient increase in incidence as more cases are detected quickly. See also *primary prevention*.

Selection bias – the introduction of bias into the results of a study because those selected to be in the study differ from those not selected in some systematic way. For example, those who agree to participate in a study may be more health conscious (e.g. less overweight, lower levels of smoking and alcohol consumption, higher levels of physical activity) than those who refuse to participate. If this affects recruitment of controls (but not cases) for a *case-control study* then comparisons between cases and controls will be biased.

Sensitivity – usually a measure of the performance of a screening test; the sensitivity of the test is the probability that someone with the condition of interest will return a positive test result. See also: *specificity, positive predictive value, negative predictive value*

Sensitivity analysis – the process of repeating the analysis of a study to see how the results are affected if different assumptions are made. If the results are similar regardless of the assumptions then we can be more confident in them; if they differ greatly then we would be less confident that we were seeing a real effect.

Significance, clinical – an observed difference between two groups that is of clinical or public health importance, irrespective of whether it is, or is not, statistically significant.

Significance, statistical – an observed difference between two groups that is unlikely to have arisen by chance. Conventionally, an association is considered statistically significant if is likely to have occurred by chance less than 1 in 20 times (or $p < 0.05$).

Simpson's paradox – where the crude association observed in a study is in the opposite direction to the true association due to *confounding*.

Source (of infectious agent) – the person, animal or object from which the host acquires the infection.

Specificity – usually a measure of the performance of a screening test; the specificity of the test is the probability that someone without the condition of interest will return a negative test result. See also *sensitivity, positive predictive value, negative predictive value*.

Standardisation – see *direct standardisation, indirect standardisation*.

Standardised incidence (morbidity) ratio (SIR, SMR) – the number of new cases of disease observed in a study population over a specified period of time compared with the number that would have been expected if the study population had had the same incidence rates as a standard or comparison population (often the general population). Calculated by the process of *indirect standardisation*. Note: confusingly, both standardised morbidity ratios and the *standardised mortality ratio* (see below) are sometimes abbreviated as SMR.

Standardised incidence (mortality) rate – an incidence or mortality rate that has been *adjusted* by the process of *direct standardisation* to remove the potential *confounding* effects of another variable, usually age. In practice, the standardised rate is the rate that would have been seen in a population with a pre-defined distribution of the factor of concern (e.g. age). See also *age-standardised rate*.

Standardised mortality ratio (SMR) – the number of deaths observed in a study population over a specified period of time compared with the number that would have been expected if the study population had had the same mortality rates as a standard or comparison population (often the general population).

Stationary population – a population that does not change in size over time i.e. the number of people entering the population (e.g. by birth or immigration) approximately equals the number of people leaving the population (death or emigration).

Statistical significance – see *significance, statistical*.

Stratification – a process in which we divide or stratify the study participants into two or more separate groups or strata and calculate measures of association separately in each group. Used to assess whether an association (or effect) varies among different subgroups of the population, i.e. there is *effect modification*. For example, if an association differs between smokers and non-smokers (stratification by smoking status).

Study population – the individuals sampled from the *target population* who actually participate in the study.

Sufficient cause – a *component* cause or group of causes that will inevitably lead an outcome to occur.

Surveillance – the systematic and continuous collection, analysis and interpretation of data, closely integrated with the timely and coherent dissemination of the results and assessment so that action can be taken. *Indicator-based surveillance* is when selected indicator conditions are under surveillance for specific purposes, such as evaluating an intervention or detecting outbreaks; *event-based surveillance* is when the main focus is to identify events of public health significance.

Survival rate – proportion of patients in a group who are still alive a specified period after diagnosis.

Systematic error – occur when observations in a study differ from the truth in a non-random way. For example, if those who agree to take part in a study are less likely to be smokers than those who do not agree to take part; or if cases are more likely to overestimate their past exposure to second-hand smoke than non-cases. See also *random errors*.

Target population – the population that we want to study.

True negative – a negative test result in a person who is truly free of the condition being tested for.

True positive – a positive test result in a person who truly has the condition being tested for

Type I error – the error that occurs when the results of a study suggest there is a relationship between exposure and outcome but the truth is that there is none (also called alpha error).

Type II error – the error that occurs when the results of a study suggest there is no association between exposure and outcome when, in truth, there is an association (also known as beta error).

Validity – see *internal validity, generalisability.*

Vector – a living organism that transmits an infectious agent, for example mosquitoes that transmit malaria and dengue, ticks.

Vehicle – something that transmits an infectious agent from one host to another. It may be inanimate (e.g. food, water, the soil) or it may be alive in which case it is called a *vector.*

Verbal autopsy – an interview method sometimes used in the absence of medical information or formal death certification to ascertain information from family members or other third parties about the circumstances of death of an individual. It is often used in situations where vital registration systems do not exist, but can also be used in epidemiological studies of mortality to obtain information on study exposures.

Virulence – the ability of an organism to produce serious disease; measured by the proportion of those who are infected (determined by immunoassay) who develop severe overt disease.

Volunteer bias or volunteerism – bias introduced because people who volunteer for a study or attend for screening are likely to be different from those who do not volunteer.

Years of life lost (YLL) – the number of years of expected life lost due to a death at a given age, equal to the life expectancy at that age. See also *potential years of life lost.*

Years of potential life lost (YPLL) – see *potential years of life lost.*